Hospital Paediatrics

For Churchill Livingstone

Commissioning Editors: Timothy Horne, Inta Ozols
Copy Editor: Pat Croucher
Page Make-up: Gerard Heyburn
Cover Design: Sarah Cape
Sales: Susan Jerdan-Taylor

Hospital Paediatrics

Anthony D. Milner MD FRCP DCH

Professor of Neonatology,
Department of Paediatrics,
United Medical and Dental School of Guy's
 and St Thomas's Hospital,
London, UK

David Hull BSc FRCP

Emeritus Professor of Child Health,
Medical School,
University of Nottingham,
Nottingham, UK

THIRD EDITION

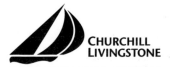

CHURCHILL
LIVINGSTONE

EDINBURGH LONDON NEW YORK PHILADELPHIA SAN FRANCISCO SYDNEY TORONTO 1998

CHURCHILL LIVINGSTONE
A Division of Harcourt Brace and Company Limited

Robert Stevenson House
1–3 Baxter's Place, Leith Walk,
Edinburgh EH1 3AF

First edition 1984
Second edition 1992
Third edition 1998

ISBN 0 443 053928

British Library Cataloguing in Publication Data
A catalogue record for this book is available from the British Library.

Library of Congress Cataloging in Publication Data
A catalog record for this book is available from the Library of Congress.

Note
Medical knowledge is constantly changing. As new information becomes available, changes in treatment, procedures, equipment and the use of drugs become necessary. The volume editors, contributors and publishers have, as far as it is possible, taken care to ensure that the information given in this text is accurate and up to date. However, readers are strongly advised to confirm that the information, especially with regard to drug usage, complies with latest legislation and standards of practice.

The
publisher's
policy is to use
**paper manufactured
from sustainable forests**

Produced by Longman Asia Ltd, Hong Kong
EPC/01

Preface

This latest edition of *Hospital Paediatrics* has been revised to take account of changes that have occurred in the management of paediatric problems presenting to the hospital-based paediatrician over the last 5 years.

The format has been altered, and we believe improved, to bring it in line with *Essential Paediatrics*. The three chapters on the Abused Child, the Shocked Child and the Poisoned Child have been replaced by one chapter on Accidents and Emergencies and one on Intensive Care. We have split two other chapters which we considered to be rather unwieldy: one on Brain, Nerve and Muscle and the other on the Newborn have been split into shorter sections entitled Muscle and Movement, Brain and Special Senses, Care of the Newborn and Intensive Care of the Newborn. We have included a new chapter on Abnormal Form (dysmorphology) as many paediatricians in training find this a particularly challenging area.

If this edition proves as successful as its predecessors, it will be very largely due to our contributors, including our 10 new authors, who we welcome.

London   A.D.M.
Nottingham   D.H.

Contributors

C. P. J. Charlton
MBChB BMedSci MRCP MRCPCH
Consultant Paediatric Gastroenterologist, University Hospital, Queen's
Medical Centre, Nottingham

David A. Curnock
MA MB BChir FRCP DCH DObstRCOG
Consultant Paeiatrician, City Hospital, Nottingham

Jonathan H. C. Evans
MBBS MRCP
Consultant Paediatric Nephrologist, Children and Young People's Kidney
Unit, City Hospital NHS Trust, Nottingham

Kathleen M. Forman
FRCPath
Consultant Haematologist, University Hospital, Queen's Medical Centre,
Nottingham

Kevin P. Gibbin
FRCS
Consultant Otolaryngologist, Queen's Medical Centre University Hospital
NHS Trust, Nottingham

Anne Greenough
MD FRCP DCH
Professor of Clinical Respiratory Physiology and Clinical Director,
Department of Child Health, King's College Hospital, London; Honorary
Consultant Paediatrician, Children Nationwide Regional Neonatal Intensive
Care Centre, King's College School of Medicine and Dentistry, London

E. Joan Hiller
BSc FRCP
Former Consultant Paediatrician, City Hospital, Nottingham

David Hull
BSc FRCP
Emeritus Professor of Child Health, Medical School, University of
Nottingham, Nottingham

Derek I. Johnston
MA MD FRCP DCH
Consultant Paediatrician, Children's Department, University Hospital,
Nottingham

David H. Mellor
MD FRCP
Consultant Paediatric Neurologist, University Hospital, Nottingham

Anthony David Milner
MD FRCP DCH
Professor of Neonatology, Department of Paediatrics, United Medical and
Dental School of Guy's and St Thomas's Hospital, London

Venkateswaran Ramesh
MRCP DCH
Consultant Paediatric Neurologist, Children's Department, Newcastle
General Hospital, Newcastle upon Tyne

Nicholas Rutter
MD FRCP
Professor of Paediatric Medicine and Honorary Consultant Paediatrician,
University of Nottingham, Nottingham

Stephanie A. Smith
BM BS MRCP
Consultant Paediatrician, University Hospital, Nottingham

Terence Stephenson
BSc DM FRCP
Professor of Child Health and Honorary Consultant Paediatrician, University
of Nottingham, Nottingham

Helen Venning
BMedSci BM BS MRCP
Consultant Paediatrician, Nottingham

Harish Vyas
DM FRCP
Consultant Paediatrician, Intensive Care and Respiratory Units, Queen's
Medical Centre, Nottingham

David A. Walker
BMedSci FRCP
Consultant, Senior Lecturer, Department of Child Health,
University of Nottingham, Nottingham

Alan R. Watson
MBChB FRCP
Consultant Paediatric Nephrologist and Unit Director, Children and Young
People's Kidney Unit, City Hospital, Nottingham

Hywel C. Williams
BSc MBBS(Hons) MRCP MSc PhD
Senior Lecturer and Honorary Consultant in Dermatology, Queen's Medical
Centre, Nottingham

Lynn Williams
FRCS FFAEM
Consultant in Paediatric Accident and Emergency, Queen's Medical Centre,
Nottingham

Ian D. Young
MD MSc FRCP
Professor of Paediatric Genetics, City Hospital, Nottingham

Contents

Hospital

Children are sent, brought or come to hospital because they are ill and in need of care. They may arrive as an emergency at the accident and emergency (A&E) department or attend out-patient clinic by appointment. Admission to hospital for ward care is avoided if at all possible but if it is necessary then the length of time in the ward is kept as short as possible. Infants and children get better faster if they are in familiar surroundings. Love and comfort may be the most important 'medicine'.

We see a hospital as a community resource, rather than a sickness castle where soldiers demonstrate their martial arts. The challenge is not only to make the right diagnosis and give the correct treatment, it is also to make wise decisions in the sequence of events from first contact to admission and discharge. These decisions will depend in part on the doctor having a knowledge of the people and the characteristics of the population served by the hospital, and the services within the community to care for the child in their home and school.

Geographical concentration of disease excites interest because it suggests an aetiology. However most problems appear to be distributed at random and the demands on health services within like communities are similar. Health inequalities relate more to disadvantage due to family and social collapse, violence and poverty, which can be found to varying extents in every society.

Disadvantage by social class starts from the beginning!

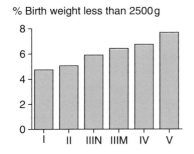

% Birth weight less than 2500 g

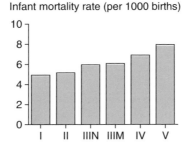

Infant mortality rate (per 1000 births)

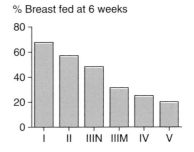

% Breast fed at 6 weeks

To give a rough guide to the work of the hospital services for children we have used information about our service. Nottingham is a city in the middle of England. The two large general hospitals both have neonatal units, out-patient and in-patient facilities and serve a population of around 800 000 with a local birth rate of around 11 000 births per year. The children's A&E service is at the University Hospital. The hospitals also provide a full range of specialist services except for cardiac surgery.

Attendance to the children's A&E services is increasing, which indicates a growing demand for an expert children's medical and nursing service available 24 hours a day. With the changing patterns of primary care, this trend seems set to continue.

Attendances at A&E departments in the UK are increasing year on year, the range of problems are similar

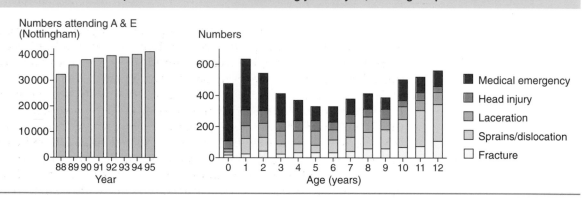

The majority of attendances are 'self-referrals'. About 25% are emergencies and the rest are accidents. Medical emergencies are commoner in infants and younger children whilst accidents occur across all age groups but increase with age. The decision-making begins at the point of reception. By far the majority are attended to and discharged, some are referred back to the care of the GP and others are brought back to the out-patients clinic for further appraisal. Around 10% are admitted for in-patient care.

In our hospital all emergencies are seen first in the A&E department. The number of children admitted to the wards had for a time been increasing. Enquiries were made to find out why. The number of children labelled as 'asthma' was an important contributor, but it is uncertain whether this was due to an increase in the illness, a change in management and family expectation or a change in 'label' or a mixture of these! The admission rate now seems to have levelled off. The average length of stay gets shorter and shorter. Between 60 and 70% only stay for one night; for them the necessary investigations have been performed, the results obtained, and the child has recovered or the illness has abated within 24 hours. As a result the number of 'occupied bed-days' has not increased but the work involved per 'bed-day' has.

The common causes of emergency medical admissions — seizures, respiratory infection, asthma, poisoning and gastroenteritis — account

The common 'reasons' why children are admitted to hospital as given by Hospital Activity Analysis

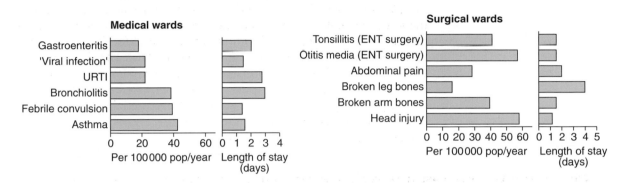

for over 70% of the whole. In children's general surgical wards 50% of admissions are for emergencies, with abdominal pain and head injury being the majority. As many children are admitted for elective surgical procedures as are admitted with an acute emergency.

The challenge for the hospital services is not these common problems where the care is usually straightforward, but the management of the children with rare, unexpected and life threatening illnesses. It is the latter group which require awareness, knowledge, skill and commitment. Strategies (guidelines, protocols, etc.) can be in place for some, for example the child in shock with septicaemia or ketoacidosis, or with respiratory failure from whatever cause, or with the first suspicion of cancer or deliberate injury. The number of times a unit will meet such problems can be predicted with fair confidence from the size of the population served. But in paediatric practice the totally unexpected occurs with surprising frequency, for example an excited child poisoned with an aphrodisiac, swelling of the tongue, talking nonsense, a discharging sinus, foreign bodies in the strangest of places. Then there is no alternative but to make a thorough enquiry, seek advice, search the literature and manage using sound general principles. For some problems there are no answers, and that to some extent will always be so.

Neonatal and infant statistics. The number of babies born with abnormalities is falling

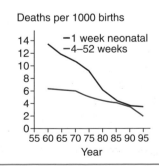

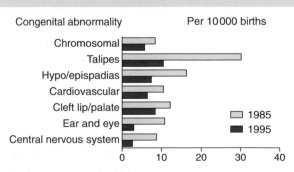

National statistics

A brief glance at national statistics puts the work of doctors, nurses and other members of the ward, out-patients clinic and A&E team in hospital into the wider context of the national health provision for child health. Neonatal and infant mortality rates continue to fall. The commonest cause of infant death is extreme immaturity! The number of infants born with congenital abnormalities has also fallen impressively, and this has made a considerable impact on the mortality figures. Only a part of this improvement can be ascribed to monitoring for fetal abnormalities with a view to early destruction.

Postneonatal mortality rates (1–12 months) have shown a dramatic dip in the last few years. They began to fall before the 'back to sleep' campaign, so we cannot be absolutely sure of the reason for the improvement. It appears reasonable to conclude that at least some of the continuing improvement is due to the change from nursing infants on their fronts to their backs. When infants are nursed on their backs, their nose and mouth are not obstructed, their cry is louder and they are more able to make physiological and behavioural responses to over-heating.

Death in childhood is rare. Happily one of the commonest causes, accidents, is becoming less common. More children with cancer are now surviving. From this brief examination of the data it is clear that targets aimed at improving these figures are not sensible outcome measures of hospital services, or indeed of the health provision as a whole. They are determined more by the way we choose to live and government policies and priorities for service provisions and the distribution of the national wealth.

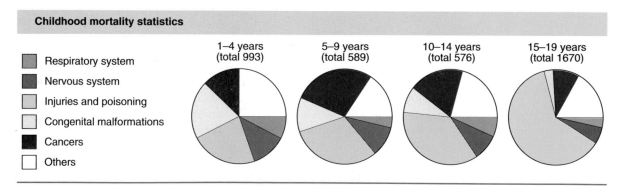

Childhood mortality statistics

Respiratory system
Nervous system
Injuries and poisoning
Congenital malformations
Cancers
Others

1–4 years (total 993) 5–9 years (total 589) 10–14 years (total 576) 15–19 years (total 1670)

Care as well as cure

An important aim of the Child Health Service is to support the family and to enable parents of infants and younger children to provide all the care whenever that is reasonable and possible. It also aims to help children to look after themselves within their understanding and abilities. If admission is necessary then parents should be encouraged to spend as much time as they are able, looking after their child in the ward. The task of the ward team is to re-inforce the family's understanding of the child's illness and to support them in the care of their child.

Those of us working in the Child Health Service should find nothing surprising or original in the fashionable health care notion of 'patient centred care'. In general hospitals we will often have to point out to colleagues and managers that services designed for adults may not suit children. If children use the service then the service must be suitable for children.

In the UK the current moves to develop primary care, to strengthen community services, to redirect health service resources to meet the targets of the 'Health of the Nation' are all important for child health. Their success, oddly enough, depends on an efficient, effective, safe, reliable, readily available hospital service for children.

FURTHER READING

Annual Report of the Chief Medical Officer of the Department of Health for the year 1995. On the state of public health. 1996 HMSO, London
Barker DJP 1994 Mothers, babies, and disease in later life. BMJ Publishing Group, London
Botting B (ed) 1995 The health of our children. OPCS, London
Forfar JO (ed) 1988 British Paediatric Association, Child health in a changing society. Oxford University Press, Oxford
Smith R (ed) 1991 The health of the Nation the BMJ view. BMJ Publishing Group, London
Spencer N 1996 Poverty and child health. Radcliffe Medical Press, Oxford
Woodroffe C, Glickman M, Barker M, Power C 1993 Children, teenagers and health. Open University Press, Milton Keynes

2

Ill children

For a child a hospital is a place full of strangers. A confusing number of health professionals come to talk and do things to them. In an atmosphere of adult concern the child's feelings and interests are easily overlooked. The child in an unfamiliar environment will turn to their parents or guardians for protection and understanding. The parent will also be distressed and may be uncertain and we must do what we can to help them care for their child.

HISTORY

Over 90% of paediatric hospital admissions enter through the A&E department. The A&E department may not be an ideal situation in which to take a careful history. Fortunately history taking can be expanded or repeated when the child is reviewed later on the ward but this should not be used as an excuse for a cursory or inaccurate history in the first instance. It is the history which largely determines the differential diagnoses, while the examination and investigations help to confirm these. Taking a thorough history is an essential discipline.

The majority of hospital paediatric admissions are young children. Two-thirds are under 3 years of age. The history is therefore usually obtained from an accompanying guardian rather than directly from the child. This makes the history more difficult to interpret as it is 'second hand', but detailed questions about the onset, duration, frequency and site of symptoms should still be asked. Parents are often assiduous observers of their children and the parent, acting as an interlocutor on the child's behalf, may give a history which is strikingly comprehensive. Unfortunately, a minority of parents can only offer a brief and vague account of the child's illness and these parents should be pressed for details, if necessary by direct and therefore leading questions. Taking a complete history on every child in a busy casualty or out-patient department is a counsel for perfection. In this context, the concept of a 'rationalised' history of the most relevant facts is pertinent.

Here we only emphasise those aspects of the paediatric history which are different from adult practice. If the symptoms are chronic, try to determine their impact on the child, his/her family, development and schooling.

Birth history

The younger the child, the more relevant the history of the pregnancy, delivery and newborn period. The amount of detail required varies depending on the presenting complaint, but certainly if the infant has previously been admitted to a neonatal unit, a detailed account of the perinatal history is required. Obviously, the perinatal history remains very relevant in older children presenting with seizures, developmental delay, or physical or mental handicap.

Nutrition

Again the younger the child, the more relevant the dietary history. Non-organic failure to thrive is commonest under a year of age and is most commonly due to a failure to offer enough food, usually through parental ignorance or neglect. A nutritional history is relatively straightforward in a formula fed baby (provided you remember that 1 fluid ounce is 28 ml) but much more difficult in a breast fed or older child. A history of dietary intake is most important when there are gastrointestinal symptoms, particularly in conjunction with chronic diseases such as cystic fibrosis or cancer. Anorexia nervosa and chronic fatigue syndrome are not uncommon in teenagers. Food intolerance is much more often claimed by parents than substantiated.

Developmental history

This is essential in all children under 2 years of age. In an older child with behavioural problems, enquire about educational difficulties and neurological symptoms. Parents may have difficulty recalling the exact age of distant developmental milestones in an older child but a favourable recollection in comparison with healthy siblings may suffice. Parent Held Records record development. Remember that any given developmental milestone will be passed later than average by 50% of all children. This is sometimes a source of misunderstanding leading to inappropriate referral. Average ages of acquisition of skills are therefore not very relevant in terms of screening for delayed development. A recognition of 'action' times (the age by which 90% of normal children will have passed a developmental milestone) is much more useful in practice and aids such as the Denver developmental assessment charts should always be available in out-patient departments.

Immunisation

A history of immunisations against a particular disease can never completely exclude the possibility of the child currently having, or previously having had, the disease. In reality, the immunisation history is more important in directing parent education than in narrowing the differential diagnoses. The reasons which parents give to explain why immunisation has been declined or withheld are rarely genuine contra-indications. A hospital attendance is an opportunity for 'opportunistic' vaccination.

Family history

This can give clues to inherited diseases but only a small fraction of the children presenting to paediatric services suffer from diseases which follow strict mendelian inheritance. Disorders such as 'migraine' and 'allergy' are sufficiently common in the community, and the terms so loosely used by the public, that a positive family history is unlikely to help clarify the child's symptoms. The symptoms currently 'in vogue' in the household may influence a child's complaints and behaviour. A child with recurrent headaches may have a grandparent who has recently suffered a stroke or the onset of enuresis may be triggered by illness in a close relative.

Contact with infections

The family history should include enquiries about contact with infectious diseases, fevers or rashes, travel abroad and contacts with recent travellers from abroad, and recent symptoms in other members of the family. These questions are relevant to the many children who attend casualty with a febrile illness or gastrointestinal symptoms. It is surprising how often the parents of an ill child have failed to recognise a pattern of self-limiting symptoms passing through the family.

Social history

This overlaps with the family history considerably and is often the most neglected aspect of history taking. Many children now are in single parent families and it is important to note the other household members, their relationship to the child, and the degree of support available in the home. The presentation of a moderately well child to a hospital A&E department is often a cry for social support rather than medical treatment.

Medicines

A list of drugs which the child is currently taking should always be sought. Drugs taken in the preceding week may also modify the illness and drugs taken in the previous months may indicate the chronicity of the problem. Parents are more familiar with a child's 'medicines' than 'drugs' and may assume that the hospital paediatrician is automatically informed about medicines prescribed from out-patient clinics or from the general practitioner. True drug allergy is rare but all alleged reactions should be noted.

EXAMINATION

Details of abnormal physical signs are given in the chapters on individual systems but some general comments apply to the examination of all children. Examining children is a challenge and the younger the child, the greater the challenge. A baby or young child should be examined on a parent's lap if possible. Standing menacingly over a small child can be avoided by getting down on your knees. A parent may helpfully distract a child and a ready supply of toys and books appropriate to different ages should be available in out-patient and casualty departments. It is not advisable to ask a toddler's permission before carrying out any part of the examination as often the response will be a refusal. Explain what you intend to do in simple terms, for the parents' sake as much as for the child, and proceed in a firm but gentle manner. Anticipate and thereby avoid hurting a child by asking about tenderness and noting the sites of bruises, swelling or erythema, and plasters or bandages. Warm your hands and your stethoscope and remove rings or watches.

The unpleasant parts of the examination should always be deferred until as much information as possible has been obtained. Young infants object to measurement of head circumference, measurement of blood pressure and testing hips. If a rectal examination is indicated, it must be done. Stethoscopes are only marginally less unpopular than auroscopes whilst fundoscopy usually ends in tears in infants. The dreaded tongue depressor is best left until the bitter end. Why not use a spoon handle, a child knows that a spoon goes in the mouth. If the child opens his or her mouth wide enough so that you get a good view, why use a depressor at all? Older children are more co-operative, unless distressed or in pain, but may be reluctant to be undressed in front of a stranger. Teenagers should be asked whether they wish their parents to be present during the examination but a pubertal girl should not be examined by a male doctor without the presence of a chaperone, except in an emergency. All children with chronic problems must have their height, weight and head circumference measured and plotted on an appropriate centile chart. Always measure the blood pressure in a child with neurological or renal problems.

One aspect of examination which is often performed badly in the casualty department is the assessment of the child with altered consciousness. A brief note of 'conscious' or 'unconscious' is rarely appropriate and the terms comatose, drowsy and obtunded are insufficiently informative and should be avoided. The Glasgow Coma Scale (see Ch. 3) is a quick, simple and reproducible technique and should be used to document level of consciousness. The initial examination of the unconscious child should also include observations of pupillary, corneal and gag reflexes, the presence or absence of doll's eye movements, deep tendon reflexes, plantar responses, and muscle tone or posturing. These simple observations are often overlooked in the acute situation but they are the only clinical parameters in an unconscious child which can provide a definite baseline against which subsequent neurological progress can be gauged.

Record the history and findings carefully with date, time and sign. It is in the interests of the patient, the hospital and yourself. We live in litiginous times. Good records suggests a thorough and careful doctor.

INTRODUCTION TO PROCEDURES

Anxiety is readily transmitted from both mother and medical staff, which may result in an upset, inconsolable child prior to any procedure. A relaxed but firm approach is required. Experienced nursing staff will facilitate this.

Restraint. For an infant, even a minor procedure, such as a finger prick or venepuncture, requires considerable restraint. The method should be as pleasant as possible for the child and easy for the doctor also. This may involve the infant's mother holding her child tightly with the nurse acting as a tourniquet. Alternatively, a towel or sheet may be wrapped around the child to isolate everything except for the limb required for venesection.

Pain relief and sedation. A topical pain relieving cream is now available. EMLA (a eutectic mixture of local anaesthetics) cream should be applied to the site of venesection or intravenous cannula insertion 1 hour before the procedure. The child then feels just pressure instead of pain. Widespread use of pain relief cream may reduce sensitisation to recurrent procedures. A local anaesthetic will help with procedures such as lumbar puncture.

Full blood picture

Blood may be obtained by finger prick sampling. A drop of capillary blood contains at least 50 µl. A heel prick is the most useful source in the newborn. If more blood is required in the older child, the antecubital veins are a useful site. In the younger child, particularly the plump, struggling toddler, venesection can be far more difficult. Sites worth examining for veins include the dorsum of the hands, wrists and feet. If the veins are poorly visualised, immersing the limb in warm water for a few minutes may be time well spent. In difficult circumstances it is worth inserting a butterfly needle into the vein, connected to a syringe once blood has flowed back down the cannula; the needle is less likely to become dislodged during the blood collection and, if necessary, can be used as an i.v. fluid line. In difficult cases the hub of a 20 gauge needle may be broken off and the needle passed through the skin along the line of a vein. Once punctured, the blood will drip back quickly through the end of the needle. Other possible sites include the neck (wrap the infant's arms and trunk in a sheet and tip him or her head down to make the neck veins more prominent) and, more rarely, femoral veins. If these procedures fail, or if the child's blood is too viscous, for example a polycythaemic child with cyanotic congenital heart disease, blood can be obtained from either a radial or brachial artery stab.

The radial artery is the preferred site for arterial puncture as this is usually not an end-artery. If there is not an indwelling arterial cannula, capillary blood gases from heel prick can provide information on pH and CO_2 retention and non-invasive pulse oximetry gives beat by beat oxygenation. Pulse oximetry should now be used routinely in the initial assessment of acute asthma and bronchiolitis.

Problems with collection of blood. If a tourniquet is applied for more than a short time, raised intravenous pressure and hypoxia of the vessel wall results in passage of water and small molecules from the lumen. This may result in high plasma calcium, protein and haemoglobin concentrations. Prolonged local hypoxia may result in leakage of intracellular constituents such as potassium and phosphate, causing falsely high plasma levels. If the child is receiving an intravenous infusion, blood should not be taken proximally from the same limb.

Correct containers for blood are important. For example, blood for glucose estimation is placed in a flouride tube to inhibit glycolosis in erythrocytes. Failure to do this will result in a falsely low glucose estimation. Sodium heparin is often used as an anti-coagulant for the collection of 'blood gases'. If this sample is also used for measurement of sodium a falsely high level may be obtained. Potassium is released from cells during clotting and hence blood for most biochemical tests is heparinised. With haemolysis, the release of haemoglobin colours the plasma red and gives falsely high potassium levels. Plasma should always be separated from blood cells within a few hours or a falsely high potassium and falsely low glucose level will be recorded.

Urine

Urinalysis is quick, cheap and should be routine in all children, in-patient or out-patient, but tends to be neglected, whereas too many specimens are sent routinely for microcopy and culture. The urine should be dip-sticked for the presence of protein, glucose and blood. These are sensitive but not specific tests.

Normal urine is yellow due to urobilinogen. Dark urine may be normal but concentrated, or may be due to blood, free haemoglobin, myoglobin or conjugated bilirubin. Brightly coloured urine is often due to drugs. Cloudy urine is most commonly benign, due to innocuous crystals, but may also be due to pyuria. Specific gravity gives an idea of concentrating ability. Urine pH normally ranges from 4.6 to 8.0 depending on diet, but is usually acidic (pH 5–6). Alkaline urine suggests infection with proteus or pseudomonas, respiratory or metabolic alkalosis, or renal tubular acidosis. Acidic urine occurs in starvation, urine infection, and respiratory or metabolic acidosis. Microscopy may show red cells, white cells, epithelial cells, casts or crystals.

Correct urine collection and analysis is important. In the older child it may be possible to collect a mid-stream urine in the standard way. More often it is necessary to rely on a bag specimen to obtain a sample. Unfortunately, this may take a considerable time and the sample may be contaminated and results difficult to interpret. In many cases it is justifiable to collect urine samples suprapubically using a needle and a 2–5 ml sterile syringe. If an ultrasound machine is available to check that the bladder is full with urine, successful suprapubic aspiration is ensured. The sample obtained should be sent immediately for microscopy for cells, casts, crystals and organisms and for culture if infection is suspected, or if there are renal problems. Urine osmolality, electrolytes and chromatography for amino and organic acids may be relevant in neurological, renal or metabolic problems.

If urinalysis shows excessive pus cells, elevated protein (i.e. greater than 1 +), organisms on microscopy (usually *E. coli* but occasionally other organisms such as pseudomonas) and positive culture (i.e. greater than 100 000 organisms per ml), the diagnosis is acute urinary tract infection. A growth of greater than 100 000 organisms per ml without associated fever, pyuria, proteinuria or organisms on microscopy is still diagnostic of urinary tract infection in a suprapubic aspirate but may be due to infection or contamination in a bag specimen.

Imaging

Radiology. The younger the child, the more difficult it is to exclude chest pathology on auscultation. An infant with fever, tachypnoea and cough, even with no abnormal signs on auscultation, should be presumed to have lower respiratory tract infection unless excluded by X-ray. When screening a child for an infection of unknown cause, chest X-ray is mandatory. Often the chest X-ray findings are not striking on admission and it is only after a further 12–24 hours that the classical picture of widespread consolidation becomes apparent radiographically. In a series of 42 cases of childhood pneumonia in Nottingham in the last 12 months, blood culture was positive in only one out of 33, serology was positive in five out of 13, and nasopharyngeal aspirate positive in four out of seven. Full blood count was unhelpful.

Chest X-ray is useful in any child with recurrent chest symptoms: for example, with wheeze or stridor to exclude congenital abnormalities such as lung cysts, foreign body (inspiratory and expiratory films needed) or evidence of persistent collapse following previous infection.

Chest radiograph showing an upper mediastinal widening and thoracic CT showing the right paratracheal mass to be a benign bronchogenic cyst—same patient

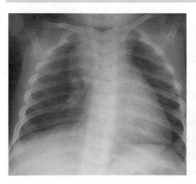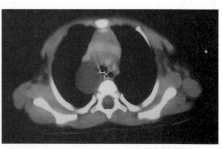

If a child has stridor and is suspected of having acute epiglottitis, the child should be transferred immediately to the intensive care unit. Sending the child to an X-ray department is dangerous as complete obstruction may occur at any time.

Diagnostic ultrasound provides cross-sectional imaging without the use of ionising radiation. Major areas of use include the heart, abdomen, pelvis, urinary tract, vertebral canal, and the intracranial contents in infancy while the fontanelle remains open. Ultrasound may be of value in the early assessment of congenital dislocation of the hip at a time when the diagnosis cannot be made radiographically. Ultrasound scanning is operator dependent and unreliable in detecting vesico-ureteric reflux and renal scarring and, alone, is inadequate for investigating urinary tract infection in young children.

Computerised tomography produces high quality images of the brain. At present it is the radiological investigation of choice for central nervous system disease once the fontanelle has been closed. Other major uses are in evaluation of masses in the thorax, abdomen and in primary bone malignancies. Thoracic CT has replaced contrast bronchography as the first line investigation in suspected bronchiectasis. Disadvantages include the need for sedation or general anaesthesia and a high radiation dose.

Magnetic resonance imaging does not use ionising radiation. A magnet induces a change in alignment of ions which produce an electromagnetic signal when returning to their normal position. This signal can be converted into a sagittal or cross-sectional image. No adverse side effects have been reported. In many cases MRI images are equal to, and in some instances superior to, CT scans, such as in the diagnosis of a posterior fossa mass. In demyelinating disease and certain spinal pathologies it is the examination of choice.

Lumbar puncture

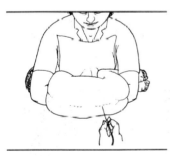

CSF microscopy

- Gram-negative intracellular diplococci—meningococci
- Gram-positive diplococci—pneumococci
- Gram-negative coccobacilli—*Haemophilus influenzae*
- Gram-negative bacilli—*Escherichia coli*; this is almost entirely limited to the first year of life

This is often required in severely sick and shocked children unless the cause of the illness is apparent. Signs of meningitis may be masked by previous administration of oral antibiotics and may not be present in children under the age of 18 months with meningitis. In a first febrile convulsion in a baby under 12 months, lumbar puncture is mandatory. In 328 children with a first febrile convulsion, lumbar puncture was done in 96% and four cases of unsuspected meningitis were identified. Another four convulsions were secondary to urinary tract infection. In contrast, blood tests were unhelpful.

All except the very co-operative older child needs restraint. It is important to ensure that the child's back is at right angles to the couch. Gowning up is probably unnecessary for the procedure, but hands must be well scrubbed and sterile surgical gloves worn. Sterilise the skin overlying the lower lumbar spine and avoid touching the area to be punctured. An imaginary line joining the highest points on the iliac crests passes over the fourth lumbar spine. Try to obtain CSF from the lumbar spaces immediately above or below the fourth lumbar spine. In an infant, the spinal cord may extend to the third lumbar spine. Unless the child is unconscious, it will help to anaesthetise the skin and tissues between the spinous processes, down to the dura with local anaesthetic. The canal is usually easy to locate providing the needle is kept at right angles to the skin. Sometimes a frankly bloody tap ensues due to puncture of the vascular plexus around the cord. Under these circumstances, attempt further puncture in the space above. It is usually not necessary to remove more than 1 ml of fluid. This should be sent for microscopy, bacterial and viral cultures, and glucose and protein estimation. Never disregard seemingly bloody CSF as this may be the only sample of CSF that is obtained. The clinical situation may indicate which blood samples are required. If unsure, it is advisable to take the following if an acute infection warrants a lumbar puncture: glucose, blood culture, viral titres, FBC and electrolytes.

Contraindications to lumbar puncture. Cerebral herniation is a rare complication of lumbar puncture. Contraindications include suspicion of an intracranial mass lesion, cerebral oedema, obstructive hydrocephalus, spinal cord mass or spinal cord swelling. However, no single sign is consistently present in any of these conditions, so clinical judgement is required. Warning signs of cerebral herniation include larger than expected head size, papilloedema, loss of retinal venous pulsation, abnormal head posture and a cracked pot percussion note over the coronal sutures. In the acute situation, when bacterial meningitis is suspected, deterioration in the Glasgow Coma Scales score or tonic fits are danger signs. Failure to localise to a painful stimulus to the head is a contraindication. If a child is thought clinically to have meningitis and raised intracranial pressure, broad spectrum antibiotics to cover common pathogens should be started (e.g. intravenous cefotaxime) and arrangements made for the child to be seen immediately in a hospital skilled at management of raised intracranial pressure. Cerebral herniation is an extremely rare complication of lumbar puncture if the fontanelle is still open and most infants should have a lumbar puncture if meningitis is suspected. In a recent series of 445 children with bacterial meningitis, only two infants under 12 months had cerebral herniation confirmed by imaging or post-mortem.

When symptoms such as headache, vomiting or fever are present over 2–4 weeks the differential diagnosis may include tuberculous meningitis, 'partially treated' meningitis following oral antibiotics, brain abscess and posterior fossa tumour. Other organisms, which less commonly produce meningitis include *Haemophilus influenzae* (rare since the introduction of the Hib vaccine), listeria (neonatal period), klebsiella, streptococci, tubercle and fungal organisms. The diagnosis will usually be confirmed on culture and identification. Previous antibiotic therapy may prevent growth.

CSF colour. Bright red blood may be due to damage to a blood vessel during lumbar puncture or a recent haemorrhage involving the subarachnoid space. Xanthochromia is a yellow discoloration of the CSF and may be caused by altered haemoglobin (following subarachnoid haemorrhage), a large amount of pus, jaundice, or very high protein levels, for example with cerebral or spinal tumours. Turbidity is usually due to increased numbers of white cells and normally indicates infection. Spontaneous clotting of the CSF due to an excess of fibrinogen may occur with tuberculous meningitis or with CNS tumours.

CSF glucose. An abnormally low glucose may occur with bacterial or tuberculous meningitis but is not found with viral infection. However, glucose may be normal in any form of meningitis. Hypoglycaemia will result in an equivalently low CSF glucose and blood glucose should always be taken simultaneously. The normal CSF glucose is two-thirds of the blood glucose. Widespread malignant infiltration of the meninges may also cause low CSF glucose levels. Persistently low CSF glucose occurs after subarachnoid haemorrhage and may occasionally be seen with chronic multisystem inflammatory disorders.

CSF pressure. This is measured by a manometer or pressure transducer attached to the needle at the onset of the procedure. Normal CSF pressure in the neonate has a range from 0 to 8 cmH$_2$O with a mean of 3 cmH$_2$O. The upper limit of CSF pressure in older children is similar to the adult value of 19 cmH$_2$O.

Typical CSF findings in various forms of meningitis

	Bacterial	Bacterial (Early or ? partially treated)	Viral	Tuberculous
Appearance	Turbid	Usually clear	Clear	Hazy
Cells (1 mm^3)	50–50 000 Polymorphs. May be a few lymphocytes	25–1000 Polymorphs. May be up to 50% lymphocytes	25–1000 Lymphocytes. May be 50% polymorphs in early stages	50–1000 Lymphocytes. Up to 50% polymorphs in early stages
Microscopy	Organism often seen in CSF. + ve culture by 24 hours	No organism seen. Culture may be sterile	No organism sterile culture	Organisms may be found in coagulum.+ve culture after several weeks
Protein (g/l)	0.8–4.0	0.8–2.0	0–1.5	0.6–6
Glucose	Low/absent	Normal/low	Normal	Very low

CSF protein consists mostly of albumin, but other proteins are present (e.g. immunoglobulins). Total protein is high in the neonatal period (upper limit 1.2 g/l) falling to adult levels (0.25–0.4 g/l) by 6 months of age. CSF protein concentration will increase in the presence of pus or blood. The CSF protein is increased by around 0.01 g/l for each 1000 red blood cells per microlitre. Non-purulent cerebral inflammation (or radiculitis as in Guillain–Barré syndrome) may also cause an increase in total protein concentration. Blockage of the spinal canal by tumours, vertebral fractures or tuberculosis may cause very high protein concentrations (Froin syndrome).

FURTHER READING

Addy D (ed) 1994 Investigations in paediatrics. WB Saunders, London

Joint Working Group of the Research Unit of the Royal College of Physicians and the British Paediatric Association 1991 Guidelines for the management of convulsions with fever

Buys H, Pesad L, Hallett R, Maskell R 1994 Suprapubic aspiration under ultrasound guidance in children with fever of undiagnosed cause. British Medical Journal 303: 634–636

Jadresic L, Cartwright K, Cowie N, Witcombe B, Stevens D 1993 Investigation of urinary tract infection in childhood. British Medical Journal 307: 761–764

Mellor, DH The place of computed tomography and lumbar puncture in suspected bacterial meningitis. Archives of Disease in Childhood 67: 1417–1419

O'Callaghan C, Stephenson T 1992 Pocket paediatrics. Churchill Livingstone, Edinburgh

Rennick G, Shann F, deCampo J 1993 Cerebral herniation during bacterial meningitis in children. British Medical Journal 306: 953–955

Rotbart HA 1990 Diagnosis of enteroviral meningitis with the polymerase chain reaction. Journal of Pediatrics 117: 85–89

Smellie JM, Rigden SPA, Prescod NP 1995 Urinary tract investigation: a comparison of four methods of investigation. Archives of Disease in Childhood 72: 247–250

Stephenson T, Wallace H Clinical paediatrics for postgraduate examinations, 2nd edn. Churchill Livingstone, Edinburgh

vanDeuren M, vanDijke BJ, Koopman RJJ, Horrevorts AM, Meis JFGM, Santman FW, derMeer JWM v 1993 Rapid diagnosis of acute meningococcal infections by needle aspiration or biopsy of skin lesions. British Medical Journal 306: 1229–1232

Accidents and emergencies

For most children, the accident and emergency department (A&E) is their first experience of hospital, though perhaps not of doctors and nurses. The circumstances surrounding the attendance are often frightening for the child and worrying for the family. The joy children have in the excitement of an ambulance's siren and flashing lights may turn to fear if the child is ill or injured.

The paediatric accident and emergency service is the 'shop window' of the hospital. The Patient's Charter requires that every patient presenting to an A&E department will be seen immediately and their need for treatment assessed. This process of triage ensures that children with life threatening conditions are treated ahead of those with less serious problems. Children require their own accident and emergency facilities, staffed by appropriately trained medical and nursing staff preferably linked to their own observation area. Liaison with general practitioners, school nurses, health visitors, community nurses and child health specialists helps to improve the service offered and to avoid unnecessary attendances and admissions. A philosophy of family centred care is fundamental to a successful service for children.

The gold standards for the care of the most seriously ill and injured children have been established by the introduction of Advanced Trauma Life Support (ATLS), Advanced Paediatric Life Support (APLS) and Paediatric Advanced Life Support (PALS) courses. Training on such a course should be considered by all providing emergency treatment for children.

EMERGENCIES

To remain in control in an emergency situation it is necessary to develop and practise a number of skills. Basic resuscitation skills should be second nature and there should be familiarity with advanced life support.

A Airway   **B Breathing**   **C Circulation**

BASIC LIFE SUPPORT—when faced with an unresponsive child

		Infant <1 year old	Child >1 year old
A Airway	**Check** responsiveness	Shake—pinch gently Shout for help	Shake—pinch gently Shout for help
	open airway	Head tilt to neutral position Chin lift/jaw thrust	Head tilt to sniffing position Chin lift/jaw thrust
B Breathing	**Check** breathing	Look—listen—feel	Look—listen—feel
	breath for child	Mouth to mouth and nose, 5 breaths	Mouth to mouth, 5 breaths
C Circulation	**Check** pulse	Feel brachial pulse Start CPR if <60/min	Feel carotid pulse Start CPR if no pulse
	chest compression	2 fingers applied 1 cm below nipple line to depth of 2 cm	Heel of one hand applied to lower sternum to depth of 3 cm

- CPR Cardiopulmonary resuscitation, 100 compressions per min at 5 : 1 breath (20 cycles per min).
- After 1 minute go for help if none has arrived.
- Remember cervical spine control in the presence of any injury.

ADVANCED LIFE SUPPORT — establish definitive airway (intubation), ventilate, active cardiac stimulation

A Airway	Failure of basic airway manoeuvres may necessitate using an oro-(Guedel) or nasopharyngeal airway. A Guedel airway can be sized by lying it from the centre of the mouth to the angle of the jaw, and it should be inserted the 'right' way up in infants and young children. A nasopharyngeal airway may be better tolerated in conscious patients but should not be used if there is any suspicion of a basal skull fracture to avoid confusion of any nasal discharge with possible CSF rhinorrhoea
B Breathing	When ventilatory support is needed, administer oxygen by bag-valve-mask and consider intubation in order to maintain a protected airway. A child can be oxygenated adequately by bag and mask in most instances until experienced help arrives. The diameter of endotracheal tube required can be estimated in an emergency by matching internal diameter to the width of the child's little fingernail or by the formula: diameter of endotracheal tube = age in years /4 + 4. Monitor by means of pulse oximetry and ECG leads
C Circulation	Most Cardiac arrest in children will be respiratory in origin. Following satisfactory institution of basic life support the absence of palpable pulses necessitates assessment of the rhythm. See section on Cardiac Arrest below

- **Estimate weight**. Weight helps with choice of tube size and drug dosages. The Broselow tape uses length to give an estimate of weight; or use the formula: weight in kilograms = [age in years + 4] × 2.
- **Start** the clock.
- **Nominate** a team member to record information on all drugs administered.

Problem

Respiratory arrest

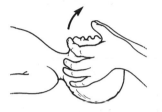

**Jaw thrust:
2nd & 3rd fingers under
angle of the jaw and lift**

The most frightening situation for anyone to face is that of the child who is not breathing and who may or may not have a cardiac output. It is frightening because it happens infrequently, but basic management principles apply as in all emergency situations.

A Airway. A child in respiratory distress will assume the position of comfort. Do not try to *improve* the situation unless facilities for advanced life support are to hand. If there is any suspicion of a cervical spine injury the safest airway opening procedure is a jaw thrust without head tilt. Do not use a finger sweep technique as this may damage the soft palate or push a foreign body down the airway.

B Breathing. A tidal volume of 7–10 ml/kg is necessary to achieve adequate ventilation but in practice normal chest expansion should be observed. Failure of adequate ventilation despite appropriate airway opening techniques suggests the presence of a foreign body.

C Circulation. A circulatory arrest is diagnosed when the pulse is absent for 5 seconds or more. For satisfactory resuscitation the child should be lying supine on a firm flat surface. An alternative technique for infants is to encircle the chest with both hands placing the thumbs over the correct landmark .

Problem

Cardiac arrest

**Chest compression:
infants — 2 fingers
children — heel of hand**

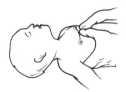

There are three basic cardiac arrest rhythms in children:

Asystole. This is by far the commonest. It usually follows a progressive bradycardia and is the response to prolonged, severe hypoxia and acidosis. On seeing an almost straight line on the monitor first check that all the leads are connected and that the gain is turned up.

Management

1. Intubate — ventilate with 100% oxygen
2. Establish intravenous (i.v.) or intraosseous (i.o.) access
3. Give adrenaline 1:10 000 0.1 ml (10 µg)/kg
4. 3 minutes cardiopulmonary resuscitation (60 cycles)
5. Consider i.v. fluids (20 ml/kg) and alkalising agents
6. Give i.v. or i.o. adrenaline 1 : 1000 0.1 ml (100 µg)/kg
7. 3 minutes cardiopulmonary resuscitation and repeat adrenaline

Notes: The routine use of alkalising agents has not been shown to be of any benefit.
    If giving adrenaline via ET tube give × 10 dose.

Unfortunately the outcome is generally poor if there is no response to the second dose of adrenaline.

Ventricular fibrillation. This rhythm is rare in childhood but may occur in those who are hypothermic, poisoned by tricyclic antidepressants or who have cardiac disease.

Management

1. Precordial thump, but only if collapse witnessed
2. DC shock 2 J/kg and repeat once
3. DC shock 4 J/kg
4. Intubate — ventilate with high flow oxygen
5. Establish intravenous (i.v.) or intraosseous (i.o.) access
6. Give adrenaline 1 : 10 000 0.1 ml (10 µg)/kg
7. DC shock 4 J/kg × 3
8. Adrenaline 1 : 1000 0.1 ml (100 µg)/kg
9. Minute cardiopulmonary resuscitation and repeat last 3 steps

Electromechanical dissociation (EMD). This is the absence of palpable pulses despite recognisable complexes on the ECG monitor and it is usually due to severe hypovolaemia. In trauma consider tension pneumothorax or cardiac tamponade. The management is the same as for asystole plus the treatment of any underlying cause.

Ongoing management of all those who survive should be in a paediatric intensive care unit and continued monitoring and intubation is vital in the early post-resuscitation period. Children have low glycogen stores and may become hypoglycaemic during an arrest situation, therefore recheck the *blood sugar*.

Problem	Choking

As soon as a foreign body is suspected decisive action is needed — back slaps or chest thrusts depending on the size of the child. The use of abdominal thrusts (heimlich manoeuvre) is contraindicated in infants as the potential for damage outweighs the possible benefits.

Back slapping and chest thrusts; for infants on your thigh, for older children across your knee or kneeling

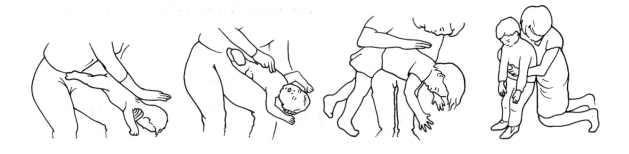

SHOCK

This can be defined as the failure of the circulatory system to perfuse tissues adequately. Early recognition and aggressive treatment are important because the loss of a relatively small amount of fluid may represent a high percentage of a child's intravascular volume. A child's circulating volume is normally 80 ml/kg and they usually compensate well until more than one-third of this volume is lost. Decompensation is late, sudden and profound. Detection of shock is based on the vital signs:

	Respiratory rate (breaths per min)	Pulse rate (beats per minute)	Systolic blood pressure (mmHg)
Infant	50	160	
Toddler	35	140	80 + (age in years x 2)
School child	25	120	
Adolescent	20	110	

Values are upper limits of normal.

There are three recognised phases of shock:

Phase 1: Compensated shock. In this oxygen to the vital structures — brain and heart – is maintained by sympathetic reflexes at the expense of non-essential tissues. The systolic blood pressure remains normal whereas the diastolic pressure may be elevated due to increase in the systemic arterial resistance.

Phase 2: Uncompensated shock develops when this mechanism begins to fail. Inefficient anaerobic metabolism supervenes in poorly perfused areas leading to the production of lactate and subsequent systemic acidosis. Late or preterminal signs of shock include falling systolic blood pressure, central cyanosis and bradycardia.

Phase 3: Irreversible shock is the result of natural progression if treatment is not effective. It is usually a retrospective diagnosis.

	Compensated	Uncompensated	Irreversible
Heart rate	↑	↑↑	↑↓
Systolic BP	normal	normal/↓	↓↓
Pulse volume	normal/↓	↓	↓↓
Capillary refill time	normal/↑	↑	↑↑
Skin colour	pale	mottled	white/grey
Skin temperature	cool	cold	cold
Mental status	agitation	lethargic/uncooperative	reacts to pain
Respiratory rate	normal/↑	↑↑	sighing
Fluid loss	<25%	25–40%	>40%

Maintenance of adequate tissue perfusion depends on a pump delivering the correct type and volume of fluid through vessels without any obstruction to flow. Shock may result from defects of the pump (cardiogenic), loss of fluid (hypovolaemic), abnormalities of vessels (distributive), flow restriction (obstructive) or inadequate oxygen-releasing capacity (dissociative), or a combination of these as is seen in most seriously ill children. The immediate treatment of shock is the same irrespective of its cause. Administration of 100% oxygen via a face mask is followed by rapid intravenous fluid replacement (20 ml/kg of crystalloid or colloid) as often as required.

Causes of shock

Cardiogenic	Arrhythmias, cardiomyopathy, heart failure, valvular disease, myocardial contusion, myocardial infarction
Distributive	Septicaemia, anaphylaxis, vasodilator drugs, anaesthesia, spinal cord injury
Dissociative	Tension pneumothorax, haemopneumothorax, flail chest, cardiac tampanade, pulmonary embolism, hypertension
Hypovolaemic	Haemorrhage, diarrhoea and/or vomiting, burns
Obstructive	Profound anaemia, carbon monoxide poisoning, methaemoglobinaemia

Problem	Anaphylaxis

This is an immunologically mediated condition which may progress to shock and is characterised by itching, flushing, urticaria, facial swelling, bronchospasm, arrhythmias, abdominal pain and diarrhoea or any combination of these. It is a Type 1 (immediate) hypersensitivity reaction mediated by IgE or IgG leading to vasodilatation. It occurs in response to an allergen such as drugs (e.g. penicillin), insect stings, blood products, radiographic contrast media or certain foods (e.g. nuts, eggs, strawberries). Anaphylactoid reactions may be triggered by the first exposure because they occur in the absence of a specific antigen.

Stop allergen

1. Assess ABC and act accordingly
2. Give 100% oxygen
3. Adrenaline 1 : 10 000 0.1 ml/kg (10 μg/kg) i.m. (i.v. or i.o. if local policy recommends)
4. Hydrocortisone (4 mg/kg)
5. Chlorpheniramine (0.2 mg/kg)
6. Consider nebulised salbutamol (2.5–5 mg)
7. Repeat adrenaline

Successful emergency treatment should be followed by a detailed documentation of events preceding the symptoms. The patient's family should be given a clear explanation and advice on management of any future episodes. The patient should be advised to wear a medic alert disc and they should have access to an emergency kit. Investigations in the form of radioimmunassay for specific IgE or cutaneous testing may be helpful but history is the best way to identify a precipitant.

Problem	Septic shock (see Ch. 4)

This is due to a mixture of causes: hypovolaemia — from inadequate fluid intake and inappropriate polyuria; obstructive — from increased pulmonary resistance; cardiogenic — from myocardial dysfunction; and distributive — from an increased microvascular permeability and peripheral blood pooling. It usually results from infection with gram-negative bacteria but gram-positives, fungi, viruses and rickettsiae can produce an identical picture. In addition to the basic supportive measures previously described, it is important to monitor blood sugar and treat with appropriate intravenous antibiotics. It may also be necessary to institute inotropic support.

POISONING

Around 40 000 children attend A&E departments annually with suspected poisonings and up to 22% of these children are admitted to hospital. Children who are poisoned fall into three broad categories:

Accidental. These are typically children of 1–4 years with boys representing 66% of cases. There is an increased incidence after household disruption like a new baby, moving house and the presence of maternal depression. In 60% of cases the substance was not in its usual storage place. Deaths are uncommon, those which occur being due to tricyclic antidepressants, household products and rarely to plants. A decline in deaths followed the introduction of child-resistant containers in 1976, though 20% of 5 year olds *can* open them!

Intentional. These are typically teenage girls and they need hospital admission for assessment and occasionally treatment. There are a worrying few in this group who are 8–12 years of age, clinically depressed and at risk of suicide unless identified.

Deliberate. The child's parents may not volunteer any relevant history, therefore deliberate poisoning should be suspected if the signs cannot be explained in any other way. Münchausen syndrome by proxy is characterised by:

— Illness in a child which is faked and/or produced by the 'carer'.
— Multiple medical opinions/presentations.
— Denial of knowledge by the 'carer' of the cause of the child's illness.
— Disappearance of acute signs when the child is separated from the 'carer'.

Most poisoned children remain asymptomatic (85%) and need little in the way of treatment or observation but up to 10% may require intensive care. Poisoning still results in a number of childhood deaths annually (10 in 1992) and therefore prevention initiatives are essential. Poisoning should be suspected in any child who presents with unexplained symptoms.

There is usually some history or indication of what may have been taken but it is often more difficult to know exactly how much has been ingested. A careful history including an assessment of how many tablets or how much medicine is missing is therefore essential and identification of remaining drugs from packaging or colour charts and natural substances from comparison with illustrated books may be helpful.

In the UK the adverse effects of the less common poisons can be obtained by ringing one of the regional poison centres which are manned 24 hours a day. They are necessarily pessimistic and will list all the known side effects of the poison and the minimum lethal dose. They will advise whether specific removal of the poison is indicated and whether an antidote exists.

Signs suggesting specific poisons

Pinpoint pupils	Opiates, organophosphates
Dilated pupils	Atropine, tricyclics
Drowsiness	Alcohol, sedatives, opiates, hypnotics, aspirin, tricyclics
Confusion, ataxia, excitability	Alcohol, tricyclics, antihistamines, salbutamol, solvent abuse
Convulsions	Alcohol, tricyclics, theophylline, lithium
Dystonic reactions	Phenothazines, metoclopramide
Cardiac arrhythmias	Tricyclics, theophylline, salbutamol, digoxin, potassium
Tachypnoea	Salicylates
Hypotension	Sedatives, hypnotics, iron
Hypertension with tachycardia	Sympathomimetics
Haematemesis	Iron, salicylates

Principles of management

Most children will not have taken a dangerous amount of a substance or indeed a dangerous substance and telephone reassurance in these circumstances is all that is required. Some aspects of the management of suspected poisoning remain unchanged, namely maintaining an airway and managing any complications. Limitation of drug absorption is dependent on local policy which may advise contacting a regional poison centre.

Activated charcoal should be considered within 1 hour of ingestion of a significant amount of a toxic substance but is not appropriate after acids or alkalis. This may need to be repeated, for example, after ingestion of significant amounts of digoxin, carbemazepine, aspirin or theophylline. The dose is 1–2 g/kg given orally (or nasogastrically as it is fairly unpalatable).

Gastric lavage is indicated if a patient presents within 1 hour of ingestion of a life-threatening quantity of a toxic substance. It is never appropriate after ingestion of corrosives or hydrocarbons. If the patient has a compromised airway then intubation should be carried out first.

Ipecacuanha is not indicated in the treatment of ingestion as there is no evidence that it alters absorption and the side effects are undesirable.

The availability of observation facilities will dictate whether a child is admitted as most can be discharged after an initial period of observation. Always admit those who are symptomatic or have ingested iron, antidepressants, digoxin or aspirin in significant amounts.

Paracetamol

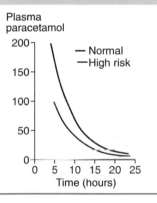

Paracetamol normogram. Patients on enzyme-inducing drugs are at higher risk. Note: 150 mg = 1 mmol

Plasma paracetamol

This is available as a junior elixir, 120 mg per 5 ml, which is rarely dangerous, or as adult tablets, 500 mg, which are large and therefore not easily swallowed by children. The clinical features depend on the amount taken and range from none at all to acute hepatic failure — confusion, drowsiness, bleeding tendency and jaundice. The plasma paracetamol level should be measured at least 4 hours after ingestion and the result compared with the normogram.

Treatment. If the level is below the toxic line discharge is appropriate unless the paracetamol was taken deliberately. Otherwise admit and treat with N-acetylcysteine as an intravenous infusion. It is useful up to 24 hours after ingestion. The side effects of this treatment include rashes, bronchospasm and, occasionally, anaphylaxis. Toxicity can occur at lower levels if the liver is induced by the simultaneous ingestion of substances like phenytoin, carbamazepine, phenobarbitone, rifampicin or alcohol. If signs of liver failure develop such as deranged liver function and clinically abnormal clotting, consider transferring the child to a specialist centre. Children are remarkably resistant to hepatotoxic effects but complacency would be inappropriate.

Tricyclics

Because of their devastating effects, this group is responsible for most deaths due to poisoning. Preparations include amitryptilline, nortryptilline and imipramine in either tablet or liquid form — sustained release capsules are especially dangerous. They will be found in the home if an adult is being treated for depression or if an older sibling is being treated for enuresis. Absorption is rapid and therefore clinical features occur soon after ingestion and are a better guide to severity than measuring blood levels. An excitatory phase of restlessness, agitation and hallucinations may be followed by a phase of depressed consciousness. The anticholinergic effects, for example a dry mouth, fixed dilated pupils and urinary retention, are less dangerous. They are useful indicators of ingestion.

Treatment. This is a serious form of poisoning and children should *always be admitted* and monitored. Cardiac monitoring and a 12 lead ECG must be instituted at the time of presentation. If the child is symptomatic admission to an intensive care unit is advisable. Treatment with gastric lavage within 1 hour of ingestion is recommended as gut motility is impaired. The mainstay of management is supportive therapy including protecting the airway. Convulsions are managed with diazepam intravenously (0.25–0.4 mg/kg) or rectally (0.5 mg/kg), and hypotension by positioning and volume expansion. Cardiac arrhythmias can be suppressed by an alkalosis (pH 7.4–7.5) induced by mechanical hyperventilation and a sodium bicarbonate infusion.

β-Blockers

These drugs result in significant arrhythmias especially profound bradycardias. They have long half-lives and therefore admission for observation is required. Intravenous glucagon will treat overwhelming cardiogenic shock unresponsive to atropine and the hypoglycaemia of hepatic suppression.

Salicylates

Since aspirin was withdrawn from paediatric treatments, overdose has been less frequent but still occurs, predominantly in the intentional group. The clinical features of salicylate poisoning are frightening and include nausea, vomiting, deep sighing respirations, tinnitus, fever and dehydration as the early features, with coma later and the possibility of bleeding due to prolongation of the prothrombin time. The salicylate level should be checked 4–6 hours after ingestion.

Salicylate poisoning	
Plasma level	Management
<45 mg/dl in the first 6 hours	Discharge with instructions to return if any symptoms develop [unless deliberate self-harm]
45–65 mg/dl at 6 hours	Admit, ensure adequate fluid intake and if necessary give i.v. dextrose 4% and saline 0.18% with potassium at a rate of 5ml /kg hour
>65 mg/dl at 6 hours	Admit to intensive care, induce an alkaline diuresis (urine pH of 8) by a dextrose saline infusion with added sodium bicarbonate. Accurate fluid balance is essential. Vitamin K may be required

In the symptomatic child check urea, electrolytes and blood sugar plus blood gases if they are comatose or very unwell. Clinical deterioration is common and later investigation may demonstrate metabolic acidosis and hypoglycaemia which in children is found more commonly than the respiratory alkalosis expected of a respiratory stimulant.

Treatment. This is determined by the relationship between the plasma salicylate level and the time from ingestion unless symptoms require immediate management.

Iron

Iron tablets are attractive to children and they are readily available in many households being prescribed in pregnancy and for treatment of iron deficiency. As little as 2 g of elemental iron may prove fatal.

Gastrointestinal bleeding and vomiting are the initial symptoms followed by a symptom free period and then cardiovascular collapse, acute encephalopathy and hepatic failure. An abdominal X-ray may show residual iron and help with management decisions. A plasma level of > 5 mg/l within 6 hours of ingestion suggests serious poisoning requiring treatment.

Treatment. Desferrioxamine by slow i.v. infusion at a rate of 15 mg/kg/h to a total dose of 80 mg/kg/day; beware of hypotension.

Alcohol

The chief problems in children are altered consciousness level and hypoglycaemia. Symptomatic children should be admitted and their blood glucose monitored hourly until the consciousness level improves. In the meantime, attend to ABC.

Narcotics

Always consider these drugs as a history of ingestion is rare, especially if they have been taken 'recreationally'. Signs include respiratory depression, pinpoint pupils, coma, convulsions, hypotension and arrhythmias. Reversal by naloxone is diagnostic. It is given i.v. in a dose of 0.2 mg (< 1 year), 0.4 mg (1–12 years) and 0.8 mg (>12 years). It has a short half-life and may need to be repeated every 15–20 minutes.

Lead

This poisoning is chronic and there is no history of ingestion. Lead can be ingested from lead piping, lead-based paint, the lead-based cosmetic *surma* or inhaled from polluted fumes. Constipation, colicky abdominal pain, tiredness and anaemia may be followed by encephalopathy — headache, disturbed consciousness, vomiting, ataxia and fits. Papilloedema may be found and X-rays may show increased density at the growth plates (lead lines) or lining the bowel. The classic haematological finding is of anaemia with basophilic stippling. A blood lead level of >50 µg/100 ml is found in symptomatic children and >80 µg/100 ml if there is encephalopathy.

Treatment. This is in order of priority starting with the treatment of raised intracranial pressure, then removal of lead from the body and finally identification and removal of the source of the lead. Raised intracranial pressure is treated with dexamethasone plus mannitol in severe cases. Lead removal is enhanced by chelating agents such as dimercaprol and calcium EDTA with penicillamine once symptoms have resolved. The child should not return home until the source of the lead has been eliminated.

Carbon monoxide

Common sources of carbon monoxide are car exhausts, poorly maintained and ventilated heating systems, smoke from all types of fires and coal gas. Carbon monoxide has a much higher affinity for haemoglobin than oxygen. It causes a left shift in the oxygen dissociation curve. Its toxic effects are the result of tissue hypoxia. Headaches, nausea, vomiting, confusion, coma and death are the central nervous system effects. There is no central cyanosis and the classic cherry red skin caused by carboxyhaemoglobin is a sign of severe poisoning and usually a terminal finding. Oxygen saturation is not reliable and it is necessary to measure carboxyhaemoglobin directly. A level over 25% suggests severe poisoning.

Treatment. Remove from the source of the gas and administer 100% oxygen. Hyperbaric oxygen therapy enhances the removal but is not readily available and local policy determines access to this facility.

DROWNING/NEAR DROWNING

Every year around 15 children in a million drown and half of them die. It is the third commonest cause of accidental death in children after road traffic accidents and burns. Near drowning is diagnosed if there is any recovery, however brief, following immersion. If basic life support is given at the waterside 70% of cases will survive. Of those that require cardiorespiratory resuscitation in hospital, 70% will make a full recovery, 25% will have a mild neurological deficit and 5% will be severely disabled or remain in a persistent vegetative state.

Breath-holding occurs on submersion leading to bradycardia (the diving reflex). Subsequent hypoxia leads to tachycardia, an increase in blood pressure and acidosis. Breathing movements occur between 20 seconds and 2.5 minutes later, causing laryngeal spasm when fluid touches the glottis. Secondary apnoea follows eventually, giving way to involuntary breathing efforts, bradycardia, arrhythmias, cardiac arrest and death. Management assumes the presence of hypothermia, electrolyte imbalance and/or injury.

Treatment follows the ABC principles together with rewarming which can be passive — removal of wet clothing, wrapping, use of radiant heat; or active — use of warm intravenous fluids, ventilator gases, gastric, bladder or peritoneal lavage or extracorporeal blood rewarming. Resuscitation should be continued until a core temperature of 32°C has been obtained.

Investigations. Measure blood glucose, arterial blood gases, electrolytes, baseline CXR and blood cultures. A fever is common in the first 24 hours, but thereafter assume infection is present and treat accordingly.

Good prognostic features include: a short time, between 1 and 3 minutes to the first gasp (there is little chance of intact survival if it takes 40 minutes or more unless hypothermia is present); a rectal temperature <33°C on arrival; an improving conscious level; a pH >7.0 with continuing treatment; a Po_2 >8.0 kPa (60 mmHg). The type of water does not affect the prognosis.

THE ABUSED CHILD

A child is considered to have been abused if he or she is treated by another person in a way that is unacceptable in a given culture at a given time. There are recognised patterns of abuse, physical, emotional, sexual and neglect, but these commonly overlap and should all be considered.

Physical abuse. Experienced accident and emergency staff will see many accidental injuries and should be in a good position to recognise those that do not fit the normal patterns. The following features should alert the examiner to the possibility of an injury being non-accidental:

— Delay in seeking medical help.
— A previous history of abuse in child or a sibling.
— Inconsistency between history and injury.
— Lack of, or vague, explanation for the injury from carers.
— Differing explanations over time.
— Child said to have contributed to the injury in a manner not possible at their current stage of development.
— Parents' behaviour gives cause for concern — disinterested or unexpectedly hostile.
— Child's relationship with parent seems abnormal — the child is frightened, withdrawn, or shows 'frozen watchfulness'.

Emotional abuse and neglect are more difficult to identify and subjective assessment is required. Features which may suggest this (or any other) type of abuse are: general neglect, poor hygiene, unkempt clothing, failure to thrive.

Sexual abuse. Girls are more often sexually abused than boys and about half of the cases occur in children under 5 years of age. The perpetrators are usually male although sadly not infrequently with the collusion of the child's mother. Presentation may be with: an allegation, a urinary tract infection, a vaginal discharge, abdominal pain, pruritis ani, anal fissure, constipation or encopresis and altered behaviour like 'acting out' or doing less well at school.

A hospital is generally not an appropriate environment for the diagnosis and management of these children who should be assessed by a paediatrician, police surgeon and social worker in privacy in a suite of rooms designed for the purpose. Many areas now manage cases of suspected child abuse almost entirely in the community, especially those relating to sexual abuse. Cases do, however, present unexpectedly in hospital without the prior warning provided by an allegation.

Action   *Record* who accompanies the child to hospital, take a detailed history and write down important quotes verbatim so that subsequent inconsistencies will be apparent. Accept what the parents tell you and avoid an adversarial situation. A detailed family and social history is important as many features are common in families of abused children. Child abuse occurs in all sections of society.

Examination. The child should ideally be fully undressed for the examination but this may not be appropriate in an accident and emergency setting when alternative arrangements should be made. The findings must be detailed, signed and dated. Features which may suggest that an injury is non-accidental are: multiple injuries, injuries of different ages, injuries which are regular in shape like belt or slipper marks, patterns of injury like bruising on the trunk or head, suggestive injuries like finger-tip bruises, black eyes, torn frenulum, or human bite marks which tend to be crescent-shaped as opposed to U-shaped animal bites. It is important not to forget examination of the mouth and fundi during the procedure. The latter may be especially important in a small child presenting with a decreased consciousness level where retinal haemorrhages may be suggestive of a shaking injury.

Responsibilities. It is the responsibility of anyone involved in the care of children who suspects that a child may have suffered abuse to report it to one of the statutory agencies. This will normally be Social Services but the NSPCC and the Police are also statutory agencies. It is important to be familiar with the local procedures documented in the Area Child Protection Committee Guidelines. If child abuse is suspected then a senior opinion must be sought. Never accuse the parents or state categorically that the child has been abused. Obtain all previous medical records and enquire whether the child is on the 'at-risk' register. If there are other children 'at risk' then social services will also arrange for them to be examined. It is vital to keep accurate notes contemporaneously. Use an appropriate diagram to note all injuries, and record the size of bruises and lacerations. If possible photographs should be obtained. Do not be persuaded to estimate the age of a bruise from its colour. This has been shown to be extremely unreliable and it is better simply to state that the injury appears recent or not. Management is decided following discussions between the paediatric and social work teams involved.

Differential diagnoses requiring exclusion	
Bruising	Henoch–Schönlein purpura, leukaemia, clotting disorders, connective tissue disorders, idiopathic thrombocytopenic purpura (ITP), mongolian blue spot or other birth marks
Cigarette burns	Identified by the typical raised rim around an ulcerated lesion, impetigo or staphylococcal skin infections
Broken bones	Osteogenesis imperfecta, copper deficiency, rickets, coffey's disease, pathological fractures through a tumour or cyst

Investigations

The following may be considered depending on the particular findings:

Clotting studies — young children do bruise more easily than adults because of the laxity of connective tissues.

X-ray of an injured limb — dictated by the nature of the injury.

Skeletal survey — this will look for multiple injuries of different ages. Periosteal new bone formation, depressed skull fractures and spiral fractures of long bones all warrant suspicion and rib fractures in children under 18 months are non-accidental injury until proven otherwise.

CHILDREN BROUGHT IN DEAD

All children found suddenly or unexpectedly dead should be admitted to the resuscitation room. Many will have received resuscitation from the ambulance personnel en route. This should be continued by staff in the emergency department, unless there is clear evidence of death such as post-mortem rigidity or dependent skin discoloration, until there has been sufficient time to assess the situation. Parents accompanying the child may wish to stay in the resuscitation room and an experienced nurse should be allocated to stay with them and explain the proceedings. They may alternatively be taken to a quiet room nearby and kept in touch with events. It is useful if one member of the team can obtain a detailed history at this stage.

The decision to discontinue resuscitation is difficult. If there has been no detectable cardiac output or any signs of cerebral activity after 30 minutes of cardiopulmonary resuscitation, it is reasonable to withdraw — some authorities recommend 20 minutes. If hypothermia is present, resuscitation should continue until the core temperature is at least 32°C.

Once the child has been certified dead do not keep the parents waiting in false hope. The responsibility for breaking the bad news rests with the most senior member of the team. There should be privacy for the initial period of distress. The parents must be told of the legal requirement to inform the coroner, and that the police will wish to visit the place of death and take a statement. It is safest not to assume a cause of death as a post-mortem will almost certainly be performed and may show something unexpected.

Careful records of all clinical findings and resuscitation measures should be made, noting particularly the state of nutrition, hydration, rectal temperature on arrival and any injuries or rashes. The following investigations should be considered depending on local policy:

— Bacterial swabs from the nose, throat and rectum.
— Urine via a suprapubic aspirate for culture, toxicology and/or metabolic analysis.
— Virology samples from nasopharynx, throat and rectum.
— Blood from the right ventricle for culture.
— A small skin biopsy for analysis.

Checklist

It is important to notify all the relevant people as soon as possible of the child's death and this is best ensured by the use of a checklist:

— GP	— Paediatric consultant on call
— Coroner	— Outpatients' department
— Local police	— Liaison health visitor

Some areas may recommend a social services register check on all children who die unexpectedly, as a significant number will have died under suspicious circumstances. The family should be offered an appointment to come and talk about the circumstances surrounding their child's death approximately 6 weeks afterwards.

Causes of sudden unexpected death in infants and children: it depends on the age of the child	
Under 1 year of age	Over 1 year of age
Sudden Infant Death	Trauma, e.g. road traffic accidents, fires, choking, poisoning, falls
Infection	Infection
Congenital abnormalities	Sudden deterioration in chronic condition, e.g. asthma, epilepsy, diabetes, heart disease
Non-accidental injury	Non-accidental Injury

Sudden unexpected death in infancy (SUDI)

Over 85% of deaths are in babies between 1 and 6 months of age. There is a preponderance amongst boys and significant associations with prone sleeping, overwrapping, social deprivation, multiple births, prematurity, maternal smoking and smoky environments. Breast feeding has many benefits but there is no direct evidence that it protects against sudden infant death. It is advised that the infants should *not* be:

— Laid on their fronts (except following medical advice).
— Exposed to cigarette smoke either before or after birth.
— Overwrapped or overheated especially when they are feverish or unwell.
— Inadequately dressed when taken out of doors in cold weather.

Recent advice to parents also recommends placing babies at the bottom of the cot to prevent them wriggling down under the covers during the night. Breast feeding is encouraged wherever possible and parents and others in charge of children are encouraged to seek medical advice promptly if an infant is thought to be unwell.

Many health authorities have follow-up arrangements such as the CONI (care of the next infant) scheme and it is important to be familiar with what is available locally.

INJURIES

Approximately 70% of children presenting to A&E departments have suffered an injury. The majority receive treatment in the department and are discharged to primary care. Up to 10% are reviewed in A&E clinics and others are admitted to hospital, or attend specialty outpatient clinics. Injury kills around 800 children each year, more than infectious diseases and malignancies combined. Over 50% of these deaths occur in road traffic accidents, the victims usually being pedestrians. It is estimated that in a class of 30 children, two will be injured in a road traffic accident before adulthood. Some 10 000 of children are disabled as a result of injury each year. Injuries occur more commonly in boys, children from poor socio-economic groups and single parent families.

With increasing mobility and independence, the environments in which children are injured increase from the home and its immediate surroundings to schools, roads, sports venues and the outside world in general. At the same time, children assume increasing control over their own actions without necessarily having developed an understanding of the concept of danger. It ought to be possible to prevent many childhood injuries and deaths by improved housing, vehicle and road designs, as well as instituting informed legislation relating to safety. Health education and accident prevention initiatives are equally important, supported by organisations such as the Health Education Council, the Child Accident Prevention Trust (CAPT) and the Royal Society for the Prevention of Accidents (RoSPA). In the UK the 'Health of the Nation' initiative established a national target to reduce the death rate for accidents in children under 15 by at least 33% by 2005 (from 6.7/100 000 in 1990 to less than 4.5/100 000).

Serious injury

Log rolling

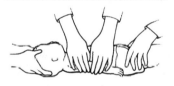

Head   Trunk   Pelvis-legs

for older children four pairs of hands required

The child should be received in the resuscitation area and managed according to Advanced Trauma Life Support principles. The *primary survey* is directed at the recognition and treatment of immediately life-threatening problems to ensure adequate oxygenation, ventilation and tissue perfusion. The ABCDE approach should be followed.

A Airway. Oxygenation is achieved via an airway which is patent and protected using a mask with a reservoir bag attached, or an endotracheal tube. Manual in-line immobilisation of the cervical spine or the application of a semi-rigid cervical collar, sandbags and tape, should be simultaneous with airway management in all seriously injured children.

B Breathing. Look for chest wall movement and injuries, feel for crepitus and listen for air entry. It is vital to exclude chest injuries posing an immediate threat to life which include:

— Tension pneumothorax; treat by needle decompression and intercostal drainage.
— Open pneumothorax; treat initially with a sterile dressing occluded on three sides to form a flutter valve, and then by intercostal drainage.
— Massive haemothorax (more than 20 ml of blood/kg body weight); treat with intravascular volume replacement and intercostal drainage.
— Flail chest; treat with oxygenation and, where indicated assisted ventilation.

Suspicion of cardiac tamponade may be raised during assessment of the breathing but is not treated before adequate ventilation and circulation are established. Less than 15% of all chest injuries will require a thoracotomy.

Intraosseous cannulation

1 finger width

45°-60°

C Circulation. Management should achieve intravenous access with two large bore cannulae ideally placed in the antecubital fossae. Blood is obtained for a full blood count and cross-match. The intraosseous route should be considered in children under 6 years following two failed attempts at intravenous cannulation. Volume replacement should be rapid, initially with 20 ml/kg body weight of *warmed* crystalloid repeated once as indicated by monitoring. The need for blood replacement is determined by the child's response to initial fluid therapy. In the presence of severe injury, haemorrhage may have occurred into the thorax, peritoneal cavity, retroperitoneal space, fracture sites or externally from wounds. In the latter case external pressure should be applied and tourniquets and clips avoided. Appropriate surgical expertise is sought early when ongoing haemorrhage is apparent.

D Disability. An assessment of conscious level and pupillary size and reaction gives a baseline for further examinations. The conscious level can be assessed by the Glasgow Coma Scale for children or categorised in the following simplified fashion:

> **A**lert
> Responds to **V**oice
> Responds to **P**ain
> **U**nresponsive

E Exposure facilitates thorough examination of the child and allows access for monitoring and treatment, but may lead rapidly to hypothermia. The resuscitation area should be warm and the child covered as soon as is practical.

Monitoring

The assessment of the child's response to resuscitation should be continuous and include pulse rate, blood pressure, oxygenation, conscious level, temperature, blood glucose and urine output. The cause of any deterioration must be vigorously sought, with re-evaluation of the Airway, Breathing and Circulation. Placement of a urinary catheter and a nasogastric tube should follow exclusion of a urethral injury and a basal skull fracture. A minimum urine output of 1 ml/kg/h is ideal for most children and 2 ml/kg/h for infants. X-rays of the chest, pelvis and lateral cervical spine should be performed on completion of the primary survey.

The events resulting in the child's injury must be sought, together with details about previous illnesses and injuries, medications and allergies, and tetanus status. The secondary survey can only be performed on a child in whom immediately life threatening conditions have been excluded or treated. A complete examination of the child from head to toe, front and back, identifies potentially life threatening injuries as well as less severe and minor ones. Log rolling the child and protecting the spine is essential prior to the exclusion of a spinal injury. Definitive care is directed by the findings of the secondary survey and by further investigations. The child's recovery following definitive care will determine the need for rehabilitation.

Problem	Head injury

CT of head

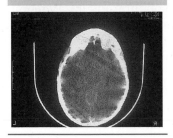

This is responsible for more children dying than any other injury. Death may be caused by the primary injury to the brain or by secondary injury caused by hypoxia, poor perfusion, hypothermia or raised intracranial pressure. Treatment must ensure that secondary brain injury is prevented or minimised by prompt oxygenation, ventilation and maintenance of circulating blood volume. The mechanism of injury, history of loss of consciousness, and the presence of neurological symptoms should be noted. The pupillary size and reaction, the central and peripheral nervous systems, and the Glasgow Coma Scale need to be examined frequently in order that deterioration is not overlooked.

A deterioration of 2 or more points on the Glasgow Coma Scale is significant and requires neurosurgical evaluation. Infants whose cranial sutures are still open may develop very large focal lesions or severe oedema of the brain before neurological deterioration becomes evident. The child's ears and nose should be inspected for bleeding or a cerebrospinal fluid leak. A child presenting with a reduced Glasgow Coma Scale may be unable to protect his/her own airway or spine. A Glasgow Coma Scale of 8 or less identifies the child as being in a coma and requiring urgent protection of the airway by endotracheal intubation.

Paediatric Glasgow Coma Scale

Glasgow Coma Scale (4–15 years)		Children's Coma Scale (<4 years)		
Response	Score	Response		Score
Eyes		Eyes		
Open spontaneously	4	Open spontaneously		4
Verbal command	3	React to speech		3
Pain	2	React to pain		2
No response	1	No response		1
Best motor response		Best motor response		
Verbal command:		Spontaneous or obeys verbal		
Obeys	6	command		6
Painful stimulus:		*Painful stimulus:*		
Localises pain	5	Localises pain		5
Flexion with pain	4	Withdraws in response to pain		4
		Abnormal flexion to pain		
Flexion abnormal	3	(decorticate posture)		3
		Abnormal extension to pain		
Extension	2	(decerebrate posture)		2
No response	1	No response		1
Best verbal response		Best verbal response		
Orientated and		Smiles, orientated to sounds,		
converses	5	follows objects, interacts		5
Disorientated and		*Crying*	*Interacts*	
converses	4	Consolable	Inappropriate	4
		Inconsistently		
Inappropriate words	3	consolable	Moaning	3
Incomprehensible				
sounds	2	Inconsolable	irritable	2
No response	1	No response	No response	1

Following resuscitation and the treatment of immediately life-threatening injuries, CT of the head is necessary to demonstrate the exact nature and severity of the injury. Neurosurgical advice should be sought to guide subsequent treatment, including that of convulsions. Injuries may be focal, including extradural, subdural and intracerebral haematomas, or diffuse, including diffuse axonal injury.

Where injury to the head is less severe, the need for X-rays of the skull will be dictated by local policy. Any child should be admitted if:

— History of loss of consciousness for more than 5 minutes.
— Unusual or unexplained behaviour.
— Amnesia of more than a momentary nature.
— Neurological symptoms or signs, including convulsions.
— Persistent vomiting.
— Penetrating injury.
— Clinical or radiological signs of a skull fracture, including a depressed fracture.
— Concomitant disease, including bleeding disorders and the presence of a neurosurgical shunt.
— Suspected cases of child abuse.

The majority of children sustain minor head injuries and do not require observation in hospital. Parents and carers require written advice on caring for a child with a minor head injury.

| Problem | Spinal injuries |

Odontoid peg fracture

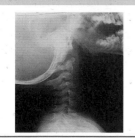

These are relatively uncommon in children but should be suspected and excluded in all seriously injured children and in those where the injury mechanism transmits abnormal forces through the spinal column. Injury may involve the spinal cord, the vertebral column or both, and the consequences of injudicious movement before such injury is excluded may be catastrophic for the child. Where a spinal injury is suspected, the entire spinal column must be immobilised in a neutral position, ideally on a spine-board, with manual in-line immobilisation of the cervical spine or the use of a semi-rigid cervical collar, sandbags and tape.

In children, the cervical spine is more frequently injured than the thoracolumbar spine. The mobile nature of a child's spine allows forces to be transmitted more widely through it and the possibility of injury at more than one level should be remembered. During examination of the spine, the child should be log rolled and the entire spinal column inspected for deformity, swelling and bruising. Palpation should exclude tenderness and gaps in the continuity of the bony contours. Examination of the peripheral neurological system should include an assessment of anal tone and perineal sensation.

Investigation involves X-rays of part or all of the spine. Those taken of the cervical spine must include the upper border of the first thoracic vertebra. Interpretation of radiological findings may be difficult in the presence of normal developmental features, particularly ossification centres. A well practised system of reading the X-rays must be followed and should include an assessment of vertebral alignment, the presence of fractures, the appearance of the intervertebral discs and joint spaces, the presence of soft tissue swelling. Normal X-rays do not exclude the presence of spinal cord injury in children, therefore spinal immobilisation must be maintained if spinal cord injury is suspected clinically. Further investigation, including computerised tomography or magnetic resonance imaging, may be necessary.

Definitive treatment is determined by the nature and stability of the injury and the guidance of paediatric spinal, orthopaedic and neuro-surgical specialists may be necessary. Rehabilitation for children with spinal cord injury is of necessity multidisciplinary.

Problem	Chest injury

X-ray of chest: pulmonary contusion

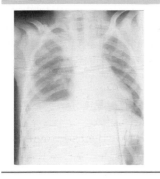

Serious intrathoracic injury may exist in a child who has no external evidence of chest wall injury. The child's compliant chest wall trans-mits energy, primarily to the lung tissue, without necessarily causing fractures of the bony skeleton.

Life-threatening chest injuries. Conditions which compromise the ability to breathe efficiently and to maintain an adequate cardiac out-put need to be considered in all children with a chest injury and include: tension pneumothorax, large open pneumothorax, massive haemothorax (more than 20 ml/kg body wt), flail chest and cardiac tamponade.

Potentially life-threatening chest injuries. These include: pulmonary contusion — which is common in children but may not be apparent at the time of the initial examination or chest X-ray, ruptured hemidi-aphragm and tracheal or bronchial tears. A high index of suspicion is required to ensure that such injuries are not missed. Constant re-evalu-ation of the chest, together with monitoring of the respiratory rate, res-piratory effort and arterial blood gases, will guide the need for ventilatory support.

Adequate pain relief must be administered to children sustaining injuries to the chest, and the type and route should be tailored to the individual. Advice should be sought from a paediatric surgeon or car-diothoracic surgeon if, following the insertion of an intercostal drain, there is a continued large air leak or bleeding. The presence of pene-trating trauma to the chest and evidence of a resulting cardiac tamponade is an absolute indication for a thoracotomy and definitive surgery.

Problem	Abdominal injury

The child's relatively protuberant abdomen makes it susceptible to injury. Clinical signs suggesting injury must be actively sought as

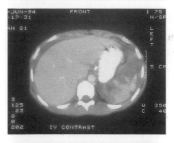

CT of abdomen: fragmented spleen

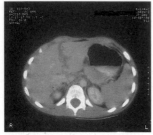

shock resulting from haemorrhage into the abdominal cavity may be insidious. Injury may involve intraperitoneal structures, those in the retroperitoneal space and pelvis, or both. A precise diagnosis is not required during the primary survey, but a high index of suspicion is vital if intra-abdominal injury is not to be missed.

The abdomen should be completely exposed and inspected for signs of injury and distension. Palpation should be gentle and exclude the presence of tenderness and peritoneal irritation. Gastric and intestinal dilatation resulting from swallowed air or an ileus requires decompression with a nasogastric or orogastric tube. When the child is log rolled, the flanks should be inspected and palpated, and a rectal examination performed if indicated by the mechanism of injury. Inspection of the urethral meatus and the genitalia, and radiology of the pelvis, should precede urinary catheterisation.

Investigation is dictated by the findings. Any child with signs of intra-abdominal haemorrhage who does not respond to attempts to restore the circulating volume needs immediate assessment by a paediatric surgeon and, in the presence of a pelvic fracture, by an orthopaedic specialist. Immediate laparotomy or stabilisation of the pelvis is indicated. Further investigations may include an ultrasound scan, computerised tomography or radiology of the urinary tract. Retrograde urethrography can be performed in the resuscitation room when urethral injury is suspected. Diagnostic peritoneal lavage as a means of excluding intraperitoneal bleeding should be reserved for older children.

Some children with intra-abdominal injury, particularly of the spleen, can be managed conservatively, but the input of paediatric surgeons and intensivists is mandatory to the decision making process.

Problems	Musculoskeletal injuries

Musculoskeletal injuries

Musculoskeletal injury

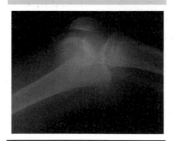

Injuries to the skeletal system are very common in children, accounting for approximately 15% of all childhood injuries. The child's skeleton is immature, much of it being cartilaginous in the small child. The appearance of ossification centres can make X-ray interpretation difficult. If a fracture is suspected, then it is assumed until confidently excluded by further assessment and investigation. Some fractures, including those at the growing end of bones, are unique to children and require recognition and appropriate treatment if the bone is to develop normally. Children's bones are generally very forgiving and remodel well. Healing is more rapid than in adult fractures and complications such as delayed or non-union are relatively uncommon. Severe ligamentous injuries and major joint dislocations are less common.

In the seriously injured child, only those skeletal injuries which are immediately life threatening are managed in the primary survey. These include open long bone fractures and traumatic amputations, where bleeding should be controlled by external pressure and volume replacement, and pelvic fractures in which stabilisation may be indicated.

In *the secondary survey* the entire musculoskeletal system is examined. Signs suggesting the presence of an underlying fracture or dislocation are sought, including bruising, swelling and deformity. The distal neurovascular function should always be examined. If this is found to be compromised, for example in a displaced supracondylar fracture of the humerus, orthopaedic advice should be sought **immediately**. A Polaroid photograph should be taken of any wound overlying or in close proximity to a long bone fracture or major dislocation, after which a sterile dry dressing is applied to the wound and an intravenous antibiotic, usually a cephalosporin, given.

Fractures should be splinted and dislocations reduced as soon as is practicable. Splintage of a fracture reduces blood loss at the fracture site, helps to prevent fat embolism and offers some pain relief. Severe pain in a splinted limb should raise the suspicion of a developing compartment syndrome and urgent orthopaedic input must be sought.

Definitive fracture treatment depends upon factors such as the site and type of the fracture, the presence of angulation or rotational deformity and whether the fracture is open or closed. Some children's fractures, for example buckle (torus) fractures and undisplaced greenstick fractures, require no more than the application of a plaster of Paris. Other fractures, and particularly displaced fractures around the elbow and ankle, may require manipulation or open reduction and internal fixation.

Dislocations. Reduction of a dislocation may need to be performed under general anaesthetic. More usually, as with finger joint dislocations, a regional nerve block is required. Some dislocations, like that occurring in a pulled elbow in a small child, simply require gentle manipulation to achieve reduction.

Injuries to tendons and nerves, while uncommon in small children, must be excluded by careful examination, especially in the hand. If a small child is unable to co-operate with examination, exploration of the injury under general anaesthetic may be required. Appropriate analgesia should be offered to all children who sustain musculoskeletal injury, the route of administration depending on the nature of the injury.

Salter–Harris fractures

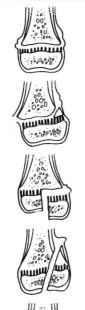

Problems

Cuts, bruises and abrasions

Very large numbers of children require treatment for superficial injuries including lacerations, bruises and abrasions. The mechanism of injury should raise suspicion of the likelihood of injury to underlying structures, which must be thoroughly examined. All injuries caused by glass must be X-rayed, as should those suspected of having a retained metallic foreign body. Bruises in themselves do not usually require specific treatment; associated swelling may require elevation of the affected part.

Abrasions should be cleaned to ensure tattooing does not occur. The presence of dirt and gravel may require administration of a local or general anaesthetic. If a dressing is required this should be of a non-adhesive type. Wound toilet must precede closure of lacerations. Alternatives to sutures, including histoacryl glue, steristrips and hair ties, should always be considered. Immunisation against tetanus must be confirmed.

Problems	**Eye injury**

In the presence of suspected or obvious ocular trauma the involvement of an ophthalmic specialist should be obtained early.

Problems	**Maxillofacial injuries**

Immediate treatment is required only in the presence of airway compromise resulting from bleeding or oedema caused by fractures of the facial skeleton. In all other circumstances diagnosis and treatment is reserved until the secondary survey or later.

If found, a displaced permanent tooth should be reimplanted in its socket at the earliest opportunity, or saved in milk. Following trauma an unaccounted for tooth should be sought on a chest X-ray.

BURNS

In the UK burns are responsible for up to 100 childhood deaths and some 50 000 paediatric attendances to A&E departments each year. Smoke inhalation occurring at the same time as a burn, usually in house fires, is responsible for the majority of deaths. A child presenting with serious burns must be managed according to Advanced Trauma Life Support principles and the burn injury should not distract from this. Facial burns or soot, particularly around the nose and mouth, should raise suspicion of burns to the airway and associated oedema. It is vital to anticipate that airway patency will be compromised and needs early protection by endotracheal intubation.

DO NOT PROCRASTINATE

Arterial blood gases are helpful together with the carboxy-haemoglobin level, as a normal oxygen saturation does not exclude carbon monoxide poisoning. Following the establishment of intravenous access, blood should be obtained for a full blood count including haematocrit, urea and electrolytes and cross-matching. Fluid replacement depends upon the extent of the burns and is required in children sustaining burns of 10% or more of their body surface area.

Calculation of the burn size is assisted by the use of a Lund and Browder chart or by remembering that the child's hand, including the fingers, represents 1% of the body surface area. An initial bolus of 20 ml/kg of fluid is given.

Fluid replacement for the next 24 hours is calculated as follows:

$$\text{Volume (ml)} = \% \text{ burn} \times \text{weight (kg)} \times 4$$

and half is given over 8 hours from time of injury.

Assessment of burns

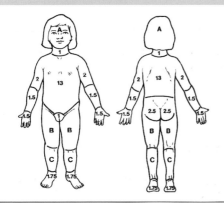

Area indicated	Surface area at				
	0	1 year	5 years	10 years	15 years
A	9.5	8.5	6.5	5.5	4.5
B	2.75	3.25	4.0	4.5	4.5
C	2.5	2.5	2.75	3.0	3.25

The choice of fluid depends on local policy; human albumin, a colloid solution or a crystalloid are all suitable. Urine output refines this further and guides subsequent fluid therapy.

First aid measures such as the application of cold water or the removal of burning clothing may have led to hypothermia in the child. This should not be compounded further and intravenous fluids should be warmed. The depth of a burn can be difficult to determine accurately immediately following the injury. Partial thickness burns are exquisitely painful when exposed to air and should be dressed at the earliest opportunity, with a sterile towel or clingfilm if the patient is to be transferred to a burns unit, or with paraffin gauze if the child is to be allowed home. Full thickness burns, with the exception of very small burns, should be reviewed by a burns specialist, as should any burn of more than 10% body surface area. Circumferential full thickness burns may threaten life, limb or digit depending on their site and require urgent escharotomy and sometimes fasciotomy. Intravenous access needs to be established prior to performing this procedure.

Burns may be one part of the injury spectrum seen in a child and the history may suggest the presence of other injuries, caused for example by falling masonry. Antibiotic prophylaxis against the possibility of toxic shock syndrome should be given according to the local policy and immunisation against tetanus confirmed.

Adequate analgesia, titrated against the child's needs, should be given via the intravenous route. The place of oral analgesia is determined by the severity of the burn.

PAIN MANAGEMENT

When dealing with ill or injured children it is easy to forget that their distress may be caused by pain. Those involved in their initial assessment should be trained to recognise the need for analgesia and in the use of pain assessment tools. It is often easier to examine a child whose pain has been alleviated. The choice of analgesia is dictated by the circumstances of each child but the following guidelines are useful:

— Oral analgesia, e.g. paracetamol, codeine phosphate or oral morphine, is usually acceptable to children but has a delayed onset.
— Intramuscular analgesia should be avoided as it is painful and absorption is unpredictable.
— Intravenous analgesia, e.g. morphine, needs to be titrated slowly against response.
— Regional anaesthesia including digital and femoral nerve blocks are useful and should be considered. Calculation of the maximum safe dose of local anaesthetic on a 3 mg/kg basis is essential.
— Topical anaesthetic creams are available and widely used in paediatric practice but their use should not delay urgent investigations and management.
— Entonox is a useful adjunct in the absence of significant injury to the head and chest.

Assessment of pain

| 0 | 20 | 40 | 60 | 80 | 100 |

REFERENCES

The American College of Surgeons 1993 ATLS manual. Chicago, Illinois
An Introduction to the Children Act 1989 HMSO, London
APLS: the practical approach 1993 BMJ Publishing Group, London
Audit Commission 1993 Children First
Butler-Sloss 1987 Report of the inquiry into child abuse in Cleveland. HMSO, London
Carty H, Ratcliffe J 1995 The shaken infant syndrome. British Medical Journal 310: 344–345
Craft A W 1988 Accidental poisoning. Archives of Disease in Childhood 63: 584–586
Department of Health Circular 1993 Recommendations of the Chief Medical Officer's Expert Group on Sleeping Position of Infants and Cot Death. Dept of Health, HMSO, London
Fisher M 1995 Treatment of acute anaphylaxis. British Medical Journal 311: 731–733
Fleming P J, Cooke M, Chantler et al 1994 Fire retardants, biocides, plasticisers and SIDS. British Medical Journal 309: 1594–1595

The Health of the Nation Targets for Accidents 1992 Dept of Health, HMSO, London

Meadows 1989 ABC of child abuse. BMJ Publishing Group, London

Morton RJ, Phillips BM 1992 Accidents and emergencies in children. Oxford University Press, Oxford

OPCS Mortality Statistics in Childhood 1992 OPCS, London

OPCS Population Trends, a review 1994 OPCS, London

Samuels M R, Southall D P 1992 Munchausen syndrome by proxy. British Journal of Hospital Medicine 47: 759–762

Sibert J R, Routledge P A 1991 Accidental poisoning in children. Can we admit fewer? Archives of Disease in Childhood 66: 263–266

Southall D P, Samuels M R 1992 Reducing risk in SIDS. British Medical Journal 304: 265–266

Wigfield R E, Fleming P J, Berry J et al 1992 Can the fall in Avon's sudden infant death rate be explained by changes in sleeping position? British Medical Journal 304: 282–284

Intensive care

The best place to treat a critically ill child is in a hospital staffed and equipped to provide intensive care for the children. Critical care begins in the emergency department or the referral hospital and must be maintained by the transport team, which should include a physician skilled in airway management, a nurse trained in children's intensive care and a technician to assist with the equipment.

Intensive care involves the management of children with various forms of shock, respiratory failure and unconsciousness due to brain disorder; usually a mixture of all three.

Case mix of 380 children admitted in 1995 to a PICU

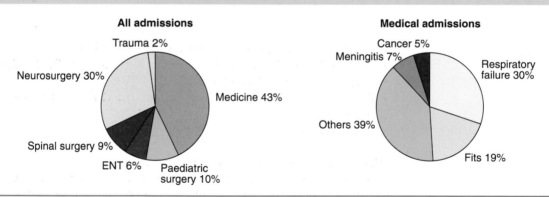

If the infant or child needs artificial ventilation during transfer or in the unit, sedation is required unless the child is unconscious. Ventilation without sedation and analgesia is uncomfortable; an agitated child may inadvertently dislodge the endotracheal tube. Neuromuscular blocking agents are often useful in combination with sedation where a patient is 'fighting the ventilator' or to reduce oxygen utilisation to a minimum in a sick patient.

Respiratory failure and brain disorder are considered in other chapters. Shock is failure of adequate perfusion of tissues. It leads to cellular dysfunction and, if inadequately treated, cellular death. In shock, whether due to cardiogenic, hypovolaemic or obstructive mechanisms, there is a compensatory increase in the systemic vascular

Sedation and neuromuscular blocking drugs		
Drug	Loading dose	Maintenance
Morphine	250 µg/kg	5–40 µg/kg/h
Midazolam	200 µg/kg	1–2 µg/kg/min
Atracurium	500 µg/kg	300–600 µg/h

resistance to maintain blood pressure, increased oxygen extraction of oxygen at cellular level and a reduction in pulmonary artery oxygenation.

SEPTIC SHOCK

In septic shock, an endotoxin induced cascade of inflammatory mediators leads to low systemic vascular resistance, a reduction in the oxygen use in the peripheral tissues (in children intense vasoconstriction is a common feature), myocardial depression, capillary leak and a coagulation disorder. Septic shock may be initiated by gram-positive organisms, fungi, viruses and rickettsiae but it is commonly due to gram-negative bacteria.

Problem

- A prodromal febrile illness with malaise for 24 hours.
- Followed by high fever, loss of appetite and occasionally diarrhoea.
- Followed by rigors and chills.
- Followed by progressive restlessness and drifting into state of unconsciousness.
- A purpuric rash.

Diagnosis — Presumed meningococcal infection

The management of septic shock is essentially the same whatever the cause apart from the selection of antibiotics. In meningococcal sepsis despite powerful antibiotics and very aggressive intensive care, the overall mortality remains around 10–20%. The mortality increases to over 50% in those children presenting with shock. We have therefore used this as our example for septic shock.

Meningococci can be present with a meningeal illness or sepsis, or occasionally both. Recognition of the specific form of illness is vital to initiate appropriate management plans. The rash may appear at any time and is usually petechial, ecchymotic or necrotic in nature, but it may be macular or maculopapular. It may appear anywhere on the body — face, palate, conjunctiva, trunk or pressure sites and the palms and soles of the feet. A thorough examination is essential. If there is associated intense vasoconstriction and coagulopathy then purpura fulminans may develop. The petechial areas coalesce and produce areas of necrosis especially at the periphery, fingers, toes, tip of the nose or the foreskin in males. Gangrene often follows.

Early assessment

In an infant or child with a fever and a petechial rash intramuscular penicillin (600 mg) is recommended prior to transfer to the hospital. In the hospital casualty department, an intravenous (or intraosseous) access should be established and blood obtained for blood cultures and further benzylpenicillin (75 mg/kg) given i.v. before transfer to the PICU. Initial assessment includes:

Heart rate. Tachycardia is the normal response in shock. The increase in the heart rate maintains the cardiac output in the presence of a reduction of stroke volume. Although at the onset a lower heart rate is predictive of survival, bradycardia is an ominous sign and is often pre-terminal.

Blood pressure. In the initial phase blood pressure is maintained, however the onset of hypotension is a sign of decompensation and is again pre-terminal.

Peripheral pulses and perfusion. In early sepsis the pulses are bounding due to high cardiac output and low peripheral vascular resistance. With progression, the cardiac output becomes compromised and the pulses are thready and low volume. The capillary refill time, normally less than 2 seconds, becomes prolonged. Mottled cold skin with pallor and peripheral cyanosis indicate severe shock. Wide core–peripheral skin temperature difference suggests poor peripheral perfusion.

Respiratory rate. Tachypnoea or pre-terminally air hunger may be seen.

Level of consciousness. Restlessness, agitation and confusion indicate hypoxia and diminished cerebral perfusion. Coma is a grave sign.

Blood gases. Metabolic acidosis is common is shock. Capillary or venous blood gas analysis will reflect tissue hypoxia.

Blood glucose. Hypoglycaemia has serious consequences in shocked patients, especially young infants with limited glycogen stores.

Initial management

Initial resuscitation should follow the established ABC order of priority.

Maintain optimal oxygenation. Oxygen is administered via a face mask with as high an oxygen concentration as possible. Any secretions are cleared with a yankauer sucker, using a laryngoscope to visualise the larynx. If respiration is adequate but there is partial airway obstruction, causing noisy breathing and excessive chest movement (assess tidal volume by feeling for warm expired air at the mouth), then insert an oropharyngeal airway provided this is tolerated. Most children do not tolerate this unless severely obtunded.

If unconscious, the child should be nursed in the recovery position to prevent regurgitation and aspiration of stomach contents. He/she should be intubated if the airway is difficult to maintain.

Circulation. Vascular access must be obtained immediately. In children under 5 years if a venous access is not obtained within 2 minutes of admission, an intraosseous needle should be placed. The easiest position is at the level of the tibial tubercle on the medial portion of the tibia. Since the intramedullary space is contiguous with the venous compartment, fluids as well drugs will readily pass into the circulation following this route. Prior to fluid infusion, blood should be obtained for culture and penicillin or a third generation cephalosporin should be injected. Initially between 20 and 40 ml/kg body weight of plasma or 4.5% albumin can be infused rapidly over 10–20 minutes. If given via the intraosseous route, the fluid may require manual pushing. If there is improvement, the volume of colloid can be repeated, however, there is a need to observe the child for onset of pulmonary oedema.

Hypoglycaemia. If the child is hypoglycaemic 25% glucose is given.

Antibiotics. Our current practice is to commence all patients on cefotaxime (200 mg/kg/day) and await culture reports and sensitivities before changing over to penicillin.

Subsequent management

Ventilation. In severe shock there is continued loss of fluid from capillary leak and the volume loss may be grossly underestimated. If the volume requirement exceeds 80 ml/kg, it is safer to electively intubate and ventilate to prevent sudden onset of pulmonary oedema. Ventilation will also optimise oxygen delivery and reduce oxygen utilisation.

A rapid sequence intubation should be performed with pre-oxygenation with 100% oxygen. A nasogastric tube should be passed and gastric contents sucked out. The child should lie supine with the head in the 'sniffing the morning' air position (i.e. the neck flexed but the head extended at the atlanto-occipital joint). A pillow under the occiput is useful to achieve this position in older children. Cricoid pressure should be applied and sedative and muscle relaxant infused rapidly followed by intubation with full relaxation. It is important to avoid

Selecting an endotracheal tube

Internal diameter (mm)	Oral length (cm)	Nasal length (cm)	Age
2.5	9.5	13.0	Preterm
3.0	10.0	13.0	Preterm
3.5	10.5	14.0	0–6 months
4.0	11.5	14.5	6–12 months
4.5	13.0	15.0	1 year
5.0	13.5	16.5	2–3 years
5.5	14.0	17.0	4–5 years
6.0	14.5	17.5	6–7 years
6.5	15.5	18.5	8–9 years
7.0	16.5	19.0	10–11 years
7.5	17.5	19.5	12–13 years
8.0	18.0	20.0	> 14 years

Sniffing position

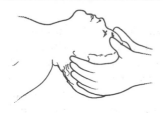

drugs producing hypotension. In severely moribund child 'awake' intubation may have to be performed. The child is initially intubated orally since this is easier and quicker than nasal intubation. Uncuffed tubes are used prior to puberty when the narrowest part of the airway is the cricoid ring which gives a good seal. After puberty the vocal cords are the narrowest part and so a cuff is necessary to form a seal. Following intubation both lung fields should be auscultated to exclude intubation of the right main bronchus and a chest X-ray should be carried out to ascertain the position of the tube and also evaluate the lungs and the heart. The child should be commenced on maintenance infusion of analgesia (morphine), sedative (midazolam) and a paralytic (atracurium).

Circulation. By this stage invasive monitoring of central venous pressure and arterial blood pressure is vital. Central venous cannulation via the internal jugular, subclavian or femoral vein should be considered. The internal jugular approach in particular is much easier in an intubated, ventilated and sedated child. Learn from an experienced practitioner! Many approaches have been described, one of which is as follows. The child is tipped head down 20–30 degrees to fill the neck veins. The site of insertion is the apex of the triangle formed by the two heads of the sternocleidomastoid muscle, lateral to the carotid pulse. The needle is inserted towards the ipsilateral nipple, care being taken to advance the tip no further than the superior border of the clavicle, and at an angle of only 10–20 degrees to the skin. Persistent attempts should be avoided as there is a significant risk to pneumothorax. The use of ultrasonic devices have made insertion of central lines relatively easy. In children femoral venous access is easy and safe. The multiple lumen catheters allow invasive monitoring of central venous pressures as well as administration of drugs, inotropes and colloid.

Circulatory support

Further colloid support. The degree of hypovolaemia is often underestimated. It is not unusual for some children to require colloid replacement of over 200 ml/kg over the first 24 hour. This is only possible with full ventilatory support and central venous monitoring.

Inotropic support. If despite volume replacement and an adequate preload (central venous pressures of between 12 and 15 mmHg) the patient remains underperfused, then inotropes should be commenced. The inotropes introduced early will restore minimum tissue perfusion pressure. Initially dopamine (5–10 µg/kg/min) or dobutamine (5–10 µg/kg/min) can be used, however, if shock persists then higher dosages of dobutamine (up to 30 µg/kg/min) can be infused. Adrenaline (at 0.01–5 µg/kg/min) infusion may improve coronary artery perfusion. Once the peripheral perfusion improves noradrenaline may be used to increase mean arterial pressure.

Vasodilators. In severe vasoconstriction, peripheral perfusion is reduced and blood flow to the limbs may be compromised. Vasodilators such as nitroprusside or prostacyclin can be infused, with caution, to improve circulation. Prostacyclins being both vasodilators as well as inhibitors of platelet aggregation appear ideal for improving peripheral circulation.

Monitoring in the PICU

ECG will be required to monitor heart rate and detect arrhythmias.

Blood pressure. Automatic non-invasive devices (e.g. Dinamap) based on the oscillotonometer tend to over-read in hypotension but are very useful for monitoring trends. An intra-arterial cannula connected to a pressure transducer provides beat by beat blood pressure monitoring but is difficult to site prior to initial resuscitation. Blood pressure is displayed digitally and the waveform displayed on an oscilloscope.

Central venous pressure. Blood must flow freely back to indicate that the catheter is in a central vein. A chest X-ray should be ordered following insertion to check that the tip is at the SVC/IVC–right atrial junction and to exclude pneumo/haemothorax. The CVP should be measured to the level of the atria, i.e. the midaxillary line in the supine patient.

The close physiological relationship between the right and left atrial pressures may be disturbed in some critically ill patients so that relying on it as a guide to the preload (i.e. the degree of stretch of myocardial fibres in diastole) of the left ventricle may lead to under or over transfusion. In Adult Respiratory Distress Syndrome (ARDS) the left atrial pressure may be low in relation to the right as a result of pulmonary hypertension and right ventricular failure. Left ventricular failure complicating trauma or sepsis causes a relatively high left atrial pressure. The catheter is inserted via a central vein, the right atrium, right ventricle and finally the pulmonary artery where it can be made to wedge by inflating a balloon at the tip. The pressure measured here, the wedge pressure, distal to the balloon, closely approximates to the left atrial pressure. At present the safety of pulmonary artery catheters has not been carefully evaluated in children. These catheters can also be used to measure cardiac output using the Fick principle by injection of a small volume of cold saline into the right atrium and measuring the fall in temperature in the pulmonary artery. Oxygen delivery and utilisation, systemic and pulmonary vascular resistance and other derived variables can be computed, allowing more precise treatment of the shock. It has been shown, for example, that increasing oxygen delivery until utilisation reaches a peak is beneficial to the shocked patient (in terms of mortality statistics) and that to achieve this supranormal values for cardiac output are required in septic shock. These catheters are associated with many complications, however, and the size of the available catheters (smallest is 5FG) precludes their use in infants.

Temperature. Core to peripheral temperature difference is monitored using a two-channel temperature recorder. This provides an extremely useful assessment of the peripheral perfusion. Core temperature is measured rectally, through a bladder catheter with a temperature probe or in the oesophagus. The peripheral temperature is measured on the dorsum of the hand or foot. The difference should not exceed

3°C (less in neonates) unless the patient has been exposed to a low environmental temperature. If the gap is greater than 3°C then peripheral perfusion is reduced, usually because of hypovolaemia, and should narrow in response to infusion. If the gap is greater than this, and the CVP is high or rising, inotropes or vasodilators are indicated.

Urine output. Urinary catheterisation allows monitoring of hourly urine output. This should normally be greater than 1 ml/kg/h. Less than this indicates either persistent hypovolaemia or incipient renal failure.

Blood gases. Arterial blood gases should be monitored in all children who require supplemental oxygen. Normal values are the same as adults (i.e. Pco_2, 5.3; Pao_2, 12.3 kPa; pH, 7.4). The frequency of their estimation should depend on the severity of the illness but as a general guide they should be taken 4 hourly in ventilated children, 12 hourly in children requiring supplemental oxygen and checked 20 minutes after changing ventilator settings. Their frequency can be reduced when using pulse oximetry and end tidal CO_2 monitoring.

Pulse oximetry is a non-invasive method of monitoring arterial haemoglobin saturation which uses the principle of differential absorption of red and infra red light by haemoglobin and oxyhaemoglobin. It should be used to monitor all patients who may require supplemental oxygen. Arterial oxygen saturation should be maintained between 90 and 100% as far as possible.

End tidal CO_2. End tidal values correlate well with arterial CO_2 in most circumstances except where there is a significant alveolar dead space. Unfortunately this occurs in shock so it is not an accurate measure of arterial Pco_2 until the patient has been resuscitated.

The following have been identified with poor prognosis in meningococcal sepsis.

— Presence of shock with hypotension and coma.
— Extremes of age.
— Rapidly spreading purpuric rash.
— Absence of meningism/meningitis.
— Neutropenia — neutrophil count <10 000.
— Thrombocytopenia.
— Coagulopathy.

Complications

Adult Respiratory Distress Syndrome (ARDS). Ventilatory support during colloid resuscitation reduces the risk of catastrophic pulmonary oedema secondary to capillary leak. Rapidly rising oxygen requirement and higher airway pressure are the earliest signs of onset of ARDS. It occurs between 24–48 hours after admission. The pathophysiology of ARDS is multifactorial. Poor myocardial function, pulmonary oedema, pulmonary haemorrhage and aggregation of neutrophils and platelets are some of the possible contributory factors. The management of ARDS includes aggressive ventilation with pressure limited mode, reversed inspiratory to expiratory ratio and addition of positive end expiratory pressures. Barotrauma may be a complication and the high airway pressures further compromise cardiac output. Recently inhaled nitric oxide, ECMO and high frequency oscillation have been evaluated for the treatment of ARDS. Diuretics and fluid restriction may be beneficial.

Fluid and electrolyte problems. Continued capillary leak is suggested by the development of severe peripheral oedema, pulmonary oedema as well as oliguria. In this state intravenous infusion of colloid and crystalloid fail to maintain intravascular pressures. The development of peripheral oedema may be reduced by controlling infusion of crystalloid to two-thirds maintenance requirements. Severe fluid restriction may produce oliguria of pre-renal origin which may respond to further colloid challenge and inotropes. When the renal perfusion is severely jeopardised then renal failure will follow requiring early dialysis. Peritoneal dialysis will not only correct the electrolyte and acid base imbalance, often seen in shock, but also reduce the extravascular fluid and reduce oedema and ascites. Hypocalcaemia, hypophosphataemia and hypomagnesaemia are frequently seen. Correction of calcium and magnesium may improve myocardial function. The other major metabolic derangement is hypoglycaemia, seen especially in young infants. Following resuscitation and aggressive inotropic therapy hyperglycaemia may follow.

Coagulopathy. In sepsis there is coagulopathy and severe thrombocytopenia. There is often clinical as well as laboratory evidence of disseminated intravascular coagulation (DIC) which may be combined with Protein C and S deficiency. In purpura fulminans Protein C levels have been observed to be low and associated with increased mortality. Treatment with Protein C concentrate appears to reduce mortality. Similarly Protein S and antithrombin III with concurrent prostacyclin infusion have shown some promise in children with impending gangrene.

CARDIOGENIC SHOCK

In cardiogenic shock there is pump failure with marked reduction in cardiac output to meet the metabolic demands of tissues. Compensatory increase in systemic vascular resistance (increase in afterload) adds to the work load further depressing cardiac output.

Causes of cardiogenic shock

Heart failure secondary to congenital heart disease
Cardiomyopathy
Valvular disease — rare in western children
Myocardial infarction — in Kawasaki disease
Arrhythmias
Septic shock

Clinical features

- Pallor and cold clammy skin.
- Fainting and altered mental status (? reduction in cerebral perfusion).
- Collapse.
- Oliguria.
- Hepatomegaly, peripheral oedema and raised jugular veins.

Diagnosis — Cardiac shock? Cause

Investigations. Carry out an ECG to identify any arrhythmia. In children, congenital heart block and supraventricular tachycardia are the two commonest abnormalities. Cardiac enzymes, which may be elevated in Kawasaki disease or in congenital anomalous coronary arteries. Echocardiography, which is useful for identifying congenital heart diseases, aberrant coronary arteries and coronary artery aneurysms. It is a useful help to evaluate cardiac function and assess therapy.

Management. Inject antiarrhythmics if the shock is due heart rate abnormalities. Currently adenosine is the drug of choice for supraventricular tachycardia. Pacing may be required in a few patients with heart block. Then 'Optimise preload' with salt and fluid restriction, augmentation of preload with fluid challenge, and give diuretics. Improve cardiac output with oxygen, correction of metabolic derangement and give inotropic support. Dobutamine is currently the catecholamine of choice. 'Reduce afterload' with sedation and analgesia — morphine has been tried and tested for years and remains the drug of choice. Add vasodilator drugs — currently angiotensin-converting enzyme inhibitors are the drugs of choice.

HYPOVOLAEMIC SHOCK

This is the commonest cause of shock in infants and children. In hypovolaemic shock there is a sudden drop in the intravascular volume so that effective tissue perfusion cannot be maintained. Healthy children can well tolerate acute losses of 10–15% blood volume by vasoconstrictive mechanisms and reactive tachycardia. Any further losses will result in decompensation.

Clinical features

- Persistent tachycardia, pallor, clammy cold mottled skin with poor capillary refill, oliguric but normotensive.

Diagnosis — Compensated hypovolaemia ? Cause

- Lethargic, acidotic, hypotensive and in coma.

Diagnosis — Uncompensated hypovolaemia ? Cause

Causes of hypovolaemic shock

Haemorrhage	Trauma — blood loss
	Bleeding from long bones
	Rupture of liver/spleen
	Intracranial bleed
	Major vessels
	Gastric bleeding
Loss of plasma	Burns
Fluid and electrolyte loss	Diarrhoea and vomiting
	Diabetic ketoacidotic crisis with dehydration
	Renal loss/diabetes insipidus

Investigations

Those performed depend very much on the history. In children involved in trauma, the cause of haemorrhage needs to be identified. The modalities available are: radiography, ultrasound, computed tomography, angiography for vascular or organ injury. Investigations for hypovolaemic shock include, full blood count, clotting profile, electrolytes, calcium and liver function tests, blood sugar, serum and urinary osmolality, urine electrolytes and blood for cross-matching.

Management

In hypovolaemic shock, successful resuscitation depends very much on aggressive fluid therapy. If there is trauma, obtain surgical consultation at the beginning of the resuscitation. Circulatory access is urgent: time should not be wasted trying to find a peripheral vein. If within 2 minutes of admission an intravenous line is not inserted then an intraosseous cannula should be used. Blood for the investigations should be taken and an initial bolus of 20 ml/kg body weight of colloid is given rapidly. If there is no improvement in the vital signs then another bolus of 20 ml/kg should be repeated. Failure to respond at this stage warrants elective intubation and control of the airway.

In life threatening haemorrhagic shock, type specific non-cross-matched blood can be given. O-negative blood should be reserved for females to avoid rhesus sensitisation. In patients requiring massive transfusion (>100 ml/kg), administer calcium to replace the chelated calcium. In severe burns continuous infusion of colloid will be necessary to replace the fluid losses. Check for hypoglycaemia.

Monitoring

Vital signs should be monitored, especially peripheral perfusion, urine output and central venous pressure. The femoral venous line is the preferred route as internal jugular line insertion is not without risk.

Fluid replacement

The choice of fluid for use in the treatment of hypovolaemia requires an understanding of the pharmacology of those available, although in an emergency any fluid is preferable to none. Colloid solutions are far superior to crystalloids, since crystalloids have much less (one-third to one-fifth) effect on blood volume. For resuscitation human plasma protein fraction (HPPF), given with enough blood to maintain the haemoglobin level at around 10 g/dl, is the ideal volume expander because of its long plasma half life and low incidence of allergic reactions. Fresh frozen plasma should be substituted if there are clotting abnormalities. Gelatin solutions (e.g. Haemacell, Gelofusine — chemically modified solutions of degraded gelatin) are second choice, although they may be first choice for the short term treatment of a previously fit patient, where the albumen concentration is known to be normal. Gelatins are thought to protect the kidneys in low flow states and do not interfere with cross-matching or coagulation. However, they only have a short plasma half-life of around 2–3 hours. Haemacell contains calcium and may cause clotting of citrated blood if infused in the same giving set. Dextrans (glucose polymers available in preparations of various molecular weights) are third choice. Dextran 40 enters the renal tubules and may cause acute tubular necrosis in hypovolaemic shock. Dextran 70 in excess of 30 ml/kg may cause capillary oozing and cross-matching is made difficult. All colloid solutions increase the blood volume by the volume infused, except for Dextran 40 which increases the plasma volume more by its oncotic effect.

Colloid solution is given with blood to maintain a packed cell volume (PCV) of around 25–30% which corresponds to a haemoglobin concentration of around 10 g/dl. At this level plasma viscosity is reduced, improving red cell passage through the capillaries, increasing cardiac output and thus oxygen delivery to the tissues. Below this figure the decreasing availability of red blood cells impairs oxygen availability. Normally the first 10–20% blood volume loss should therefore be replaced with colloid solution, and thereafter a mixture of blood and colloid solution aiming to maintain this optimum PCV.

Having initially corrected any hypovolaemia, associated dehydration should be corrected over the following 12–24 hours with crystalloid solution. Here again 7–10 ml/kg can be given over 15–30 minutes in severe hydration, or over 2 hours in a less severe state. When rapid rates of replacement are required, close monitoring, preferably with a CVP line, is necessary, with reassessment after every bolus. The total volume required will obviously be somewhere between 50 ml/kg for mild (5%) dehydration and 150 ml/kg in severe (15%) cases. The choice of fluid depends on the patient's electrolyte balance but if this is within normal limits then normal saline should be used. This is given in addition to maintenance fluids.

Other shock syndromes

Haemorrhagic shock encephalopathy syndrome. Profound shock associated with convulsions, coma and bleeding may represent the haemorrhagic shock encephalopathy syndrome (HSES). About 90% of the children are aged less than 1 year. There may be a mild prodromal illness. Other features of the condition are anaemia, disseminated intravascular coagulation (DIC), bloody diarrhoea and impairment of renal and hepatic function. No definite aetiological factor or agent has so far been identified. A low level of circulating alpha-1-antitrypsin has led to speculation that there may be a release of proteolytic enzymes which overwhelm the natural protease inhibitors and induce the sequelae. With this in mind the early use of fresh frozen plasma may be beneficial but the treatment is essentially supportive. The condition carries a high mortality and most survivors are neuro-logically handicapped.

Reye syndrome. Shock may be associated with encephalopathy and fatty degeneration of the liver in Reye syndrome. Following a prodro-mal illness (chicken pox and influenza B in particular) the child, who may be of any age between infancy and adolescence, develops vomit-ing, drowsiness and often convulsions. There is often hypoglycaemia at presentation and a raised blood ammonia helps to differentiate Reye syndrome from HSES (normal or slightly elevated). The blood ammo-nia is very high early in the course of the illness but often returns towards a normal level by day 3 or 4. The liver transaminases are raised and prothombin time prolonged but the bilirubin is often nor-mal. Neutrophilia is to be expected. The diagnosis can be confirmed by liver biopsy but this should be reserved for cases where the diagnosis is in doubt because of the associated bleeding diathesis. The encephalopathy is due to cerebral oedema and CSF is normal. Aggressive treatment of low cerebral perfusion pressure has been shown to lower mortality and morbidity and we favour early intracra-nial pressure (ICP) monitoring. Aspirin has been implicated as a cause of Reye syndrome and is contraindicated in children except for specific conditions. Inborn errors of metabolism may present with a Reye-like illness, most notably medium chain acyl-Co A dehydrogenase defi-ciency, and it is prudent to collect urine for organic acid assay at the time of acute illness in all cases.

Toxic shock syndrome. High fever, watery diarrhoea, pharyngitis, conjunctivitis and erythroderma (with subseqent desquamation) may be associated with shock in the toxic shock syndrome. Neutrophilia and DIC are common. Children of school age are typically affected and the cause is a toxin released from *Staphylococcus aureus* phage type 1 which arises from a local infection such as osteomyelitis, empyema or skin abscess. Blood cultures are negative. The treatment is supportive and antibiotics directed against the staphylococcus.

Heatstroke. Although classically a condition of hot climates, heat-stroke has been reported in an English winter due to excessive clothing and bedding. Increased evaporative loss, peripheral vasodilatation and vascular endothelial damage induce a combination of distributive and hypovolaemic shock.

Drug ingestion. This should also be considered in all young children with shock in whom there is an absence of trauma or apparent sepsis. This may be one of the features of iron poisoning. Arrhythmias due to tricyclics or peripheral vasodilatation occurring with an overdose of barbiturates or tranquillisers may result in the same picture.

COMA

In the management of coma, the advanced life support measures for the airway, breathing and circulation are the top priority. Oxygenation should be generous, normocarbia ensured and an adequate mean blood pressure established. Immediately treatable conditions such as hypoglycaemia and opiate overdose should be recognised and treated in the first hour. If the Glasgow Coma Score is 9 or less, where the airway is not secure or there are bulbar signs the child should be sedated, intubated and ventilated. In trauma cerebral hypoperfusion is likely if extracerebral injuries are left untreated — these injuries take priority.

Raised intracranial pressure. Coma, pupillary inequality, irregular or abnormally slow respiration, hypertension and bradycardia are all signs of intracranial hypertension. Whatever the initial insult, therapy is principally aimed at preventing secondary damage. A cerebral blood flow adequate for cerebral metabolism is established by the manipulation of intracranial volume and hence pressure, the cardiodynamic status and factors affecting cerebral metabolic rate.

Minimise cerebral metabolism with:

— Sedation	Midazolam infusion 100–300 µg/kg/h
— Analgesia	Morphine infusion 10–40 µg/kg/h
— Muscle paralysis	Atracurium infusion 5–10 µg/kg/min
— Anticonvulsants	It is important to have a high index of suspicion for seizures in the paralysed patient. Cerebral function anlysing monitor (CFAM) may help
— Antipyretics	Paracetamol by mouth or rectally 10–15 mg/kg/dose, max dose 60 mg/kg/day

Brain herniation. Progressive coma with bilateral pupillary dilatation and decorticate then decerebrate posture usually over hours indicates transtentorial brain herniation. Uncal brain herniation is typically more sudden with almost simultaneous coma and commonly with a unilaterally fixed dilated pupil. Herniation syndromes progress untreated to brainstem infarction. Transient hyperventilation will reduce intracranial pressure by critically reducing cerebral blood flow and a diuresis is forced with mannitol while neurosurgically amenable causes are sought.

Metabolic encephalopathy should be considered in infants and children who present with coma which may be rapidly progressive, or associated with neuronal excitability, or with focal neurological deficits that do not add up and in whom neuroimaging fails to identify an intracranial cause. Investigations include an EEG and urine and blood for metabolic screening. The therapeutic aims are to correct electrolyte disturbances, and minimise nitrogen metabolism by preventing protein intake and giving 2.5–3.5 g/kg/day of glucose with an insulin infusion if required for hyperglycaemia. Acidosis should be vigorously treated with sodium bicarbonate although if hypernatraemia results peritoneal or haemodialysis should be started, they may be indicated for hyperammonaemia at levels of 500–700 μmol/litre. Coagulopathy should be corrected with blood products and vitamin K.

BRAINSTEM DEATH

Irremediable structural brain damage may occur leading to a child being ventilated in an apnoeic coma from which there is no hope of recovery. If clinical tests show complete absence of brainstem function then all support should stop. Two senior doctors will apply the tests. They must be clear that the brain damage is a result of a condition recognised to cause such circumstances, most commonly following severe head injury or intracranial bleeding. Other important preconditions are that the coma is not due to a metabolic disturbance, poisoning or hypothermia and that therapeutic interventions are not the cause, particularly sedative and paralysing drugs. It is vital that tests are conducted without haste and that all the preconditions are met. Two sets of tests are done up to 24 hours apart. Once it is certain that there is no life in the brain of the child it is important that the parents are clear that their child entered an irreversible coma some time ago. As the child may look well this needs to be addressed as it may fuel the natural denial that is commonly observed. The family must be given time to accommodate, they may have special requests and require

Tests of 'brain death'

RESPIRATION
Was the arterial $P\mathrm{co_2}$ below 6 kPa before the ventilator was disconnected?
Are there any spontaneous respirations within 5 minutes of disconnecting the ventilator?

BRAINSTEM REFLEXES
Do the pupils react to light?
Is nystagmus or other eye movement present when each ear in turn is irrigated with ice cold water for 1 minute?
Is there any eye movement during the Doll's-eye manoeuvre?
Does any response occur when each cornea is touched in turn?
Is any movement present in the head and neck either spontaneous or in response to bilateral supraorbital nerve pressure?
Is there a gag reflex or reflex response to a suction catheter passed down the trachea?

BODY TEMPERATURE
Is the core body temperature below 35°C?

DRUGS
Have any neuromuscular blocking drugs been given during the past 12 hours?
If they have is there any residual neuromuscular blockade?
Have any other drugs which may affect consciousness been given during the preceding 12 hours?
Is there any evidence of renal failure?
Is there any evidence of hepatic failure?

METABOLIC
Is the coma due to a metabolic or endocrine cause?

unhurried, clear information about what will happen next. Enquiries about organ donation commonly arise before death, it is our practice to raise the issue in a positive fashion, if questions have not arisen, after the second set of brainstem function tests. The coroner and family doctor must be kept informed of events.

FURTHER READING

Advanced life support – the practical approach. 1996 BMJ Publishing Group, London

American College of Surgeons 1988 Paediatric trauma. In: Advanced trauma life support teachers manual

Anon 1987 Plasma substitutes: the choice during surgery and intensive care. Drugs and Therapeutics Bulletin 25(10): 18

Bone RC et al 1987 A controlled clinical trial of high dose methylprednisolone in the treatment of severe sepsis and septic shock. New England Journal of Medicine 317: 653–658

Clarke GM 1987 Septic shock. Medicine International 38: 1582–1586

Jenkins JG et al 1987 Reye's syndrome: assessment of intracranial monitoring. British Medical Journal 294: 337–338

Levin M et al 1983 Haemorrhagic shock and encephalopathy: a new syndrome with high mortality in young children. Lancet ii: 64–67

The Veterans Administration Systemic Sepsis Cooperative Study 1987 Effect of high dose glucocorticoid therapy on mortality in patients with clinical signs of systemic sepsis group. New England Journal of Medicine 317: 659–665.

Wetzel RC 1987 Shock. In: Rogers MC (ed) Textbook of paediatric intensive care. Williams & Wilkins, Baltimore

Yates DW 1987 Volume replacement: the choice of fluid. Hospital Update 1987 297–306

5 Care of the newborn

Parents hope for and expect healthy normal children, reflecting the better outcome of pregnancy and the reduction in child deaths over the past 50 years. But one in 40 pregnancies still results in a baby with serious congenital abnormalities or problems, and about nine babies per 1000 are stillborn or die in the first week of life, and another three per 1000 die after the first week but before their first birthday. Neonatal care is provided in the delivery room and by the mother's bedside as well as the neonatal unit where the staff are based.

In the labour suite. The normal newborn who has started to breathe should be handed up to the mother. The wet delivery sheet is replaced by a warmed dry towel because avoidance of cold stress is important. The 1-minute Apgar score is recorded together with an accurate weight and head circumference. The temperature is checked before the mother and baby are transferred up to the postnatal ward, and if this is done rectally anal atresia will not be missed. The aim should be to keep mother and baby together whenever possible, and simple special care can be provided on the postnatal wards by close co-operation between the midwives and the paediatrician. This will include observations of temperature and of respiratory rate and pattern, blood sugar recordings when needed and the assessment of jaundice and its treatment with phototherapy. When staffing levels are satisfactory some well preterm babies can be kept with their mothers on the postnatal ward, even if some tube-feeding is included in the care. In this way admissions to the neonatal unit can be reduced to 5% of births and 8–10% should be the aim of all delivery units.

On the postnatal wards. Vitamin K, 1 mg, should be given to all babies orally with the first feed to prevent haemorrhagic disease of the newborn. The current recommendation in the UK is that two further doses at 1 and 6 weeks are given to breast fed infants, but this may change now that there is a licensed oral preparation available. There are no contra-indications at this dosage. It is the rarer late onset vitamin K deficiency bleeding which causes brain damage or death.

Breast feeding is the best method of feeding healthy full-term babies and encouragement and education begins in the antenatal classes. Most mothers want and need a lot of support from the midwifery staff when breast feeding. Bottle fed babies should be fed using the milk formula of the mother's choice, with the first feed within 4 hours of birth.

Fluid requirements

	Term	Preterm	Small for dates
Day 1	40	40	60
Day 2	60	60	80
Day 3	90	80	100
Day 4	120	100	120
Day 5	150	120	150
Then up to	150	180–200	200–220

Add 30 ml for phototherapy, 20–30 ml for radiant heater. In preterm infants, modify according to results of serum sodium, urine and plasma osmolarity.

Meconium and urine should normally have been passed by the time the baby has the thorough check at 24 hours of age. If there has been no bowel action, check that the anus is patent, that the abdomen is soft and not distended, and that there has been no vomiting or bile regurgitation. Re-examine in 12 hours. If vomiting or distension develop take erect and supine abdominal films to look for atresia or obstruction. If urine has not been passed, check the genitalia and the number of cord vessels, and palpate the kidneys and bladder. If they are not enlarged wait for a further 12 hours. If urine has still not been passed, arrange a renal ultrasound to check that the kidneys are present and normal in appearance.

Screening tests include examination for hip dislocation and instability, and the blood spot screening performed when the baby is on full milk feeds on about the sixth day. Galactosaemia, maple syrup urine disease and homocystinuria can also be detected in the newborn period, but screening is not routinely performed.

Screening for metabolic disease

	Prevalence	Screening test	Treatment
Phenylketonuria	1 in 10 000	Guthrie	Low phenylalanine diet
Hypothyroidism	1 in 4 000	Raised TSH	Thyroxine
Cystic fibrosis	1 in 2 000	Raised immunoreactive trypsin	Physio, antibiotics, pancreatic enzymes

Immunisation should be provided immediately after birth for two diseases. BCG gives cell-mediated immunity to tuberculosis. The vaccine must be given, 0.05 ml, intradermally above the site of the insertion of the deltoid on the left arm. The technique is difficult because subcutaneous injection must be avoided. It is offered to all babies at increased risk, including those with African, Caribbean and Asian parents and those with a recent family history of tuberculosis. Babies born to mothers with hepatitis should have both anti-HBs immunoglobulin and hepatitis B vaccine at birth.

The best care of normal newborns and their mothers depends on good communication between the mother, the midwives and the paediatrician, and then between the hospital and the community health teams.

RESUSCITATION

Newborn babies can tolerate acute total asphyxia far better than older children or adults. Nevertheless, inadequate or delayed resuscitation can lead to permanent brain damage and sometimes unavoidable death. It is essential that somebody skilled in resuscitation techniques, preferably part of the paediatric team, is present at all high risk deliveries and available within 2 minutes to resuscitate babies within low risk groups.

High risk deliveries account for approximately 25% of all deliveries and include over 60% of those who will require intubation

Caesarean section	Preterm delivery
Breech delivery	Fetal distress
Multiple pregnancy	Severe PE I
Instrumental delivery—	Maternal diabetes mellitus
Ventouse extraction	Rhesus incompatibility
Keilland rotation and	Maternal myasthenia gravis
extraction	Meconium staining of liquor

Commence timing from delivery of the baby. Dry excess fluid off the baby's skin with a warm towel. Check rapidly for severe congenital malformations, including myelomeningocoele and microcephaly. Check at 1 minute for respiratory efforts and heart rate.

Situation (1)

Baby blue and apnoeic or making inadequate respiratory efforts. Heart rate greater than 80/min

Response. Try to stimulate the baby by flicking the baby's feet or blowing cold oxygen over the baby's face from a face mask. If this fails, attempt face mask T-piece or bag and mask resuscitation. If the baby fails to improve within 30–50 seconds or the heart rate falls below 80/min, proceed to intubation.

Ventilation by face mask

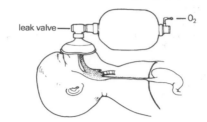

leak valve

— O$_2$

Problems:

1. Adequate face seal

2. Inflation pressure operator—dependent

3. Gas distension of stomach (pass stomach tube and apply gentle pressure)

Situation (2)

Baby blue/white, apnoeic and heart rate less than 80/min

Response. Try facemask T-piece or bag and mask resuscitation for up to 20 seconds. If there is no response, proceed to orotracheal, or if preferred, nasotracheal intubation.

If T-piece resuscitation is used limit inflation pressure to 25–30 cm H$_2$O initially. Prolonging the first inflation for 2–3 seconds will produce better lung expansion and aid in the formation of a gaseous reserve (functional residual capacity). Subsequently, ventilate at 20–30 inflations/min, allowing approximately 1 second for each inflation. Alternatively, attach the endotracheal (ET) tube to an anaesthetic rebreathing bag or self-filling manual bag system and inflate at 40–60 times/min.

Check the heart rate and listen for air entry on both sides of the chest. If there is no air entry, remove the ET tube, as it is almost certainly in the oesophagus, and reintubate. Air entry to one lung only indicates either that the tip of the tube is in the main bronchus, almost certainly the right, or alternatively that the baby has a pneumothorax or diaphragmatic hernia. Try withdrawing the tube by 1–2 cm while listening over the poorly ventilated lung. If air entry improves, the tube was too far down. It may be necessary to continue intermittent inflation until an X-ray is available to identify a pneumothorax or diaphragmatic hernia. If the baby's condition is critical and a pneumothorax suspected, the affected side can be needled.

Tracheal intubation

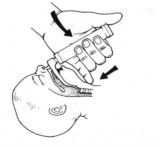
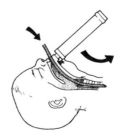

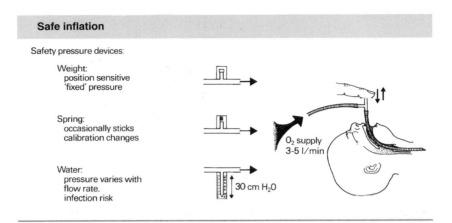

Safe inflation

Safety pressure devices:

Weight:
position sensitive
'fixed' pressure

Spring:
occasionally sticks
calibration changes

Water:
pressure varies with
flow rate.
infection risk

O_2 supply
3-5 l/min

30 cm H_2O

Situation (3)	Heart rate undetectable or falling despite adequate ventilation

Response. The baby almost certainly has a severe metabolic acidosis. Give external cardiac massage at 100–120 beats/min while continuing with lung inflation. Inject 1 ml of 1 in 10 000 adrenaline down the ET tube. If there is no response, obtain venous access via the umbilical vein or by injecting directly into the umbilical vein using a syringe and needle. Give an additional 1 ml of 1 in 10 000 adrenaline, into the umbilical vein catheter. If the heart rate fails to improve give sodium bicarbonate 8.4% intravenously, dissolved in an equal volume of glucose solution. This should be infused over 3–5 minutes, 20 ml to a large baby, 10 ml to a small baby. This cycle of adrenaline and bicarbonate can be repeated two to three times.

Other special situations

Apgar 0–1 at birth. If the baby is born without a detectable cardiac impulse, but the fetal heart was noticed up to 15 minutes before delivery, intubation, external cardiac massage, adrenaline and bicarbonate should be given without delay. These attempts should be abandoned if the baby is not improving with at least some respiratory efforts at 20 minutes of age.

The heart rate rises in response to resuscitation, ventilation appears to be adequate and the baby becomes pink but fails to make respiratory efforts. The most likely cause is respiratory depression from opiates given to the mother. Under these conditions, give naloxone i.v. 200 µg. If this produces a dramatic improvement give an additional 200 µg i.m. for a more prolonged effect.

Gestation less than 30 weeks. Try face mask T-piece or bag and mask resuscitation for 15–20 seconds. If the baby is not vigorous, breathing normally and pink, proceed to intubation.

Amniotic liquor noticed to be meconium stained. Suck out the naso- and oropharynx as soon as the head is delivered. Proceed to direct laryngoscopy immediately the baby is delivered. If meconium is present in the oropharynx airway, intubate immediately and connect the side arm of the ET tube to the suction source (50–100 cmH_2O). Occlude the

T-piece and remove the ET tube. This should be repeated until either no further meconium is recovered or the baby's heart rate falls below 80/min.

Subsequent management

After resuscitation always provide explanation and, where appropriate, reassurance to the parents. Babies who respond rapidly to resuscitation and can be extubated within 1–2 minutes are probably not at significant risk of subsequent problems and can be nursed with their mothers, providing there is adequate supervision. Those who take longer to improve, requiring repeated inflations before any obvious respiratory efforts, need to be admitted to the neonatal unit for observation, as some may develop asphyxial encephalopathy with apnoea, fitting, and feeding problems. Providing the baby does not fit and is neurologically normal within 24–48 hours the long-term prognosis is almost always good. Those who are severely asphyxiated at birth but are making some, albeit inadequate, respiratory efforts during resuscitation should be ventilated for 24–48 hours. The baby's neurological state must be carefully assessed in conjunction with intracranial ultrasound examinations. If the baby remains grossly abnormal, or if there is evidence of severe ischaemic lesions, it is reasonable to withdraw support after discussion with parents. There is no evidence that high dose barbiturate or steroid therapy have any useful effects.

EXAMINATION OF THE NEWBORN BABY

The initial examination is carried out on the labour suite shortly after birth to confirm for most parents that they have a healthy boy or girl, and to find any major or life-threatening abnormality so that treatment can be started locally or transport arranged to a referral neonatal unit. Apgar scores at 1 and 5 minutes are recorded and the baby is kept warm while the checks are made.

If the genitalia are ambiguous it is wise to say so and get expert help rather than making a guess. Birth weight and head circumference need to be recorded accurately. Assess the baby's facies and proportions; parents want to know on the first day if a syndrome is diagnosed or strongly suspected. The spine is checked to exclude *spina bifida*, the anus to exclude *atresia*, and the mucousy baby has a wide-bore tube passed to the stomach to exclude *oesophageal atresia*. For healthy babies who are pink and breathing normally, further checks are postponed until later because there are a number of misleading physical signs in the first few hours after birth. Some normal babies will have a cardiac murmur because the ductus arteriosus and the foramen ovale are still partly open, many will have fine crepitations in the lung fields due to unresorbed lung fluid, and may be neurologically shocked to some degree. Also the baby needs to be kept wrapped and warm and the mother needs to rest.

Examination of the newborn

Check	Comments
Facies, trunk and limbs	Are the baby's overall appearance, proportions and limbs normal? Check the weight and note small- or large-for-dates
Fontanelle(s) and sutures	Exclude signs of hydrocephalus, and of craniostenosis. Check the head circumference
Eyes	Exclude cataracts. Reassure the mother about subconjunctival haemorrhages
Nose	Pass a feeding tube to exclude choanal atresia if there is doubt about patency
Mouth	A cleft of the soft palate is important and easy to miss. Beware of loose supernumerary teeth, they need removing
Neck	Check for cysts and sinuses, and for shortness or webbing
Upper limbs	Check the digits and the brachial pulses. Single palmar creases are markers of possible anomalies elsewhere, not just of Down syndrome, and may be normal
Heart	If a murmur is still persisting the baby should be followed up
Chest	There should be no crepitations now, and no respiratory distress
Abdomen	The liver may be palpable up to 2 cm below the costal margin, but not the spleen. The kidneys may just be felt in the well-relaxed baby. A single umbilical artery may mean anomalies elsewhere especially in the renal tract. Meconium and urine should normally be passed within 24 hours
Genitalia	Hypospadias will always be associated with a hooded prepuce which should not be retracted because there are natural adhesions to the glans in the early years. Follow-up babies with undescended testes. Labial fusion separates spontaneously in time. White vaginal discharge is normal
Femoral pulses	Often difficult to feel. Check the blood pressure in the limbs by Doppler if coarctation is suspected
Spine	Midline dimples and sinuses over the coccyx and lower sacrum are benign, but those above S2 need a surgical opinion because communication with the spinal canal is possible. Tufts of hair and lipomas may also indicate spinal anomalies
Lower limbs	If talipes cannot be fully and over-corrected seek early orthopaedic advice
Neurological system	Check active and passive tone and the neonatal reflexes, looking for floppiness or asymmetry
Hips	Ask for any family history and use Ortolani and Barlow methods. Check persistent clicks and at-risk babies (breech especially in girls, those with positive family history) by ultrasound

At about 24 hours of age the thorough and definitive examination of the newborn should be carried out in the presence of the now refreshed mother, and with the baby warm and stable. In a good light check the baby from head to toe and explain the findings to the mother as you do them. Sum up at the end and ask if she has any questions.

Congenital infection

Specifically look for evidence of the infections which cross the placenta and may result in intra-uterine growth retardation and widespread organ damage. They are conveniently remembered by the mnemonic TORCH: *toxoplasmosis, rubella, cytomegalovirus* and *herpes virus hominis*. To these should be added syphilis in countries where this is not screened for and treated in pregnancy. Diagnosis is confirmed by the serology for each organism. The *Human Immunodeficiency Virus* (*HIV*) also crosses the placenta but is not obvious at birth. About 25% of babies born to HIV positive mothers will later develop AIDS but this can be reduced to about 8% by giving zidovudine to the mother during the pregnancy, and then to the newborn baby for 6 weeks after birth.

Minor anomalies

Most newborn infants have minor blemishes but a few have significant abnormal features like abnormal facies, abnormal body proportions, e.g. trunk to limb size, single palmar creases, single umbilical artery, limb abnormalities including polydactyly, syndactyly and curved or crossed over fingers. An accurate clinical description, photography and radiology, if appropriate, are required prior to asking for expert genetic counselling advice. The clinical features and the family history will indicate which chromosome studies and biochemical tests for metabolic diseases will need to be done. A similar approach is used for stillbirths with obvious urgency in getting the specimens.

Newborn infants have health problems like anyone else. Many follow their need to establish an independent existence. They may be due to structural defects or inherited biochemical disorders or failure of the infant to respond to the challenges of a strange and potentially hazardous environment.

BIRTH TRAUMA

The newborn examination will often reveal minor degrees of trauma which should be discussed with the mother, including scalp lesions from the fetal monitoring electrode, small lacerations from scalp blood sampling and from artificial rupture of the membranes, scalp oedema (caput succedaneum) and moulding, and forceps bruising. The risk of trauma is greater in breech deliveries, preterm births, precipitate deliveries, and when the baby is unexpectedly large. Most serious are intracranial bleeds due to tentorial tears or direct brain trauma. Happily now fractures to bones are rare but they can cause a pseudo palsy. Injury to the upper roots of the brachial plexus (*Erb palsy*) leads to adduction and internal rotation of the extended arm with the wrist and fingers flexed. This injury can be confused with cord injuries which also occur in difficult deliveries. The fractures will heal rapidly with excellent long term results and therefore the treatment is symptomatic with bandaging to the broken limb to secure some degree of immobilisation while allowing for skin care. Plexus and nerve injuries require regular physiotherapy, all involved joints are put through full movement many times each day. Recovery is difficult to forecast; it may be rapid or it may be slow and incomplete.

HEART MURMURS IN THE NEONATAL PERIOD

Asymptomatic heart murmurs are more difficult to sort out in the neonatal period than in later childhood and often the clinical signs, chest X-ray and ECG are not sufficiently helpful for a definite diagnosis to be reached. The majority will eventually turn out to be due either to a transitory patent ductus or to be innocent. The following will provide a logical approach:

Finding

- Pulses jerky and full, murmur maximum at left subclavian region.

Diagnosis — Patent ductus arteriosus

The murmur is often only systolic and ejection in character as the pulmonary and systemic diastolic pressures are similar. Chest X-ray is either normal or shows plethora, if the shunt is large. The ECG is also usually within normal limits, showing the usual RV predominance with a dominant R in V_1 and a dominant S in V_5. Many close spontaneously within days. Echocardiography will reveal a large left atrium.

Findings

- Increasing respiratory difficulty.
- Rising $P\text{CO}_2$, falling $P\text{O}_2$, falling pH.
- Pallor in the absence of anaemia.
- Apnoea (in immature infants or in an infant who is being ventilated).
- An increasing oxygen requirement.
- Difficulty weaning the infant off ventilation.

Diagnosis — Significant patent ductus arteriosus needing treatment

The chest X-ray will show marked pulmonary plethora and echo-cardiography and a left atrial/aortic ratio of 1.2:1 or greater. If fluid restriction to 70% of normal fails to improve the symptoms, use indomethacin, a prostaglandin synthetase inhibitor at a dose of 0.2 mg/kg, given three times at 12-hourly intervals. Give frusemide 1 mg/kg simultaneously to counteract the fluid retaining properties of indomethacin. Indomethacin should not be used if there is a generalised bleeding disorder, platelet count <75 000/mm³, bilirubin level sufficient to require an exchange transfusion, or creatinine level greater than 140 μmol/l.

Finding

- An ejection systolic murmur in the second to fourth left interspace radiating through to the back and femoral pulses are absent.

Diagnosis — Coarctation of the aorta

Femoral pulses can be difficult to feel in the immediate neonatal period and measurements of upper arm and calf blood pressure using a Doppler system can be very helpful. In the presence of significant coarctation, this will differ by more than 20 mmHg. Occasionally these babies develop heart failure in the first few months of life. Most remain asymptomatic and will not require any treatment apart from follow-up until surgical correction is carried out at 4–10 years of age. Chest X-ray will usually show no abnormality at birth; rib notching does not appear for several years. The normal RV dominance may be absent on the ECG but usually no abnormality is found.

Finding

- A pansystolic murmur maximum in the fourth to fifth left interspace close to the sternal edge.

Diagnosis — Probable ventricular septal defect

In the immediate neonatal period the murmur may be soft and not pansystolic; the classical murmur appears over the subsequent weeks as the pulmonary vascular resistance falls and the left to right shunt increases. The chest X-ray and ECG will be normal if the shunt is small. If the pulmonary vascular resistance has fallen and the defect is large, the heart will appear bulky with pulmonary plethora and the ECG will be more in keeping with that of an older child with a dominant R in V_5 and a dominant S in V_1. Children thought to have a ventricular septal defect need careful follow-up as there is a tendency for them to go into heart failure at 6–8 weeks of age as the pulmonary vascular resistance falls. If the chest X-ray and clinical signs suggest that there is a large defect the parents should be taught to recognise the signs of impending heart failure (rising respiratory rate, tendency to expiratory grunting, difficulty with feeds, poor weight gain and tendency to sweat profusely).

A large majority of the remaining babies with heart murmurs will have:

Findings

- A soft to moderate ejection systolic murmur maximum in the third to fourth left intercostal spaces.
- Present femoral pulses.

Diagnosis — (1) Atrial septal defect

- Fixed splitting of the second heart sound is often difficult to identify in the immediate neonatal period.

Diagnosis — (2) Pulmonary stenosis

- With a single second heart sound (usually).

Diagnosis — (3) Aortic stenosis

- The murmur radiates into the neck.

Diagnosis — (4) Innocent heart murmur

This latter makes up the large majority. If in doubt, re-examine the child in 1–2 days. If the murmur is present at the time of discharge the parents should be told of its presence and that follow-up is indicated. The frequency of innocent heart murmurs in the neonatal period should be stressed, and the parents reassured as far as possible.

NEONATAL JAUNDICE

Neonatal jaundice is a common problem in the full-term and preterm baby. The level below which the baby is entirely safe from kernicterus has yet to be defined. Most would accept that 350 μmol/l should not be exceeded in full-term babies less than 3 days of age, but that mature babies who are well can tolerate levels of up to 450 μmol/l by the fifth day without evidence of damage. Preterm babies are more susceptible and the earlier the gestational age the lower is the safe threshold, so that the bilirubin level in babies of 26 weeks or less should not be allowed to rise above 150 μmol/l. Even these levels may be dangerous if a baby of any gestation is ill, has a severe metabolic acidosis or has a low albumin level. All babies who have had bilirubins near to exchange levels should have neonatal hearing screening tests.

Problem

- Onset of clinically obvious jaundice at 2–3 days of age in a preterm or full-term baby.
- Baby otherwise well and alert and feeding or tolerating feeds normally.

Diagnosis — Physiological jaundice

By far the commonest cause of neonatal jaundice is relative immaturity of the liver's conjugating system, occurring in 65% of term and 80% of preterm infants. As long as this does not produce a management problem or persist for more than 5–7 days, no investigations other than serum bilirubin estimations are indicated. If the bilirubin approaches treatment levels, the baby should be examined carefully because physiological jaundice is a diagnosis made by exclusion. Urine should be sent for culture, and blood for group and Coombs' test, total and conjugated bilirubin, and to exclude galactosaemia.

Management. Jaundiced babies tend to be rather sleepy and to feed less vigorously and any resulting degree of dehydration exacerbates jaundice. Therefore ensure that the baby is being given sufficient fluids to maintain full hydration. In the healthy full-term baby phototherapy should be commenced when the bilirubin exceeds 350 μmol/l. In the preterm baby, particularly those with problems, it is safer to commence phototherapy at considerably lower levels. The eyes should

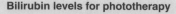

Bilirubin levels for phototherapy

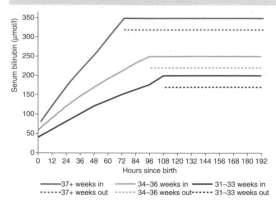

For babies of 30 weeks' gestation or less, commence phototherapy when the bilirubin level in µmol/l is 100 times the weight in kg. e.g. for a baby weighing 0.6 kg start phototherapy when the bilirubin reaches 60 µmol/l

be covered as there is a theoretical risk that exposure to bright light can damage the retina. Phototherapy tends to reduce bowel transit time producing frequent loose stools, and therefore it is often necessary to use a small napkin to limit the need for nursing care, although this reduces slightly the area of skin exposed.

Phototherapy alters the pigment in the skin so that serial bilirubin levels are crucial to determine the child's progress, rather than relying on skin colour. Giving phototherapy to a baby in an incubator may cause a pyrexia due to the heat from the lights. Phototherapy to a naked baby in an open cot may expose the child to too low an environmental temperature. This can be avoided by using a cot lid or ensuring that the room temperature is at least 30°C.

Problem

- Jaundice appearing within the first 2 days of life.
- Often with associated anaemia.

Diagnosis — Jaundice due to excessive haemolysis

Jaundice appearing in the first 2 days of life is usually associated with a haemolytic process. *Rhesus incompatibility* is now less common but obviously should be considered when the mother is rhesus negative and antibodies have been detected during the pregnancy. More commonly haemolytic jaundice is due to *ABO incompatibility*, usually when the mother is Group O and the baby is A or B. Occasionally jaundice results from abnormalities of red cell shape such as *spherocytosis*, or to instability of the red cell membrane because of *glucose-6-phosphate dehydrogenase* (G6PD) deficiency or *pyruvate kinase deficiency*.

When rhesus incompatibility is anticipated cord blood should be collected for haemoglobin and PCV, blood group, Coombs' test and bilirubin. In rhesus incompatibility Coombs' test is always positive, but it may be positive or negative in ABO problems, which can be confirmed instead by finding raised levels of anti-A or anti-B haemolysins (antibodies) in the mother's blood. The diagnosis of congenital spherocytosis can be difficult in the newborn period because of the immature red cell forms present in normal babies. It is helpful to examine the parents' blood films because the condition is inherited. When the baby is a few months old the diagnosis can be confirmed by osmotic fragility tests.

On a world scale *G6PD deficiency* is a very important cause of haemolytic jaundice. It occurs in at least three forms affecting Negro, Mediterranean and Asian races, but all are inherited in a sex-linked dominant character with variable penetrance, so that there is a wide range of clinical severity. A screening test is available, and later the actual levels of the enzyme can be measured in the red cells to give an indication of the severity. Episodes of haemolysis in neonates are usually precipitated by non-specific events such as hypoglycaemia or acidosis, but certain drugs including sulphonamides and aspirin may also be responsible.

Management. Commence phototherapy as soon as the jaundice is apparent. Measure and plot the bilirubin and haemoglobin levels 6 hourly. As rhesus incompatibility is often associated with hyperinsulinaemia, measure blood glucose 6 hourly. Ensure that the baby is well hydrated. Exchange transfusion must be carried out soon after birth if the cord blood haemoglobin is less than 10 g/dl, and subsequently if the rate of rise in bilirubin is faster than 20 μmol/h or the bilirubin is approaching the exchange level for a baby of that gestation.

Indications for exchange transfusion

Gestation (weeks)	Bilirubin levels (μmol/l)	
	well baby	ill baby
> 36	450	400
34–36	350	300
31–33	275	225
27–30	175	150
< 27	150	150

Problem

- Skin has a greenish-yellow tinge as the bilirubin is partly conjugated.
- Hepatosplenomegaly.
- Often petechiae are seen shortly after birth.
- Usually small-for-dates.

Diagnosis — Jaundice due to congenital infection

Intrauterine growth retardation may have been detected during pregnancy and special serological tests need to be taken for toxoplasmosis, rubella, cytomegalovirus and herpes virus hominis. Damage to eyes and brain may also be present, but sadly no treatment is effective.

Problem

- Onset of jaundice after 48 hours.
- Other signs of illness, e.g. lethargy, irritability, feeding poorly or vomiting.

Diagnosis — Jaundice due to acquired infection or inherited metabolic disorder such as galactosaemia or fructosaemia

These babies require more extensive investigation. Send urine for microscopy and culture to exclude UTI and for urine metabolic screen. Obtain blood culture to exclude septicaemia and examine CSF to exclude meningitis. Most will require intravenous antibiotics, e.g. penicillin and gentamicin, until the blood and urine results are known.

JAUNDICE FOR MORE THAN SEVEN DAYS

This is a frequent and troublesome problem although usually the jaundice resolves without any long term significance.

Problem

- Persistent jaundice.
- Little or no conjugated bilirubin.
- Pale urine and stools.

Diagnosis — Persisting conjugation defect

Some cases have *hypothyroidism* which is confirmed by measuring serum thyroxine and TSH. When identified and treated with thyroxine early, the prognosis for normal development is excellent, but if the diagnosis is missed in the lethargic, constipated and jaundiced baby permanent developmental delay may result. In this group *galactosaemia* should again be excluded by sending the urine for sugar chromatography and measuring the serum galactose-1-phosphate uridyl transferase. Damage will result unless the baby is nurtured on a galactose-free diet.

Very occasionally babies have persisting jaundice due to inherited enzyme defects which interfere with normal conjugation. Of these the recessively inherited *Crigler–Najjar* is potentially the most serious but one of its types improves with phenobarbitone. *Gilbert syndrome* is chronic but less severe and is probably a defect in the uptake of unconjugated bilirubin into the liver cell. The other inherited hyperbilirubinaemias, *Dubin–Johnson syndrome* and *Rotor syndrome*, give an obstructive picture with raised conjugated biliurubin.

Problem

- Breast fed.
- Jaundiced with virtually all the bilirubin unconjugated.
- Otherwise healthy.

Diagnosis — Breast milk jaundice

This poorly understood condition is relatively common. It persists for weeks but has no long term implications and does not require treatment. This is another diagnosis made by exclusion, but if there are any doubts the baby can be changed on to bottle feeds for 48 hours. The diagnosis is confirmed if the jaundice fades only to recur on recommencing breast feeds.

| Problem | • Continuous and often progressive jaundice.
• Elevated conjugated bilirubin, i.e. greater than 50%.
• Dark urine containing bilirubin and urobilinogen. |

Diagnosis — Either (a) biliary atresia, (b) inspissated bile syndrome or (c) hepatitis

These diagnoses may be difficult to unravel, but most can be sorted out by means of an isotope labelled dye test, observing first passage down the biliary tract with a gamma camera and then measuring its excretion in stools and urine, together with an ultrasound examination to try to demonstrate the gall bladder, and a liver biopsy. The differential diagnosis is important because biliary atresia needs surgical treatment with a Kasai procedure before 6 weeks of age, while in hepatitis a laparotomy should be avoided if at all possible.

Follow-up of jaundiced babies. Babies who have neonatal haemolytic episodes need to be seen at regular intervals up to the age of 2 months, to ensure that they do not become severely anaemic. A haemoglobin below 7.0 g/dl or above that associated with evidence of incipient cardiac failure (tachypnoea, tachycardia, failure to thrive) are indications for giving a top-up transfusion of fresh packed cells (20–30 ml/kg body weight). Any baby who has had an exchange transfusion, or high bilirubuin approaching exchange levels, should have a newborn hearing screening test, and follow up to confirm normal hearing at the 7-month distraction test and subsequent normal language development.

HARE LIP AND CLEFT PALATE

Hare lip never presents a diagnostic problem as the defect is obvious to all. The isolated cleft palate is more easily missed, particularly by those who do not inspect the mouth during a routine examination of the newborn baby at birth. The definitive treatment is undoubtedly that of surgery with repair of the hare lip at 3–6 months and closure of the palatal defect by formation and mobilisation of pedicles at 1 year. There is, however, a major short and long term medical role to ensure that the baby thrives satisfactorily and does not suffer from long term side effects.

Feeding. Breast feeding is difficult but can be successful in those with

Before and after

Unilateral cleft lip and palate

Bilateral cleft lip and palate

a small palatal defect. If the lesion is large the baby can sometimes be fed using a specialised teat, but most important is skilled advice and encouragement for the mother from nurses experienced in cleft lip and palate work.

Moulding of defects. The use of a T-bar strapping aids the development and closure of the lip and anterior palatal defect and should be commenced in the immediate neonatal period.

Children with clefts have an increased incidence of sensorineural hearing problems and are also at a considerably greater risk of ear infection which may lead to conductive deafness if not recognised and treated. Careful hearing tests are important, and all will benefit from speech therapy advice. It is therefore essential that the paediatrician is involved in the long term follow-up of these babies. The condition also has a familial tendency and so genetic counselling will be required.

T-bar and feeding plate

Feeding plate

wire wings

cut

3"

fold

'T' bar

long teat

SPINA BIFIDA

Spina bifida presents major management rather than diagnostic problems which are both practical and ethical. Experience over the last 30 years has shown that although surgical intervention with closure of the lesion is often possible in the immediate neonatal period, extensive lesions will be associated with hydrocephalus, urinary incontinence leading to chronic pyelonephritis and early death. For this reason many paediatricians and paediatric surgeons advise a selective intervention approach. Careful assessment is an essential prerequisite to parent counselling.

Examine the lesion to define its extent. Those associated with a good prognosis are limited to lumbar vertebrae rather than extending upwards to involve thoracic segments as well. Occasionally the lesion involves cervical vertebrae or even the occiput where there may be a very large sac sometimes exceeding the size of the head. The size of the sac is no guide to the severity of the occipital lesion as there may be only a small bony defect and no extrusion of brain substance. Examine the lower limbs. If the spinal cord is already damaged there are often

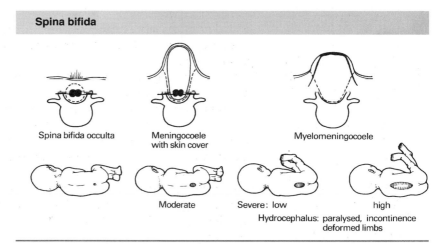

Spina bifida

Spina bifida occulta

Meningocoele
with skin cover

Myelomeningocoele

Moderate

Severe: low   high

Hydrocephalus: paralysed, incontinence
deformed limbs

striking deformities of the legs and feet. Test the lower limbs for sensation using either a pin or preferably a lump of ice. If sensory loss is present the baby will not respond below the proximal extent of the lesion. Assess anal tone using the fifth finger, a flaccid sphincter is likely to be associated with later faecal incontinence. Feel the abdomen carefully. The bladder may already be distended due to parasympathetic damage.

If sensory loss is minimal and regular leg movements can be induced, the bladder not distended and anal tone normal, the parents should be advised that operative intervention can lead to a reasonable quality of life. The child will probably walk and be continent although shunts may be required to control hydrocephalus. If these encouraging features are absent and the lesion is very extensive the parents should be advised that the long term outlook will be extremely gloomy. Under these circumstances the parents will usually not press for surgery. It is then the paediatrician's responsibility to ensure that the baby is kept comfortable and pain free. Sometimes the baby will develop an overwhelming meningitis, at other times there may be a tendency for the lesion to epithelialise followed by progressive hydrocephalus. The onset of hydrocephalus is easy to recognise in the immediate neonatal period; the baby will be lethargic, the anterior fontanelle full with clinically obvious separation of the sutures. The head circumference will increase at an abnormally high rate. Under these circumstances the paediatrician and paediatric surgeon will again need to discuss with the parents whether a shunt operation should be carried out.

Shunts require frequent refashioning as the child grows and there is also a tendency for the tubing to block and become infected. Shunt blockage is easy to miss in the older child. Suggestive features are lethargy and drowsiness, headache and vomiting. Fundoscopy may reveal changes indicating raised intracranial pressure, and CT scanning will confirm the problem. Blocked catheters represent an emergency situation, as blindness and cerebral damage may be produced in a very short period.

FURTHER READING

Connor EM et al (The Pediatric AIDS Clinical Trials Study Group) 1994 Reduction of maternal–infant transmission of human immunodeficiency virus type I with zidovudine treatment. New England Journal of Medicine 331: 1173–1180

Frenkel LD, Gaur S 1994 Perinatal HIV infection and AIDS. Clinics in Perinatology 21: 95–107

Hall SM 1993 The diagnosis of congenital infection. Current Paediatrics 3: 171–179

Milner RDG 1989 A colour atlas of the newborn. Wolfe Medical, London

Ogilvy-Stuart AL, Wilkinson AR 1993 Resuscitation of the newborn. Current Paediatrics 3: 214–219

Passmore SJ, McNinch AW 1995 Vitamin K in infancy. Current Paediatrics 5: 36–38

Peterec SM 1995 Management of neonatal rhesus disease. Clinical Perinatology 22: 561–592

Punt J 1995 Surgical management of neural tube defects. In: Fetal & neonatal neurology & neurosurgery, 2nd edn. Churchill Livingstone, Edinburgh, pp. 311–318

Redington AN 1991 Clinical assessment of the neonate and infant with suspected congenital heart disease. Current Paediatrics 1: 65–72

Roberton NRC 1988 A manual of normal neonatal care. Arnold, London

Roberton NRC 1993 Neonatal jaundice and liver disease. In: A Manual of Neonatal Intensive Care, 3rd edn. Arnold, London, pp. 238–260

Sommerland BC 1994 Management of cleft lip and palate. Current Paediatrics 4: 189–195

Stephenson T, Barbor P 1995 Ethical dilemmas of diagnosis and intervention. In: Fetal & Neonatal Neurology & Neurosurgery, 2nd edn. Churchill Livingstone, Edinburgh, pp. 709–718

Tudehope DI, Shearman AD 1995 Neonatal monitoring and equipment. Current Paediatrics 5: 195–200

Yoxall CW, Isherwood DM, Weindling AM 1996 The neonatal infection screen. Current Paediatrics 6: 16–20

Abnormal form

Dysmorphology can be defined as the study of abnormal form. In the context of paediatrics this embraces a wide spectrum of clinical presentations, ranging from the ill neonate with multiple structural abnormalities to the perfectly healthy child whose only distinguishing feature is a slightly unusual facial appearance. Unlike most medical disciplines the emphasis is on diagnosis rather than treatment. Reaching a diagnosis can be extremely difficult but it is nevertheless well worth persevering. The child may benefit by being spared the discomfort of further investigations and possible complications, such as retinal detachment (*Stickler syndrome*) and aortic dilatation (*Marfan syndrome*), can be detected and treated at an early stage. Benefit for the parents comes in the form of an accurate prognosis and the provision of information about genetic implications for future children. Contact with other families through well organised parent support groups can also be extremely helpful.

DEFINITIONS AND CONCEPTS

When assessing an infant or child with structural abnormalities it is well worth pausing to reflect on how they should best be classified. The ensuing train of thought will often help in pointing to a diagnosis as well as in providing insight into a possible cause and associated genetic implications.

First of all consider whether the abnormalities are serious or of only trivial importance. A *major* defect is one which has an adverse effect on function or social acceptability. Approximately 2–3% of all babies have at least one major abnormality. In contrast, a *minor* defect is of little if any medical or cosmetic importance. Minor defects are subdivided into *minor malformations* such as a supernumerary nipple and *minor variants* such as a single palmar crease. Minor defects are present in at least 10% of all individuals and there is little point in bringing these to a parent's attention if one is detected during a routine examination. However the discovery of more than one minor defect in a baby should prompt a careful examination to exclude a more serious underlying diagnosis. For example in a very premature baby whose features are concealed by extensive neonatal life support equipment, the diagnosis of Down syndrome may first be suspected by the astute observation of a single palmar crease and fifth finger clinodactyly.

Next try to determine whether the infant or child has a single abnormality or whether there are multiple problems. For example isolated polydactyly is not a cause for serious concern, but polydactyly in a child with mental retardation or other structural abnormalities should lead to consideration of an underlying 'syndromal' diagnosis.

The classification of congenital abnormalities has been the subject of much discussion and confusion. The following definitions have been devised to try to introduce an element of order and logic and to enhance understanding of the underlying pathogenic processes.

Single abnormality

Digital amputations and pseudosyndactyly with fenestration due to amniotic bands

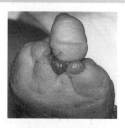
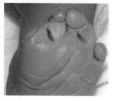

A malformation or primary defect results from an abnormal *intrinsic* developmental process. Commonly encountered examples include cleft lip/palate and neural tube defects. Most isolated malformations are thought to show multifactorial inheritance with a low recurrence risk to siblings and offspring of around 2–4%.

A disruption or secondary defect is caused by interference with normal development by an *extrinsic* factor such as intra-uterine infection or amniotic bands. Examples are cataracts caused by 'congenital' rubella infection and limb amputations resulting from amniotic band occlusion.

A deformation represents an abnormal shape or form which results from an abnormal mechanical force such as uterine constriction. Common examples include congenital dislocation of the hips and talipes. Generally deformations have a better prognosis for treatment than malformations.

A dysplasia is caused by abnormal organisation of cells within a tissue, organ or system. A dysplasia may involve only a single site as in abnormal neuronal migration leading to lissencephaly, or it may be widespread as in skeletal dysplasias such as achondroplasia. Many dysplasias are caused by single gene defects.

Multiple abnormalities

A sequence is a pattern of abnormalities which results from the consequences of a single primary insult or event. The most widely quoted example is the 'Potter sequence' of pulmonary hypoplasia, squashed facies and talipes which results from oligohydramnios due to renal agenesis or urethral outflow obstruction.

An association refers to the non-random occurrence of multiple abnormalities for which there is no clear cause. For example, the VATER association was proposed to account for the tendency of *V*ertebral, *A*nal, *T*racheo-*E*sophageal and *R*enal/*R*adial abnormalities to occur together. The finding of two or more of these abnormalities should prompt careful examination of the other relevant systems.

A field defect relates to organs or systems which respond as a unit to an embryological signal or insult. A field defect is *monotopic* if adjacent structures are affected. For example, radial hypoplasia or aplasia is often associated with abnormalities of the thumb. A field defect is *polytopic* if two or more widely separated structures are affected. For example, the cranial sutures and digits are involved together in several premature craniosynostosis disorders such as *Apert* and *Pfeiffer syndromes*.

Finally a *syndrome* is a pattern of abnormalities which are consistent, recognisable and causally related. For example, *Meckel syndrome* is consistently characterised by an encephalocoele, polycystic kidneys and polydactyly: the causal autosomal recessive gene has been mapped to chromosome 17q. In essence a syndrome can be distinguished from an association by its consistency and because it has a known cause.

To some extent these definitions are somewhat arbitrary with a degree of overlap, and in particular the term 'syndrome' is used very loosely and widely to describe almost any clinical entity. However careful consideration of the nature of a child's abnormalities based on this type of classification will often provide a useful starting point in trying to identify a cause and establish a diagnosis. Each of the three major steps needed to complete this process — the medical history, the clinical examination and special investigations — will now be considered.

THE MEDICAL HISTORY

As in every other clinical situation the assessment of a child with dysmorphic features should start with a detailed medical history. When taking the history special attention should be paid to the pregnancy and neonatal period and, if at all possible, it is important to try to review relevant maternity and neonatal records.

Pregnancy

Evidence of possible teratogenic exposure should be sought, remembering that the list of confirmed and suspected teratogens has expanded to include physical agents such as sustained hyperthermia and drugs such as valproate and warfarin.

Fetal movement is reduced or absent (*fetal akinesia*) in many disorders presenting with arthrogryposis as well as in those characterised by hypotonia whether central, such as in the *Prader–Willi syndrome*, or peripheral, such as in the congenital dystrophies and myopathies. Large fibroids or a bicornuate uterus can cause deformations, as can a multiple pregnancy which leads to fetal crowding. The incidence of prematurity is increased in connective tissue disorders such as the more severe forms of the *Ehlers–Danlos syndrome*.

Information about the placenta and umbilical cord can also be helpful. A single umbilical artery is a non-specific finding but is consistent with a diagnosis of the VATER association and sirenomelia. A fetus papyraceus would explain embolic infarction consequences, such as intestinal atresia or aplasia cutis in the surviving twin.

Proven or suspected teratogens

Agent	Effects	Agent	Effects
Drugs		**Infections**	
		Viral	
Alcohol	Cardiac defects, facies and microcephaly	Cytomegalovirus	Chorioretinitis, hearing loss and microcephaly
Chloroquine	Chorioretinitis and hearing loss	Herpes simplex	Microcephaly and microphthalmia
Diethylstilboestrol	Uterine malformations and vaginal carcinoma	Rubella	Cardiac, CNS, eye and hearing abnormalities
Lithium	Ebstein anomaly	Varicella zoster	CNS, eye and skin abnormalities
		Bacterial	
Phenytoin	Cardiac defects, cleft palate and digital hypoplasia	Syphilis	Hydrocephalus, osteitis and rhinitis
		Parasites	
Retinoids	CNS, ear and eye abnormalities	Toxoplasmosis	CNS, eye and hearing abnormalities
		Physical	
Streptomycin	Hearing loss	Ionising radiation	CNS and eye abnormalities
Tetracycline	Dental enamel hypoplasia	Prolonged hyperthermia	CNS and eye abnormalities
Thalidomide	Cardiac, ear and limb abnormalities		
Valproic acid	Facies and neural tube defects		
Warfarin	Nasal hypoplasia and epiphyseal stippling		

The neonatal period

Irritability and poor feeding can be symptoms of withdrawal from addictive agents such as alcohol. Most babies with the *Prader–Willi syndrome* require tube-feeding in early infancy because of their severe hypotonia. Hypoglycaemia occurs in the *Beckwith–Wiedemann* and *Silver–Russell* syndromes. Hypocalcaemia is a feature of the *DiGeorge* syndrome. In contrast transient hypercalcaemia is seen in *Williams syndrome*.

Family history

Advanced paternal age should raise suspicion of a new dominant mutation: this well documented phenomenon was first recognised in a study of *Apert syndrome*. Advanced maternal age is seen in all of the autosomal trisomies which survive to term, i.e. trisomy 13 (*Patau syndrome*), trisomy 18 (*Edwards syndrome*), trisomy 21 (*Down syndrome*). Parental consanguinity is suggestive of autosomal recessive inheritance.

Polite enquiries should be made about unusual parental or family illnesses. For example the mother of a boy with sex-linked recessive ectodermal dysplasia may volunteer that she has mild dental or dermal abnormalities. Similarly the mother of a boy with Lowe syndrome may give a history of lens opacities.

Behavioural characteristics

Several dysmorphic syndromes are associated with striking behavioural phenotypes. Repetitive speech (*echolalia*) is a feature of the

Fragile X syndrome. Many children with *Williams syndrome* have wonderful social skills with so called 'cocktail party manner' which conceals a quite significant underlying intellectual deficit particularly in mathematical skills. *Angelman syndrome* is characterised by happiness, inappropriate laughter and a fascination with water and mirrors. In contrast girls with *Rett syndrome* are irritable, hesitant, non-communicative and pre-occupied with compulsive hand-wringing. Many children with the *Smith–Magenis syndrome* show a very disturbed sleep pattern with disruptive behaviour which can extend to self mutilation, including the pulling out of finger nails and the insertion of foreign objects into body orifices.

THE CLINICAL EXAMINATION

This is by far the most important step in the evaluation of any child presenting with unusual physical features. The examination should not be unpleasant for the child as it relies mainly on observation, utilising the normal ploys of gaining the child's confidence and being prepared to adapt to his or her mood and choice of surroundings. Liberal use should be made of a measuring tape so that apparent abnormalities such as short digits or widely spaced eyes can be checked against standard charts. A good light source is essential and a checklist detailing all aspects of the examination is a useful *aide-mémoire*. A Wood's lamp should be used to look for pigmentary abnormalities of the skin. It can also be helpful to review photographs from infancy and early childhood, as clinical features can change quite noticeably with age to become more or less typical of the standard text-book photographs and description.

General physique

An examination should always include measurement of height, weight and head circumference. Remember that both macrocephaly and microcephaly can be familial so, if relevant, measure and record the parental head circumference: standard charts for normal adult head circumference are now available. Observe whether body size is in proportion. Is the lower segment, as measured from the symphysis pubis to the sole of the feet, significantly greater than the upper segment? The upper to lower segment ratio decreases progressively during childhood from around 1.7:1 at birth to 1.2:1 at age 4 years to 1:1 at 9 years. Span is normally less than height up to around the age of 11 years. An abnormally low upper to lower segment ratio and a relatively long span are seen in disorders associated with a 'Marfanoid' habitus.

Also note whether there is any obvious body asymmetry. If the child is obese, is this generalised or localised to the trunk? Is there absence of subcutaneous fat as in the lipodystrophies?

Causes of a Marfanoid habitus	Causes of asymmetry	Syndromes associated with obesity
Marfan syndrome	Beckwith–Wiedemann syndrome	Cohen's syndrome (truncal)
Homocystinuria	Chromosome mosaicism	Klinefelter's syndrome
Beals syndrome	Klippel–Trenauny–Weber syndrome	Laurence–Moon–Biedel syndrome
Klinefelter syndrome	Neurofibromatosis 1	Prader–Willi syndrome
Multiple endocrine adenomatosis IIB	Proteus syndrome	Pseudohypoparathyroidism
Stickler syndrome	Silver–Russell syndrome	

The skull

A long narrow skull (*scaphocephaly* or *dolicocephaly*) can be caused by premature sagittal suture synostosis. Premature bilateral coronal suture synostosis results in a short broad skull (*brachycephaly*). Unilateral coronal suture synostosis leads to an asymmetrical 'parallelogram' shaped skull (*plagiocephaly*): this can also be a consequence of intra-uterine deformation. Premature fusion of the metopic suture causes a triangular shaped head (*trigonocephaly*). Premature fusion of the lambdoid, coronal and metopic sutures causes a pointed or tower-shaped skull (*turricephaly*).

The face

The human face is an extraordinarily complex structure. Sometimes a diagnosis can be made quickly by simply looking at a child's face which triggers off recognition of a well recognised facial gestalt as in *Down syndrome*. This is one of the many situations in which medicine can justifiably be said to be more of an art than a science. On other occasions a child's face may seem a little unusual but the features do not immediately suggest any obvious diagnosis. For these children it is essential that the facial characteristics are correctly detailed and documented if diagnostic progress is to be achieved. Finally there are many children with dysmorphic syndromes who have a perfectly normal facial appearance but in whom careful examination will reveal useful diagnostic clues.

The overall size or shape of a face can help lead to a diagnosis. For example the face is round in *Down syndrome* and in young children with the *Cri-du-Chat (5p-) syndrome*. A face with a flat lateral profile is suggestive of chondrodysplasia punctata or *Stickler syndrome*. A long face is characteristic of the *fragile X syndrome* and of children with a congenital myopathy. Babies with the *Potter sequence* have a squashed facies because of intra-uterine compression. A triangular shaped face with a large head and small features is typical of the *Silver–Russell syndrome*.

The forehead

This can be prominent or bossed as in some of the craniosynostosis syndromes, such as *Crouzon syndrome*, and many of the storage disorders, such as *Hurler* and *Hunter syndrome*. Prominence of the supraorbital ridges is a feature of many of the sclerosing bone dysplasias such as frontometaphyseal dysplasia. The forehead can be narrow, as in the *Prader–Willi syndrome,* or receding as in microcephaly. Furrowing of the skin on the forehead is a feature of lissencephaly.

Eye-lids, palpebral fissures

The eyes can be widely spaced (*hypertelorism*) as in frontonasal dysplasia, or close together (*hypotelorism*) as in holoprosencephaly. This can be assessed by measuring the inter-pupillary distance and comparing this with standard charts. Lateral displacement of the inner canthi (*telecanthus*) with normal positioning of the eyes is seen in one of the two forms of *Waardenburg syndrome.* The palpebral fissures slope upwards from inner to outer canthi in disorders associated with poor forebrain development such as microcephaly. They slope downwards in disorders associated with maxillary hypoplasia such as the *Rubinstein–Taybi* and *Treacher–Collins* syndromes. The palpebral fissures are short in the horizontal axis in the fetal alcohol syndrome and long in the *Kabuki make up syndrome.* They are short in both the horizontal and vertical axes (*blepharophimosis*) in the *Marden–Walker* and *BPES (Blepharophimosis, Ptosis, Epicanthus inversus, Syndrome) syndromes.* Drooping of the eye-lids (*ptosis*) occurs in the *Noonan* and *Smith–Lemli–Opitz syndromes.* Notches (*colobomata*) in the eye-lids are seen in the *Treacher–Collins syndrome.* Fusion of the eye-brows in the midline (*synophrys*) is a feature of the *Cornelia-de-Lange syndrome.*

The eyes

It is important to try to determine whether these are abnormally large or small. This can only be achieved accurately using ultrasound but an estimate can be made by determining whether the horizontal corneal diameter is greater than 13 mm or smaller than 10 mm. *Megalocornea* shows a rare association with mental retardation. *Microcornea* and *microphthalmia* are seen in many disorders such as the CHARGE association (**C**oloboma, **H**eart defect, **A**tresia choanae, **R**etarded growth and development, **G**enital anomalies, **E**ar anomalies), congenital rubella infection and trisomy 13.

Corneal opacification occurs in storage disorders, such as *Hurler syndrome,* and in primary ocular malformations such as *Peters anomaly* and *Rieger syndrome.* Blue sclerae are normal in infancy and persist thereafter in connective tissue disorders such as osteogenesis imperfecta. Scleral telangiectasia should prompt consideration of ataxia telangiectasia. Small benign scleral tumours, known as epibulbar dermoids, are found in *Goldenhar syndrome.*

The iris can provide useful diagnostic information. Small de-pigmented dots lying in an arc around the outer margin are known as Brushfield spots and are a feature of *Down syndrome.* Small pigmented heaped up patches, known as Lisch nodules, suggest *neurofibromatosis type 1.* Segments of different colour (*heterochromia*) are a feature of *Waardenburg syndrome.* A star-like pattern ('*stellate iris*') around the pupil in a blue iris is seen in *Williams syndrome.* An iris coloboma should prompt consideration of the aforementioned CHARGE association and also occurs in chromosomal abnormalities such as

Wolf–Hirschhorn syndrome (4p-), triploidy and *trisomy 13*. Absence of the iris (*aniridia*) is an important diagnostic feature of the *WAGR* (*Wilms tumour, Aniridia, Genitourinary abnormalities, Retardation*) *syndrome* and is an indication for detailed chromosome 11 analysis.

Lens opacities can be suspected by failure to elicit a normal pink reflex with the ophthalmoscope. Cataracts are found in many syndromes. Subluxation or complete dislocation of the lens occurs in homocystinuria, *Marfan syndrome*, the *Weill–Marchesani syndrome* and sulphite oxidase deficiency. Retinal examination in young children is not easy! A pigmentary retinopathy is seen in older children in the many isolated forms of retinitis pigmentosa as well as in a large number of multisystem disorders.

Syndromal causes of cataracts	Syndromal causes of a retinopathy
Chondrodysplasia punctata	Abetalipoproteinaemia
Cockayne syndrome	Cohen syndrome
Congenital rubella	Cockayne syndrome
Lowe syndrome	Hurler/Hunter syndrome
Marinesco–Sjögren syndrome	Laurence–Moon–Biedl syndrome
Pseudohypoparathyroidism	Usher syndrome

The ears

Anomalous auricle– Goldenhar syndrome

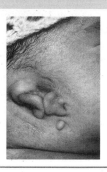

Ears are low set if an imaginary line drawn through the inner and outer canthi passes above the attachment of the uppermost part of the pinna. Low-set ears often show posterior rotation in the vertical axis as the embryonic development of the ear involves a 90 degree rotation from the horizontal to the vertical plane. Although often recorded, low-set ears are a rather non-specific finding of limited diagnostic value.

Malformed auricles are much more suggestive of a particular syndrome diagnosis. Preauricular tags, also known as accessory auricles, occur along the line of fusion between the maxillary and mandibular embryonic processes. Creases in the ear-lobe are a useful diagnostic sign in *Beckwith–Wiedemann syndrome*.

Syndromes associated with malformed auricles
Beal syndrome (crumpled)
CHARGE association
Diastrophic dysplasia (cysts)
Goldenhar syndrome
Saethre–Chotzen syndrome (prominent crus)
Townes–Brocks syndrome
Treacher–Collins syndrome

The nose

A depressed or flat nasal bridge (*glabella*) is a feature of many skeletal dysplasias and storage disorders. Nasal hypoplasia also occurs in babies whose mothers were treated with warfarin in pregnancy. If this is severe the nasal airways can be compromised. A small nose is characteristic of many disorders, including *Cornelia-de-Lange* and *Down syndrome*. If the nasal bones are short the nares are described as being 'anteverted': this is a feature of the *Smith–Lemli–Opitz syndrome*.

A large or prominent nose is found in the *Rubinstein–Taybi, Seckel* and *tricho-rhino-phalangeal syndromes*. In the *Rubinstein–Taybi syndrome* a lateral view shows that the central nasal pillar (*columella*) extends below the adjacent alae nasi and the nose has a beaked configuration. In *Seckel syndrome* prominence of the nose contrasts with microcephaly and an otherwise small face. In the *tricho-rhino-phalangeal syndrome* the nasal tip is bulbous. Notching of the alae-nasi occurs in the *DiGeorge / Shprintzen syndrome*. Absence of the nose occurs as a consequence of premaxillary agenesis in holoprosencephaly. The nose is bifid in frontonasal dysplasia: this may involve only the nasal tip or in severe cases there may be almost a complete cleavage between the two nostrils.

The lips

Prominence or fullness of the lips is seen in many of the storage disorders as a manifestation of progressive facial coarsening. It is also a major component of the characteristic *Williams syndrome* facies. A smooth philtrum is consistent with intra-uterine teratogenesis, most notably due to prolonged exposure to alcohol. This also causes the vermillion border to be thin as seen in the *Cornelia-de-Lange syndrome*. Cleft lip and / or cleft palate occur in a very large number of syndromes. When assessing a child with facial clefting it is important to look for pits in the lower lip: these are found in the popliteal web and *Van der Woude syndromes*, both of which show autosomal dominant inheritance in contrast to non-syndromal cleft lip / palate which is multifactorial.

The mouth and tongue

Lobules on the tongue: oral-facial-digital syndrome

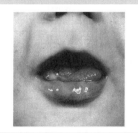

The mouth is small (*microstomia*) in trisomy 18 and the *Treacher–Collins syndrome* and big (*macrostomia*) in the *Beckwith–Wiedemann syndrome*. Asymmetry with unilateral macrostomia occurs in *Goldenhar syndrome* due to failure of normal fusion between the developing maxillary and mandibular processes. In *Beckwith–Wiedemann syndrome* the tongue is also large (*macroglossia*). Macroglossia also occurs in the later stages of the storage disorders. *Microglossia* occurs in association with a small jaw (*micrognathia*) and posterior U shaped cleft palate in the *Pierre–Robin sequence*, in which the primary abnormality is thought to be mandibular hypoplasia. This sequence is a common presentation in *Stickler syndrome*. Micro- or hypoglossia is a cardinal feature of the hypoglossia-hypodactyly syndrome in which the underlying cause is probably hypoperfusion of distal regions such as the tongue and the limbs. Controversy surrounds the recent suggestion that this combination may result from fetal vascular disturbance caused by chorionic villus sampling performed before 10 weeks' gestation. Lobulation of the tongue is seen in association with multiple oral frenulae in the *oral-facial-digital (OFD) group of syndromes*.

Causes of cleft lip/palate

DiGeorge–Shprintzen syndrome (submucous)
EEC syndrome
Meckel syndrome
Oral-facial-digital syndromes
Popliteal web syndrome (+ lip pits)
Roberts syndrome
Trisomy 13
Van der Woude syndrome (+ lip pits)
Wolf–Hirschhorn (4p-) syndrome

The neck

Webbing of the neck is usually associated with a low posterior hairline. This combination is seen in *Noonan syndrome, Turner syndrome* and the *Klippel–Feil sequence* in which the underlying abnormality is fusion of the cervical vertebrae. The neck webbing in *Turner syndrome* is a residue of the delay in maturation of the lymphatic drainage system which often results in severe hydrops fetalis and early pregnancy loss. Branchial fistulae and clefts are seen in the *branchio-oto-renal (BOR) syndrome* in association with hearing loss, preauricular pits and renal dysplasia. This disorder probably accounts for the longstanding maxim that external ear and renal abnormalities are often associated.

Chest

Hypoplasia of pectoralis major and syndactyly: Poland syndrome

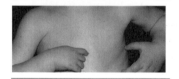

A small thoracic cage is a feature of many potentially very serious forms of skeletal dysplasia such as *Jeune thoracic dystrophy* and *spondylocostal dysostosis*. Unilateral absence or hypoplasia of the pectoral muscles occurs in the *Poland sequence* in association with ipsilateral hand hypoplasia and syndactyly. Depression of the lower part of the sternum (*pectus excavatum*) occurs in *homocystinuria* and *Marfan syndrome*. Protrusion of the sternum (*pectus carinatum*) often occurs with a kyphosis in skeletal/storage disorders such as *Morquio syndrome*. A shield shaped chest with increase in the inter-nipple distance is a feature of *Turner syndrome*.

Supernumerary, also known as accessory, nipples lie on the embryonic milk line and are relatively common and non-specific. They can usually be distinguished from other lesions by their pigmentation and by their location in a short horizontal skin crease.

The abdomen

An umbilical hernia and supraumbilical divarication of the rectus muscles (diastasis recti) are common in young children and of little diagnostic value or significance. An exomphalos, also known as an omphalocoele, can occur in isolation but is associated with an underlying syndrome diagnosis such as *Beckwith–Wiedemann syndrome* or *trisomy 18* in approximately 50% of all cases diagnosed in utero. Hepatosplenomegaly is a feature of many of the progressive storage disorders and is an unexplained finding in about 25% of children with *Noonan syndrome*.

The genitalia

Genital abnormalities occur in many dysmorphic syndromes. Hypospadias shows a high incidence in the *Opitz, Smith–Lemli–Opitz* and *WAGR syndromes* as well as in many chromosome abnormalities. Underdevelopment of the genitalia consisting of micropenis and/or bilateral cryptorchidism is also seen in many disorders.

Causes of hypogenitalism

CHARGE association
Meckel syndrome
Noonan syndrome
Prader–Willi syndrome
Robinow syndrome
Septo-optic dysplasia
Smith–Lemli–Opitz syndrome, types 1 and 2
Triploidy
Trisomy 13

Complete sex reversal with a male karyotype and a female phenotype should prompt consideration of campomelic dysplasia, the *Denys–Drash syndrome* and the severe neonatal type 2 form of *Smith–Lemli–Opitz syndrome*. A 'shawl shaped' scrotum with a fold of the scrotum extending over the shaft of the penis is a key feature of *Aarskog syndrome* in which the other common findings are hypertelorism and brachydactyly. Examination of the genitalia in girls is neither easy nor appropriate as part of a dysmorphology assessment. Presentation with a hydrometrocolpos should raise consideration of the *McKusick–Kaufman syndrome* in which the other features are polydactyly and cyanotic congenital heart disease.

The limbs

Radial aplasia: Fanconi anaemia

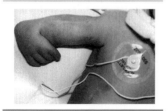

Limb shortening can involve the proximal (*rhizomelic*), intermediate (*mesomelic*) or distal (*acromelic*) segments. Significant symmetrical limb shortening is suggestive of an underlying generalised skeletal dysplasia. Specific limb abnormalities occur in many syndromes. For example radial aplasia shows a frequent association with haematological and/or cardiac abnormalities. A Madelung deformity, in which

---

Causes of radial aplasia/hypoplasia

With haematological abnormalities:
    Aase syndrome
    Fanconi anaemia
    Thrombocytopenia absent radius (TAR)

With cardiac abnormalities:
    Aase syndrome
    Holt–Oram syndrome
    Trisomy 18
    VATER association

---

the wrist shows a dinner-fork appearance due to subluxation of the ulna, is seen in the *Leri–Weill dyschondrosteosis syndrome* and in *Turner syndrome*. Hypoplasia of the patella occurs in the nail-patella syndrome, the popliteal web syndrome and trisomy 8 mosaicism.

The hands and feet

Examination of the hands provides a useful starting point in a dysmorphological assessment, as even the most timid or recalcitrant child can usually be persuaded to allow his or her hands to be visualised. Abnormalities of the fingers and toes are numerous.

Digital abnormalities

Arachnodactyly	long and thin
Brachydactyly	short
Camptodactyly	flexed
Clinodactyly	curved
Macrodactyly	enlarged
Polydactyly	extra digit(s)
Syndactyly	fused

Arachnodactyly is seen in *Marfan syndrome* and in other disorders with a Marfanoid habitus.

Brachydactyly is a feature of *Aarskog syndrome, achondroplasia* and a large group of isolated brachydactyly syndromes subdivided into types A to E on the basis of which digits are involved. Shortening of the fourth and fifth metacarpals with absence of the knuckles on making a fist occurs in pseudohypoparathyroidism and Turner syndrome.

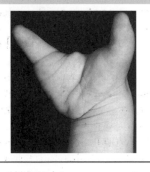

Ectrodactyly: EEC syndrome

Camptodactyly is often associated with large joint contractures in various forms of arthrogryposis. It is also a feature of *Beals syndrome* and *trisomy 8 mosaicism*.

Ectrodactyly, also known as a lobster claw deformity, can occur in isolation or as one of the three cardinal components of the *EEC* (*Ectodermal dysplasia, Ectrodactyly, Cleft lip/palate*) *syndrome*. *Clinodactyly* usually involves only the fifth fingers and is a rather nonspecific finding although it is particularly common in *Down syndrome* and the *Silver–Russell syndrome*.

Macrodactyly is very suggestive of the *Proteus syndrome*.

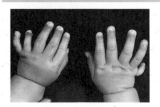

Bilateral post-axial polydactyly

Polydactyly is described as *pre-axial* if it arises from the radial or tibial aspect and *post-axial* if it arises from the ulnar or fibular aspect. It can take the form of a fully developed extra digit or consists simply of a tiny postminimus connected to the hand or little finger by a thin stalk containing its vascular supply. Isolated non-syndromal post-axial polydactyly is a common autosomal dominant trait in Afro-Caribbeans. Polydactyly occurs in association with other abnormalities in a large number of syndromes.

Syndactyly can be *cutaneous* if only skin is involved or *osseous* if the phalanges are fused. Mild cutaneous syndactyly between the second and third toes is a common harmless trait. More severe degrees of

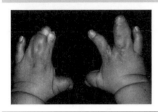

Partially repaired syndactyly: Apert syndrome

Causes of polydactyly	Causes of syndactyly
Carpenter syndrome	Amniotic bands (pseudosyndactyly)
Ellis–van Creveld syndrome	Apert syndrome ('mitten hand')
Jeune thoracic dystrophy	Greig syndrome
Laurence–Moon–Biedel syndrome	Oral-facial-digital syndromes
McKusick–Kaufman syndrome	Poland sequence
Meckel syndrome	Saethre–Chotzen syndrome
Oral-facial-digital syndromes	Smith–Leml–Opitz syndrome, types 1 and 2
Pallister-Hall syndrome (insertional)	Triploidy
Trisomy 13	

syndactyly are seen in many syndromes. A combination of polydactyly and syndactyly is referred to as *polysyndactyly*.

Ectodermal structures

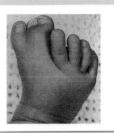

Pre-axial polysyndactyly

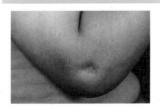

Skin dimpling over elbow: mild arthrogryposis

These consist of the skin, hair, nails and teeth. Because of their shared embryological origin all of these structures are involved in the group of disorders known as the ectodermal dysplasias.

Skin. By virtue of its easy accessibility examination of the skin will often provide valuable diagnostic clues. Traditionally the study of dermatoglyphics has been an important component in the assessment of children with a possible chromosome abnormality, but this has now largely been superseded by direct laboratory chromosome analysis. A single palmar (*simian*) crease occurs unilaterally in about 4% of all babies and in up to 50% of children with *Down syndrome*. Generally this is not a particularly helpful diagnostic feature, although it does provide some indication of early embryonic welfare as the pattern of palmar creases is a reflection of growth and movement up to 12 weeks' gestation. Absence of flexion creases on the palms and fingers is a manifestation of disorders which cause fetal akinesia and is seen in the *Pena–Shokeir phenotype*.

Punched out discrete scalp defects occur in the *Johanson Blizzard syndrome, trisomy 13* and the *Adams–Oliver syndrome*, in which the presence of distal limb defects suggests an underlying vascular aetiology. Abnormal skin pigmentation is seen in many disorders. Areas of depigmentation are often best detected using a Wood's lamp. A mosaic pattern of skin involvement following the embryonic Blaschko's lines occurs in *hypomelanosis of Ito*, which is often due to chromosome mosaicism such as diploidy/triploidy, and in females with X-linked dominant disorders such as *chondrodysplasia punctata* and *incontinentia pigmenti*.

Hair. A generalised increase in body hair (*hirsutism*) is a feature of the *Cornelia-de-Lange syndrome* and appears progressively in many of the storage disorders, most notably the mucopolysaccharidoses. In contrast sparse hair occurs in many forms of ectodermal dysplasia, including the EEC syndrome and the relatively common sex-linked recessive hypohidrotic form. The hair is 'kinky' in *Menke disease* and often 'woolly' in *Noonan syndrome*. A white forelock is characteristic of *Waardenburg syndrome*.

> **Causes of abnormal skin pigmentation**
>
> Increased (including cafe-au-lait patches):
>   Bloom syndrome
>   Fanconi anaemia
>   Incontinentia pigmenti (whorled)
>   LEOPARD syndrome (lentigines)
>   McCune–Albright syndrome
>   Neurofibromatosis 1 and 2
>   Peutz–Jeghers syndrome (mucocutaneous)
>
> Decreased:
>   Hypomelanosis of Ito
>   Oculo-cutaneous albinism
>   Piebaldism
>   Tuberose sclerosis
>   Waardenburg syndrome

Digital and nail hypoplasia: phenytoin teratogenicity

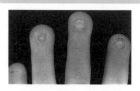

Nails. The nails are dysplastic or hypoplastic or both in many forms of ectodermal dysplasia and in many other disorders such as *dyskeratosis congenita*, the *Ellis–van Creveld syndrome* and the *nail-patella syndrome*. Nail hypoplasia can also be caused by teratogens such as phenytoin. Longitudinal nail splitting occurs in craniofrontonasal dysplasia, a rare disorder affecting only females who have craniosynostosis and the facial features of frontonasal dysplasia.

Abnormal dentition in male: X-linked hypohidrotic dysplasia

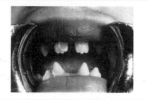

Teeth. Dental anomalies occur in many syndromes, so that although oral inspection of a young or disabled child can be very difficult a good view of the teeth can be very rewarding. Neonatal teeth are often present in the *Ellis–van Creveld syndrome* and early dental eruption occurs in association with advanced bone age in the overgrowth syndromes. Reduction in the correct number of teeth (*hypodontia*) is seen in cleidocranial dysostosis and in many forms of ectodermal dysplasia in which the incisors may be conical or pointed. Dentine hypoplasia is a diagnostic feature of some forms of osteogenesis imperfecta in which the teeth are translucent with a yellow or brown discoloration. Enamel hypoplasia is seen in pseudohypo-parathyroidism and in *Goltz syndrome*.

INVESTIGATIONS

Standard chromosome analysis. This should be undertaken in every child who presents with abnormalities of physical or mental development. Most cytogenetic laboratories require 2–5 ml of venous blood collected into lithium heparin. A minimum of 3 days is needed to obtain a result, although in a clinical emergency, such as a neonate presenting with ambiguous genitalia or a life-threatening malformation, an earlier result can sometimes be obtained. In practice most laboratories have a substantial backlog so be prepared to wait several weeks for a routine karyotype result.

Specialised chromosome analysis Several special techniques can be used to diagnose particular syndromes. It is always sensible to discuss this with the local laboratory before collecting a blood sample from the child.

Fragile X syndrome. Detection of the X chromosome fragile site associated with this disorder is facilitated by culturing the circulating lymphocytes in a folate depleted medium. Increasingly this diagnostic approach is being replaced by direct DNA mutation analysis.

Chromosomal breakage syndromes. In disorders such as *ataxia telangiectasia, Bloom syndrome, Fanconi anaemia* and *xerodermu pigmentosa,* an increase in the normal rate of in vitro chromosome breakage can be demonstrated using clastogenic agents such as mitomycin C, radiation or UV light.

Microdeletion syndromes. Recent research has shown that several well established dysmorphic syndromes are caused by tiny chromosome deletions which are often so small that they cannot be visualised using a light microscope.

Microdeletion syndromes

Syndrome	Chromosome
Williams	7q11
Langer–Giedion	8q24
WAGR	11p13
Angelman	15q11 (maternally derived)
Prader–Willi	15q11 (paternally derived)
Miller–Dieker (lissencephaly)	17p13
Smith–Magenis	17p11
Alagille	20p12
DiGeorge/Shprintzen	22q11

These 'sub-microscopic' contiguous gene deletion syndromes can now be diagnosed by applying a DNA probe from the deletion region to a chromosome spread and then observing whether it has annealed to only one or to both of the relevant chromosomes. The technique most commonly used for this type of analysis is known as 'fluorescent in-situ hybridisation' (FISH).

Syndromes in which the genetic defect has been identified

Syndrome	Gene	Locus
Achondroplasia	FGFR3	4p
Apert	FGFR2	10q
ATR-X	XH2	Xq
Campomelic dysplasia	SOX9	17q
Chondrodysplasia punctata	ARSE	Xp
Crouzon	FGFR2	10q
Fragile X	FMR1	Xq
Greig	GLI3	7p
MEN 2B	RET	10q
Pfeiffer	FGFR1/2	8p/10q
Thanatophoric dysplasia	FGFR3	4p
Waardenburg 1	PAX3	2q
Waardenburg 2	M1TF	3p
Treacher–Collins	Treacle	5q

Molecular genetic analysis. The number of dysmorphic syndromes in which the basic genetic defect has been identified is increasing rapidly.

In practice the only disorders for which this is widely available are the *fragile X syndrome* and *congenital myotonic dystrophy* which result from expansion of a triplet repeat. In addition, many laboratories can now confirm a clinical or cytogenetic diagnosis of the *Angelman* or *Prader–Willi syndromes* by demonstrating that the two number 15 chromosomes show an abnormal pattern of DNA methylation due to either a deletion, uniparental disomy or, rarely, an inherited imprinting methylation mutation.

Other laboratory tests. Specific haematological or biochemical abnormalities have been identified in a small number of genetic dysmorphic syndromes. For example, Hb H inclusions are present in red blood cells in males, and in some carrier females, with the *X-linked α-thalassaemia/mental retardation (ATR-X) syndrome.* Approximately 20% of children with *Noonan syndrome* have abnormal clotting function tests. Thrombocytopenia is a feature of both *Fanconi anaemia* and the *thrombocytopenia-absent radius (TAR) syndrome.* In the *Smith–Lemli-Opitz syndrome* a defect in cholesterol synthesis leads to low levels of cholesterol and very high levels of the cholesterol precursor 7-dehydrocholesterol.

Radiology. On the principle that X-rays should be used only sparingly, a full skeletal survey is not recommended in all children who present with dysmorphic features. However in some situations localised X-rays can provide useful confirmatory support for a diagnosis. For example, bone age is advanced in the overgrowth disorders such as *Sotos* and *Weaver* syndrome, whereas it is delayed in the *Silver–Russell syndrome* and in many skeletal dysplasias. Cone shaped epiphyses are found in the *Langer–Giedion* and *tricho-rhino-phalangeal syndromes.* Wormian bones are a feature of *cleidocranial dysostosis* and *osteogenesis imperfecta.* Dental cysts are present in *Gardner syndrome* and in *Gorlin syndrome* in which bifurcation of the ribs is another useful diagnostic sign.

MAKING A DIAGNOSIS

By this point it should be clear that the assessment of a child with dysmorphic features is a complex and painstaking process. Sometimes it is relatively easy to arrive at a confident diagnosis. The facial gestalt may be familiar, or a careful examination and appropriate investigations may reveal features which point strongly to one of the more easily recognised dysmorphic syndromes. Several of these have been mentioned briefly in the preceding clinical section. It is important to emphasise that these constitute only a very small proportion of the more than 3000 syndromes and chromosome abnormalities which have been described. Consequently it is often necessary to utilise other avenues to try to arrive at a diagnosis.

The study of dysmorphology has generated a burgeoning literature with several medical journals devoted largely or exclusively to the description and delineation of dysmorphic syndromes. Several excellent text-books can be consulted, a selection of which are listed at the end of this chapter.

Computerised data sources such as the London Dysmorphology Database provide extremely valuable diagnostic assistance. Using these it is possible to search for a diagnosis by entering a limited number of abnormal clinical features. A list of differential diagnoses is provided which can be scanned in more detail to see if any is likely to be correct. The use of 'hard' diagnostic handles, such as iris coloboma or post-axial polydactyly, is preferable to 'soft' relatively non-specific signs such as low-set ears and fifth finger clinodactyly. An indication of the extent of the existing knowledge base is provided by the London Dysmorphology Database listing of 88 syndromes featuring iris coloboma and 115 with post-axial polydactyly.

A philosophical post-script   It is rarely easy to make a confident diagnosis in a dysmorphic child so do not be discouraged. Instead be prepared to reassess the child at regular intervals and accept that even after detailed investigations and lengthy literature review a diagnosis may still not be forthcoming. Try to resist the temptation to force a diagnosis. Many parents will wish to join a support group and it will soon become obvious both to the parents and to everyone else if the proposed diagnosis is incorrect.

This is one of the most sensitive and potentially emotionally painful situations in which parents can find themselves. A much loved child becomes the unwanted focus of medical interest and attention. On occasions doctors and other professionals can quite inadvertently make comments which are perceived as deeply hurtful by the parents. Some may not be ready to accept that their child is unusual or abnormal, and even the most understanding and perceptive parents may find it very difficult to come to terms with a syndrome diagnosis. Do not be afraid to admit defeat. Parents recognise and respect the truth and some are quietly pleased that their child has bamboozled the medical experts. Unfortunately in the field of dysmorphology this is not very difficult!

FURTHER READING

Aase JM 1990 Diagnostic dysmorphology. Plenum, New York
Donnai D, Winter RM 1995 Congenital malformation syndromes. Chapman and Hall, London
Gorlin RJ, Cohen MM, Levin LS 1990 Syndromes of the head and neck. Oxford University Press, New York
Hall JG, Froster-Iskenius UG, Allanson JE 1989 Handbook of normal physical measurements. Oxford University Press, Oxford
Graham JM 1988 Smith's recognisable patterns of human deformation, 2nd edn. Saunders, Philadelphia
Jones KL 1988 Smith's recognisable patterns of human malformation, 4th edn. Saunders, Philadelphia
Schinzel A 1994 Human cytogenetics database. Oxford University Press Electronics Division, Oxford
Winter RM, Baraitser M 1995 London dysmorphology database. Oxford University Press Electronics Division, Oxford

7 Intensive care of the newborn

RESPIRATORY DISTRESS
CYANOSIS
CHRONIC LUNG DISEASE
APNOEA
BLEEDING
OEDEMA
JITTERS, TWITCHES AND FITS
FLOPPY BABIES
VOMITING

If it is at all possible neonatal care should be practised by the mother's bedside, either in the postnatal ward, or in areas designated for transitional care. When this is neither safe, nor appropriate by virtue of staff resources or maternal well being, the baby will need to be transferred to a specialist unit. The criteria for admission to a special or intensive care unit will vary from hospital to hospital but needs to be defined. Transfer of the sick newborn infant to another hospital is a major task which requires that the transfer team should be able to maintain, on the journey, the support that is provided in the intensive care unit. Whenever possible the need for intensive care should be anticipated and the mother transferred to an appropriate unit prior to birth.

In recent years techniques have been developed so that we can sustain the life of extremely immature babies, 22–24 weeks' gestation. Experience is needed to know when it is inappropriate to begin intensive care in a very immature baby, and also when to withdraw intensive care from a baby whose long term future is severely and irreversibly compromised.

The care of the family must accompany the 'high-tech' clinical care of the sick infant. The neonatal unit must be friendly and welcoming. Parents should be able to be close to their baby and get to know members of the team providing the care. Parent support meetings help. Staff must find time to talk with parents and learn about their concerns. Regular staff meetings at which problems and potential problems can be discussed are useful. It is often the unsupported and underprivileged family with least internal reserves whose baby, by virtue of prematurity, birth asphyxia or congenital abnormality, needs intensive neonatal care. The time of birth is an opportunity to try and break the cycle of disadvantage.

The staff must also become expert in the management of the dying baby, approximately 5% of the babies admitted to a referral unit will not survive, usually as result of extreme prematurity or overwhelming congenital problems.

Maturity. One of the commonest reasons for admitting an infant to the unit is a low birth weight. This may be due to prematurity or to intrauterine growth retardation resulting in a 'small-for-dates' baby — birth weight below 10th centile for gestational age. The problems likely to arise in these two groups of babies are often very different, and it is important to distinguish them in order to plan effective care. Allowance should be made for factors such as racial group and parental size. A baby who has a genetic predisposition to be large may be growth retarded and yet have a weight considerably above the 10th centile for gestational age. Asymmetrical growth retardation, that is a small body but normal head size, suggests recent onset of growth failure and if the head is also small, that the problem has been longstanding.

Thermal environment. Exposure to an inappropriately cool environment increases neonatal morbidity and mortality. Although the newborn baby can respond to cold exposure by producing extra heat in brown adipose tissue, this will only occur if the child is not hypoxic as oxygen is required for the metabolic process. Thus the baby with severe respiratory problems is at increased risk from cold exposure. Glucose is also required. Hypoglycaemia is a dangerous complication of hypothermia. The optimum ambient temperature, the thermoneutral environment, depends on maturity, postnatal age and body weight. Body heat is best conserved by nursing the baby clothed in a cot with sides which protect the baby from draughts. Under these conditions the babies can be nursed in cooler environments more tolerable for adults and there is less need for precision in the control of the room temperature.

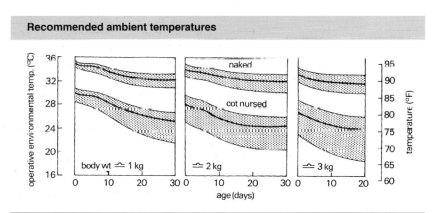

Recommended ambient temperatures

Incubator care. The small baby, weighing less than 1200 g, and larger babies with problems requiring frequent observation and medical attention are most conveniently nursed in incubators. They may be naked or partly clothed. The incubators are set to provide environmental temperatures appropriate to the baby's size and postnatal age. The figures available are based on information from healthy babies studied in metabolic chambers. They tend to underestimate the temperatures required for very preterm babies in the first few days of life and those whose metabolic responses are damaged by asphyxia or illness.

The preterm baby has high radiant as well as convective loss when nursed in a standard incubator. There are now a new generation of double-walled incubators on the market which appear to be effective in reducing radiant heat loss.

Transepidermal water loss. Very preterm babies, less than 30 weeks' gestation, have a phenomenal transcutaneous water loss (up to 120 ml/kg/day) which has a dramatic cooling effect on the baby. It is possible to overcome these losses by using environmental temperatures of 38°C or even higher. These temperatures cannot be achieved by most standard incubators, unless working in a servo-mode set to maintain the baby's skin temperature at 36.5–37°C. Servomode probes have their own hazards and are not easy to apply to very small infants. However lying on the probe or partial detachment of the probe does not produce the worrying over-heating effect that such an event would in an older or more mature infant.

Evaporative water loss can most easily be reduced by raising the relative humidity. In the past, this form of therapy has been unpopular due to worries about contamination and overgrowth with hydrophilic organisms, including *Ps. aerogenes*. The risks of infection can be greatly reduced if the incubator reservoir is drained each day and left dry for 1–2 hours before refilling with sterile water. Use of high humidity (75%+) is indicated for the first 7 days for all babies born weighing less than 1200 g. If temperature control remains a problem radiant and evaporative heat loss can be reduced by partially clothing the baby, particularly the head, covering the baby with insulating material or inserting a heat shield.

Radiant heaters provide an attractive alternative to incubators allowing free access to the baby. Unfortunately these devices exacerbate transcutaneous water loss and fluid requirements will need to be increased by 10–30%. In addition, very immature babies will require covering with insulation material to reduce evaporative water loss. Radiant heaters maintain body temperature by providing a positive radiant heat source rather than by warming the air temperature; the incubator settings do not apply. If radiant heaters are to be used for more than a few minutes the heater output must be servo-controlled from the baby's skin temperature. A potential over-heating hazard is likely to arise if the probe becomes detached and is subsequently shielded from the radiant heat. In this situation the heater will produce full output and this may be missed if the baby is not receiving continuous nursing attention. Ideally, an alarm system should be incorporated to give warning of probe detachment.

Hypothermia. Babies admitted to the neonatal unit with hypothermia, that is a core temperature of less than 35°C, are most easily warmed by placing in an incubator and selecting an environmental temperature 1°C above skin temperature. This temperature can be increased at hourly intervals until the core temperature reaches 37°C. It is essential to monitor blood sugar at 4-hourly intervals during the period of warming and in the subsequent 24 hours to detect hypoglycaemia before it becomes symptomatic.

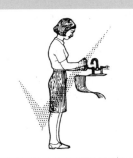

Washup hands!

Infection protection. It is crucial to protect the baby from infection as far as it is possible. Although the newborn baby derives IgG transplacentally, resistance to *Staphylococcus aureus*, the alpha and beta haemolytic streptococcus and gram-negative bacilli is low, and death can result within hours of the onset of septicaemia. There is no evidence that wearing gowns, overshoes or face mask have anything to offer. It is far more important to ensure that hands and forearms are washed prior to handling any baby. Adequate space between incubators and cots also provides a considerable degree of protection.

Nutrition. Much research has gone into the nutritional requirements of newborns. For preterm as well as full term babies, breast milk is the best and most easily tolerated food. Sometimes preterm infants need extra calories to ensure adequate growth. One approach is to use breast milk fortifiers which add calories while keeping the osmolarity of the feed to less than 240 mmol/l. However not all mothers are able or willing to express breast milk in sufficient quantities. In the past breast milk banks were established to store and supply human milk. However, boiling or pasteurising, freezing and thawing alters the characteristics of breast milk and eliminates many of the potential advantages that breast milk has over modified cows' milk feeds.

Recommended volumes of feeds for sick full-term and preterm infants

Expressed breast milk or modified cow's milk (ml/kg body weight each day)

Sick full-term infants		Premature and small-for-dates infants	
1st 24 hours	40	60	
2nd 24 hours	60	90	
3rd 24 hours	80	120	
4th 24 hours	110	150	
5th 24 hours	150	180	(if tolerated)
via 5 FG tube 4 hourly		Via nasogastric tube	
First feed 6 hours after birth		In dysmature first feed at 1 hour after birth	

Special milk formulae have been developed which are suitable for very low birth weight babies. These formula enable most preterm infants to achieve good rates of growth and development. Recent evidence suggests that the longer chain polyunsaturated fatty acids in human milk may assist membrane development, and they are now being added to the preterm formula.

Nasogastric feeding. Most full-term, small-for-dates and preterm babies born after 34 weeks' gestation can take feeds from the breast or a bottle within hours of birth provided there are no other major problems. If the babies are unable to suck, a 4–5FG nasogastric tube is preferable to an orogastric tube, as this can be left in situ for 24 hours and will disturb the baby less than frequent passage of orogastric tubes. When continuous feeding is indicated, a syringe or roller pump should be used as unassisted gravity feed systems are too inaccurate at low flow rates. The majority of preterm babies, even the most immature, are able to tolerate nasogastric feeds. In some, intake is limited by delay in gastric emptying which leads to regurgitation and possible aspiration.

If the abdomen is not distended secondary to functional ileus, nasojejunal feeding can sometimes avoid the need for total parenteral nutrition. Continuous feeding can then be maintained. This method of feeding may lead to small bowel distension and has been incriminated as a factor in the aetiology of necrotising enterocolitis. A further problem is the tendency for the tube to be displaced back into the stomach.

Positioning a nasojejunal tube

Right lateral position

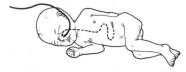
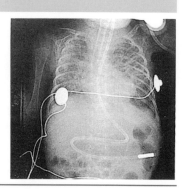

1. Pass tube into stomach (18 cm term, 12 cm preterm)
2. Advance 1 cm each hour
3. Aspirate until alkaline—then X-ray
4. Commence feed, 1 ml/hr

Parenteral fluids. In some circumstances the oral route is contraindicated; these include severe respiratory distress, intestinal obstruction or ileus, overwhelming septicaemia and shock. Babies born with severe growth retardation, particularly those with birth weights below 1000 g, are at increased risk of necrotising enterocolitis and should not receive oral feeds for the first 14 days. In all these situations intravenous fluids should be given through a peripheral vein.

Parenteral fluids

	Day					
	1	2	3	4	5	6
Dextrose 10%	10	10	10	10	10	10
Amino acid	10	15	20	25	30	30
Fat emulsion 20%	0	5	10	15	15	15
Electrolyte solution	5	5	5	5	5	5
Kilocalories (150 ml/kg)	60	68	76	84	86	88
Kilocalories (180 ml/kg)	72	80	88	96	98	101*

* Rises to 149 kcal if 20% dextrose solution given.
Electrolyte solution contains a minimum of Na 5 mmol, K 2 mmol, Ca 1 mmol, PO_4 7 mmol, Mg 0.6 mmol.

Parenteral nutrition. If the baby is extremely immature with a birth weight of less than 1200 g, parenteral nutrition should be considered. In larger babies, the decision to commence therapy can be delayed for 4–7 days until the baby's condition is satisfactory. If the baby runs into problems within the first 2–3 days of life parenteral nutrition should be commenced immediately. This form of therapy is also indicated in babies requiring extensive abdominal surgery in whom oral therapy cannot be started within 7–10 days of birth and those in whom oral feeding has to be abandoned for more than a few days for whatever reason.

Venous access. In large babies, parenteral nutrition can be maintained for several weeks using peripheral veins. In small preterm babies a central line should be set up earlier via the jugular, saphenous or brachial veins to minimise excessive handling. It is often possible to pass a fine silastic catheter into a cubital or jugular vein through a size 19 butterfly needle.The aim should be to place the tip of the catheter in the superior or inferior vena cava, close to the right atrium. Parenteral nutrition has to be introduced slowly. Computer programs are now available to calculate the constituents of the feeds which are then made up by the pharmacy department.

Complications of i.v. feeding. There is no doubt that fat emulsions may accumulate in many organs, including the liver, lungs and even the brain. Whether this leads to long term damage is not known. Current recommendations are that 3 g/kg should not be exceeded, and that in preterm babies with sepsis, this should be reduced to 2 g/kg. Amino acids may also cause liver damage, sometimes progressing to cirrhosis. The fat emulsion should be discontinued when phototherapy is

Iron and vitamin supplements

	Dose	Indication
Children's vitamin drops	0.15 ml (5 drops) once daily contains vitamin A 700 units vitamin C 21 mg vitamin D* 280 units	Given to all babies once feeding is established until 2 years of age
* Give additional vitamin D drops to babies on neonatal unit until discharge:	less than 1.5 kg: 1000 units/day more than 1.5 kg: 500 units/day	
Iron	2 mg/kg/day	Give to all babies with birth weight less than 2.5 kg or less than 36 weeks' gestation starting at 1 month and continuing until on a full soild intake
Folic acid	0.2 mg daily	Give to babies with haemolytic anaemias due to blood group incompatibilities until 8 weeks

required for hyperbilirubinaemia and amino acid withdrawn if there is evidence of obstructive jaundice with elevation of both conjugated and unconjugated bilirubin. Unfortunately it is not possible to give sufficient calories without using fat emulsion.

Vitamins. Babies born small-for-dates or preterm have limited vitamin reserves and are likely to take longer to reach a fully balanced weaned diet. They should be started on vitamin supplements once enteral feeding is established, and on an iron-containing preparation at 4 weeks of age. All babies should receive vitamin K shortly after birth to prevent haemorrhagic disease of the newborn.

RESPIRATORY DISTRESS

In the neonatal period the respiratory system responds to a wide variety of pathological processes with tachypnoea (respiratory rate 60 plus/min), recession of the chest wall and sternum, and expiratory grunting. As the child's condition deteriorates cyanosis develops, due to ventilation perfusion imbalance, right to left shunting at pulmonary, atrial and duct level, and alveolar hypoventilation. This picture can result from cardiac, neurological and metabolic causes, as well as conditions which are primarily respiratory.

Problem

- Preterm baby.
- Tachypnoea, recession with or without grunting apparent within 4 hours of birth and becoming progressively worse.
- Chest X-ray showing granular or opaque lung fields with blurring of the cardiac border and often an air bronchogram. Changes are usually symmetrical.

Diagnosis — Respiratory distress syndrome (RDS)

The diagnosis to a large extent depends on ruling out other respiratory and cardiac causes, for example transient tachypnoea, streptococcal pneumonia, pneumothorax and cardiac failure. The condition is rare in full-term babies, although it can be produced by hypothermia, maternal diabetes and familial absence of surfactant protein B. Interpartum asphyxia can produce a similar picture (Acquired or Adult RDS). In the absence of surfactant therapy, RDS tends to get worse over the first 48 hours of life. It is important to assess the baby's condition, recording colour, activity, heart rate, blood pressure and tissue perfusion, respiratory rate, respiratory effort and degree of sternal and chest wall recession. Crepitations can be present on auscultation but these should have disappeared within 24 hours of age. A baseline head circumference measurement and assessment of fontanelle tone are also useful.

Investigations

Daily haemoglobin estimations are required, as anaemia whether due to haemolysis, haemorrhage or sampling, adds to the infant's problems. If the haemoglobin falls below 12 g/dl during the acute phase of the disease, blood transfusion is indicated.

Blood gases. Although it is possible to provide appropriate respiratory support based on information from arterial stabs, these are difficult in very preterm babies and may be misleading as the additional handling involved often causes a transitory fall in the Pao_2 and thus misleading results. Blood sampling from an indwelling arterial catheter is far preferable. Blood glucose should be checked at the same time, as hypoglycaemia is likely to develop in the first 48 hours. Continuous reading oxygen electrodes are available, mounted on the tip of 4 and 5FG catheters. These need calibration in vivo and tend to drift, but provide very useful additional information.

Umbilical artery catheters. It is not usually possible to insert an umbilical artery catheter after the first 48 hours of life. The risk of arterial emboli is reduced if the tip of the catheter lies above the diaphragm. Also check that the catheter has 'gone down before it goes up', then you can be confident that it is in the artery and not the vein. Alternative sites are the radial, ulnar or posterior tibial arteries. All catheters need continuous perfusion with half normal saline containing 100 units of heparin per 500 ml at rates of 0.5–1 ml per hour to maintain patency. With catheters in position it is possible to measure blood gases as clinically indicated on samples of about 200 μmol.

Transcutaneous saturation monitors 'calculate' the percentage saturation by comparing the absorption of light at two frequencies representing haemoglobin and oxyhaemoglobin. They have internal calibration systems, a response time of less than 6 seconds and can be attached to the hand or foot of even the most immature infant. When in use the probe must be protected from light, as this often leads to malfunction. Although transcutaneous monitors have proved reliable and acceptably accurate (+/-2%), they are insensitive once a saturation of 93–94% has been exceeded due to the shape of the haemoglobin/oxygen association curve, so that babies may then be at

Position of umbilical artery catheter

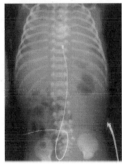

Umbilical artery catheters go down before they go up

Umbilical artery catheterisation

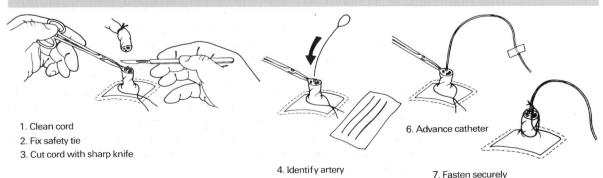

1. Clean cord
2. Fix safety tie
3. Cut cord with sharp knife

4. Identify artery
5. Dilate with dilators

6. Advance catheter

7. Fasten securely
8. X-ray to check tip is above diaphragm

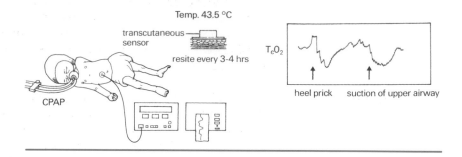

Transcutaneous oxygen monitors. The heated sensor leaves little burn marks

Temp. 43.5 °C

transcutaneous sensor

resite every 3-4 hrs

T_cO_2

CPAP

heel prick   suction of upper airway

risk of hyperoxia. They are extremely useful for detecting episodes of desaturation and should be run with alarm limits of 88% and 95%.

Transcutaneous oxygen and carbon dioxide monitors are also available. These heat the skin to 43/44°C in order to increase local blood flow and reasonably free diffusion of oxygen and carbon dioxide across the skin to the sensors. The carbon dioxide sensors provide reproducible results but tend to over-record by approximately 30%, probably due to CO_2 production by the skin. The oxygen devices often under-record as the skin matures and thickens, a problem limiting their use in babies with chronic lung disease and when perfusion is poor. They also produce grossly misleading results from time to time. For these reasons they should not be used as an alternative to blood gas sampling, but can be extremely useful as trend monitors, particularly in babies who are proving difficult to ventilate. The probes must be resited every 3–4 hours to prevent local burns.

Monitoring

It is essential to monitor the respiration of all babies with RDS using one of the systems currently available. As these babies tend to have periodic respiration, an apnoea alarm of 10–15 seconds is appropriate. Unfortunately none of the devices available will detect mixed or obstructive apnoea. However, respiratory efforts against a closed airway will often produce a striking bradycardia within seconds. For this and other reasons, the heart rate must also be monitored using a system with an ECG display and an alarm set to go off when the heart rate drops below 90/min. Unfortunately this will result in frequent false positive alarms. In practice, the most useful device for detecting significant apnoeic episodes is the oxygen saturation monitor.

Environmental oxygen must be monitored continuously whenever oxygen enrichment is prescribed. It will also be necessary for the nurse to record incubator setting temperature, air temperature, core temperature, the baby's heart rate, respiratory rate and the presence of grunting and recession, hourly initially; this can be reduced to 4 hourly as the baby's condition improves. Most babies who continue to deteriorate and require respiratory support will require regular blood pressure monitoring. Wherever possible this should be monitored continuously by connecting a perfused pressure transducer to the arterial indwelling line and ensuring that this is as close to the level of the atria as possible. Data on the minimal acceptable blood pressure are limited. Most units aim to keep the mean arterial pressure above the value provided by the gestational age expressed as mmHg. If it is not possible to carry out continuous intra-arterial blood pressure monitoring, useful information can often be obtained using an automated oscillometer device or, if necessary, obtain intermittent measurements with a limb cuff and Doppler device.

Oxygen therapy

Up to 30% can be given by feeding oxygen directly into the incubator. If more than that is required a head box is essential. As a general rule, arterial blood gases should be measured every 4 hours during the acute phase of the illness or within 40 minutes of a change in the level of respiratory support. Continuous intra-arterial oxygen catheters and transcutaneous devices are useful supplementary systems but are unfortunately no substitute for regular blood gas sampling. The aim should be to maintain the aortic (post-ductal) arterial blood between 6 and 12 kPa, as even with a large right to left shunt at duct level, carotid and thus retinal tensions will not then exceed 20 kPa. The role of hyperoxia, if any, in the aetiology of retinopathy of prematurity is still uncertain. There is no advantage to the infant to have arterial oxygen pressures above 12 kPa. Inhalation of more than 80% oxygen can undoubtedly cause damage to the lung. It is therefore better to accept a PaO_2 of 6–8 kPa rather than expose the lungs to an unnecessarily high oxygen concentration. RDS tends to get worse over the first 48–72 hours. A significant metabolic acidosis (>10 mmol/l base deficit) can produce adverse effects on oxygenation and cardiac output. This may be due to poor peripheral perfusion as a result of hypovolaemia or reduced cardiac output, from anaemia, sepsis or even the parenteral nutrition. Correction of this acidosis can often lead to a dramatic improvement. If intravenous colloid is ineffective or contraindicated, the volume of molar (8.4%) sodium bicarbonate required is calculated from the formula below:

$$\text{Volume} = (\text{body deficit}/3) \times \text{body weight (kg)} \times 0.5$$

This is best given over a 30-minute period after dilution with an equal volume of glucose solution by slow i.v. injection as rapid administration can cause massive fluid shifts which may play a part in the aetiology of intraventricular haemorrhage.

Ventilation

Continuous distending pressure almost invariably leads to an improvement in oxygenation. This is probably achieved by increasing the amount of air in the lungs at end expiration and so reducing ventilation perfusion imbalance. It usually leads to a reduction in minute volume and hence an increase in the arterial carbon dioxide level. In some units all babies born at a gestation of less than 30 weeks, not requiring ventilation, are given continuous distending pressure from birth on the assumption that this will reduce the severity of the respiratory distress syndrome. Other units commence therapy if the baby is becoming progressively hypoxic, (e.g. PaO_2 less than 6.5 kPa with a FiO_2

exceeding 0.6). Continuous distending pressure can be given via endotracheal tube, nasal prongs, a single nasal catheter or by face mask. Commence at a pressure of 5–6 cm H_2O and an FiO_2 0.6. Adjustments can be made on the results of transcutaneous saturation or oxygen tension but blood gases will need repeating at 30 minutes. Progressive deterioration on continuous distending pressure is usually an indication for commencing intermittent positive pressure ventilation (IPPV). Sudden deterioration may be due either to aspiration of stomach contents or more commonly to an air leak; including pneumothorax, pneumomediastinum or pneumoperitoneum. Such babies usually require immediate intubation and ventilatory support before other treatments such as drainage of pneumothorax are carried out. There is no generally accepted pattern for weaning babies off continuous distending pressure back to a head box system, but in view of the risk of air leak it seems sensible to reduce the pressure down to 3–4 cmH_2O before dropping the inspired oxygen below 0.5–0.6. If the baby continues to deteriorate despite continuous distending pressure, ventilatory support is required.

Ventilator settings	
Initial settings:	Rate 60/mm Inspiratory/expiratory ratio 1:1 Gas mixture 0.7 FiO_2 Inflation pressure 20 cmH_2O Positive end expiratory pressure 2 cmH_2O

Intermittent pressure. Ventilatory therapy is used to support the baby who is in severe respiratory failure, allowing time for the underlying pathological processes to improve. Ventilation therapy is in no way curative and it is crucial to ensure that this potentially dangerous technique causes the minimum of damage to the baby's lungs. The indication for using IPPV varies from unit to unit; broadly speaking those with most experience tend to commence therapy earlier than those with less. Most authorities would accept: (1) PaO_2 less than 6 kPa with inspired oxygen fraction of at least 0.6; (2) peripheral shock with a pH of less than 7.1, not responding to i.v. bicarbonate; (3) $PaCO_2$ >8 with a pH <7.25; (4) recurrent apnoea not responding to stimulation or requiring repeated intubation.

Alternative methods. Ventilators are now available which can be triggered by the baby's own respiratory efforts, either as changes in airway pressure or flow or body movements. These are often helpful when the baby is fighting the ventilator but appear to be least useful in the most immature babies, who have poorer respiratory drive. High frequency jet (rates 100–400/min) and high frequency oscillation (HFO, 500–3000/min) have also been recommended. HFO is particularly useful in infants with severe homogeneous lung disease, and may reduce the incidence of chronic lung disease.

Surfactant. There are now commercially available surfactant preparations which can be given as suspensions directly down the ET tube. Those derived from animal lung (bovine/porcine) are effective in improving oxygenation within 20–30 minutes if given early in the course of the disease and will reduce mortality by 30–50% if given at birth or as rescue therapy. Artificial surfactants are also useful but take longer to work (12–24 hours).

Oro-endotracheal or naso-endotracheal tubes can be used; the first is easier to pass, the latter easier to fix. Oro-tubes can be held in place with winged stabilising devices which fit closely around the endotracheal tubes. The wings can then be attached to a bonnet by a ribbon or by sticky tape — avoid using 2mm tube if at all possible, even in the smallest baby as these almost invariably block with secretions.

If the arterial oxygen remains low, i.e. less than 6 kPa, the following measures can be taken:

1. Increase the FiO_2 by 0.1 steps. If it is necessary to provide a FiO_2 in excess of 0.9, the baby has persistent pulmonary hypertension of the newborn (see page 112). This concentration is toxic and will produce alveolar and airway damage after 48–72 hours.
2. Increase the level of PEEP to 4–5 cmH_2O. This improves the ventilation perfusion match, probably by reducing alveolar collapse, but will reduce tidal volume and so impair carbon dioxide clearance.
3. If the baby is fighting the ventilator, raise the respiratory rate, attempting to ensure that the baby breathes in time, i e synchronous, with the ventilator. The more immature the baby, the higher the rate likely to be needed. Those less than 28 weeks' gestation often need rates of up to 100/min, those more mature babies (28–32 weeks) are often synchronous at rates of 70–80/min. Increasing respiratory rate is not likely to improve oxygenation in babies who are apnoeic or breathing synchronously at rates of 60/min. When high rates are used, it is essential to ensure that the expiratory time is at least as long as the inspiratory time to prevent inadvertent alveolar PEEP, which will not be apparent from measurements provided by the ventilator. If synchronous ventilation cannot be achieved and oxygenation remains poor, improvement can sometimes be achieved by suppressing respiratory efforts with an intravenous diamorphine trip (0.05 mg/kg/h). If this fails, the baby should be paralysed with pancuronium (100 mg/kg stat and as indicated) after increasing inspiratory pressure by 4–6 cmH_2O to compensate for the loss of the baby's respiratory efforts.
4. Occasionally the more mature baby (gestation greater than 32 weeks) is helped by using a slow rate (30–40/min) with a reversed inspiratory/expiratory ratio of 1.5 : 1 or even 2 : 1. These slow rates and reversed ratios are more likely to induce pneumothoraces if the baby has not been paralysed.

5. Further improvement sometimes results from increasing the inflation pressure to 30 cmH$_2$O or even higher. This increases the risk of pneumothorax and chronic lung disease but is preferable to keeping a baby in an Fio$_2$ greater than 0.9 for more than 2–3 days.

6. Those who remain hypoxic are likely to have persistent pulmonary hypertension with shunting, particularly at atrial but also at ductal levels due to high pulmonary vascular resistance. Ensure that the arterial CO$_2$ is in the lower normal range so that there is no respiratory acidosis. If the baby has an associated metabolic acidosis, this may be due to a number of causes including hypovolaemia, infection and anaemia. Any systemic hypotension must be corrected with i.v. plasma expander to ensure that the mean systolic blood pressure is at least equal to the gestational age expressed in mmHg. Correct any persisting metabolic acidosis with either sodium bicarbonate, or if the baby has an associated respiratory acidosis or hypernatraemia, THAM. If the baby remains cyanosed, a number of therapeutic measures can be tried. Magnesium sulphate (200 g/kg over 20–30 min, then 20–50 mg/kg/h) is sometimes helpful but may take 12 hours to produce benefit. Inhaled nitric oxide (5–40 ppm) can produce a dramatic response within minutes, but information on long term side effects is very limited. Other non-specific vasodilators can also be tried. Tolazoline 1–2 mg/kg can be given intravenously as a bolus. This sometimes produces a dramatic improvement in arterial oxygenation and can then be given as a continuous infusion. Tolazoline does, however, drop the systemic as well as the pulmonary vascular resistance and so will often lead to hypotension, often needing both an i.v. plasma expander and an inotrope, such as dopamine (3 μg/kg/min) i.v. or dobutamine. Tolazoline also tends to produce gastro-intestinal bleeding. Alternatively i.v. prostacyclin (5–20 ng/kg/min) can be given.

Arterial carbon dioxide levels are less critical. Very high levels may increase the risk of intraventricular haemorrhage, although evidence that critically ill preterm babies have effective autoregulation of the cerebral blood flow is lacking. **Measures to reduce the carbon dioxide levels are**:

1. Reduce the airway dead space, either by shortening the proximal end of the ET tube or modifying the ventilator circuit. It must be remembered that the tidal volume of the most immature babies with severe respiratory distress may be as little as 3 ml.

2. Reduce the level of PEEP. This will increase tidal volume but may lead to desaturation (see above).

3. Increase the respiratory rate while keeping the I:E ratio constant. This maneouvre will be effective whether or not the baby is making respiratory efforts against the ventilator.

4. Increase the inflation pressure. Sometimes pressures in excess of 40 cmH$_2$O will be required; this is particularly likely if the baby has an

association pulmonary hypoplasia or very severe RDS. Although they are likely to be damaging in the long-term, such high pressures are justified if the baby cannot be adequately ventilated without them, and if alternative methods of ventilation, e.g high frequency oscillation, are not available.

Deterioration

The natural history for RDS is for the condition to deteriorate over the first 48–72 hours. If the severity of the deterioration is unexpected, other causes must always be considered, particularly if the deterioration develops rapidly. Consider:

1. *Ventilator malfunction* or leak in the ventilator circuit. This would be indicated by a fall in the display pressure and will trigger the pressure alarm.
2. *Tube blocked or displacement* into the right main bronchus or oesophagus. This is suggested by reduced chest wall movement and poorly conducted breath sounds. Some of the new ventilators are attempting to identify these situations from a change in the inflation pressure wave form or reduction in tidal flow. If suspected, try sucking down the ET tube. If the baby fails to improve, replace the ET tube.
3. *Air leak*, e.g. pneumothorax, pneumediastinum and pulmonary intestitial emphysema (PIE) It is sometimes possible to identify a pneumothorax clinically, as this will tend to shift the cardiac apex and produce asymmetrical air entry. A fibreoptic cold light source tends to produce diffuse translucency on the affected side, an effect also seen with extensive PIE. If the baby's condition permits, the diagnosis can be confirmed by chest X-ray. If the baby's condition is critical, insert a butterfly needle into the pleural space on the affected side (3rd or 4th intercostal space, anterior axillary line) while keeping the open end submerged in a small quantity of water. The chest drain can then be inserted, and the distal end of the catheter connected to an underwater seal. Connect the open end of the tube from the underwater seal to a low pressure suction source (5–10 cmH$_2$O). One of the commercially available flap valves can be used for transport.

Tube in right main bronchus

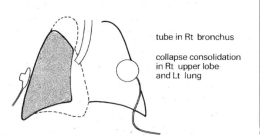

tube in Rt bronchus

collapse consolidation
in Rt upper lobe
and Lt lung

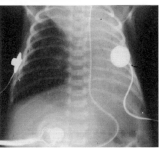

4. *Other diagnoses. Pulmonary interstitial emphysema* occurs most frequently in very immature babies and splints the lungs so that they then become very stiff and difficult to ventilate. It is then necessary to use high inflation pressures (often over 30 cmH$_2$O) and high rates. If the PIE is unilateral, it is sometimes possible to selectively intubate the opposite lung. This is relatively easy when PIE affects the left lung, more difficult on the right. Deliberate rupture of the lung with a needle (scarification) has been recommended, but there are no controlled studies on whether this alters outcome. There is some evidence that jet ventilation has a role in these babies.

Massive intraventricular haemorrhage often occurs on the 2nd to 5th day of life, particularly in very ill, severely preterm babies. Grade III and IV IVHs are often associated with a deterioration in blood gases, persistent metabolic acidosis and hypotension. These can most easily be identified by cranial ultrasound, but will also often cause distension of the fontanelle and free blood in the CSF.

Primary infection or superimposed infection. Always suspect infection in a baby who fails to improve. Beta haemolytic streptococcal infections can produce a picture very similar to RDS, although this can affect babies of all gestations. Take blood and tracheal secretion culture and review antibiotic therapy. It is now routine for neonatal units to commence all babies with significant respiratory symptoms in the immediate neonatal period on systemic penicillin and amino-glycosides or a third generation cephalosporin to combat this problem.

Heart failure, associated with cyanotic congenital heart disease, particularly transposition of the great vessels, can mimic ARDS. Cardiac ultrasound will allow these babies to be identified.

General management

It is important to ensure that the babies are nursed in a thermo-neutral environment to keep metabolic requirements to a minimum. Intravenous fluids will be needed from birth but in those over 28 weeks' gestation, it is often possible to delay i.v. alimentation for 4–5 days. Those needing ventilation for more than 1–2 weeks, but who are otherwise well, will often tolerate nasogastric feeds. ET suction leads to rapid desaturation and can be limited to every 6–12 hours providing there are not excessive secretions present.

Weaning the baby off IPPV. The aim should be to reduce the peak inspiratory pressure to below 20 cmH$_2$O and the Fio$_2$ to less than 0.4 as rapidly as possible and certainly before reducing the respiratory rate. It is also important to keep the inspiratory time short, i.e. maximum of 0.5 seconds rather than keep the I:E ratio constant. This will reduce the risk of pneumothorax and lead to more rapid weaning. Once the respiratory rate is down to 20/min the baby should be commenced on either i.v. aminophylline, oral theophylline or caffeine. The baby can then be weaned off either by reducing the rate down to 2–3/min (IMV) and then transferred to continuous positive airway pressure (3–4 cmH$_2$O) for 1 hour before attempting extubation.

Extubation is not without its hazards. There is an increased tendency to aspirate in the subsequent hours. Laryngeal stridor can be a problem. Therefore omit milk feeds and empty the stomach 4 hours prior to extubation and substitute 4% dextrose 0.18% saline. Continue this for 12 hours after extubation to eliminate the risk of milk aspiration until upper airway reflexes and laryngeal function return to normal. Suck out the pharynx and the stomach, 10 minutes before removing the endotracheal tube. Babies developing stridor can sometimes be helped by oral dexamethasone 0.2 mg/kg body weight 3 times a day for 2 days, or nebulised adrenaline (1 ml/1 in 1000). Where babies have to be re-intubated for stridor, pharyngeal continuous positive airway pressure given via a single nasal catheter may help support the upper airway following extubation.

Pulmonary haemorrhage. A number of babies with idiopathic respiratory distress syndrome deteriorate rapidly with blood stained fluid welling up the trachea. The mechanism for this condition is not understood, the blood stained fluid transfers across into the alveolar space presumably secondary to rising pulmonary venous pressure. This is associated with the dramatic deterioration in the child's condition and in the appearance of the chest X-ray. Affected infants should be paralysed and sedated, fluid restricted and ventilated with increased PEEP levels.

Problem

- Usually full term, often having been delivered by caesarean section.
- Tachypnoea from birth with some recession and grunting.
- Chest X-ray showing well expanded lungs but streaky shadows spreading out from the mediastinum.

Diagnosis — Transient tachypnoea

In this condition the respiratory symptoms appear to be secondary to delayed clearance of lung fluid after birth. The respiratory problem settles within hours or at the most within 2–3 days of delivery. Some babies need an oxygen-enriched environment and will require blood

Transient tachypnoea of newborn

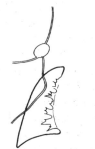
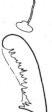
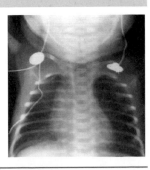

—bilateral shadowing radiating from hilar region

gas estimations. Carbon dioxide retention rarely occurs and no other treatment is required provided there is no doubt about the diagnosis. The main difficulty lies in distinguishing it from an early streptococcal pneumonia. If there is doubt take a nasopharyngeal swab, blood cultures and commence on parenteral penicillin and aminoglycosides.

Problem

- Usually a history of fetal distress.
- Meconium-stained liquor with meconium in the mouth and pharynx.
- Tachypnoea, recession and often grunting from birth.
- Barrel shaped chest.

Diagnosis — Meconium aspiration syndrome

There is little difficulty establishing this diagnosis. If direct laryngoscopy shows that meconium is present in the oropharynx at birth, the baby should be intubated immediately and the meconium aspirated from the larynx and trachea. This is best achieved by attaching the side arm of the endotracheal tube to the suction source (50–100 cmH$_2$O), occluding the free end of the tube and withdrawing it. This should be repeated until no more meconium is aspirated. There is a tendency for symptoms to get progressively worse over the next 2–3 days as meconium moves into the small airways. Usually respiratory distress is associated with gross hyperinflation with a barrel shaped chest and displacement of the liver down into the abdomen. Diagnosis is confirmed by chest X-ray. Pneumothoraces are a common complication. Oxygen may be required if severe aspiration has occurred. When IPPV is required, it is often necessary to use high inflation pressures. Alterations in the I:E ratio sometimes result in improvements and it is most important that each child should be considered individually.

Many will have persistent pulmonary hypertension. It is then often necessary to paralyse the baby and give vasodilator such as nitric oxide or tolazoline. Those with severe unresponsive disease may need extracorporeal membrane oxygenation (ECMO). Some of these babies will have an associated asphyxial encephalopathy and it will obviously be very important to assess the neurological status of these babies carefully, including intracranial ultrasound, as this may influence the level of support which it is considered ethical to provide. There is evidence from animal studies that meconium aspiration increases the risk of secondary bacterial pneumonias and therefore antibiotics, for example gentamicin 3 mg/kg 12 hourly and penicillin 25 000 units/kg 12 hourly should be prescribed. Symptoms usually settle within a matter of days so that total intravenous alimentation is rarely required.

Meconium aspiration

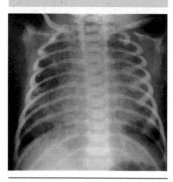

Problem

- Tachypnoea with grunting and often cyanosis.
- Barrel shaped chest.
- Diminished air entry over one side of the chest.
- Diffuse glow on transilluminating the side with reduced air entry.

Diagnosis — Pneumothorax

Although occurring most commonly as a complication of continuous distending pressure, IPPV or meconium aspiration syndrome, symptomatic pneumothoraces can occur spontaneously. The symptoms are those of respiratory distress with hyperinflation of the thorax. Displacement of the cardiac apex is often difficult to detect in small babies, but there is usually asymmetry of air entry.

Air leaks

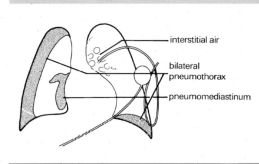
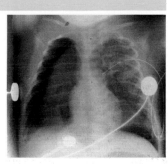

interstitial air

bilateral
pneumothorax

pneumomediastinum

Problem

- Sudden onset of tachypnoea and grunting.
- History of regurgitating feeds.
- X-ray showing generalised mottling.

Diagnosis — Aspiration of feeds

Aspiration of feeds is a common occurrence in preterm and full-term babies with neurological or other cardiorespiratory problems. Symptoms are again those of tachypnoea, recession and expiratory grunting, often following a history of coughing and cyanosis during or soon after a feed. If the episode of aspiration is noted, the damage can be minimised by prompt nasopharyngeal suction and tipping. The chest X-ray will reveal patchy shadowing not unlike that seen in meconium aspiration but without hyperinflation. On examination coarse crepitations can almost always be heard. Antibiotics such as gentamicin and flucloxacillin and physiotherapy are indicated. Aspiration occurring at the first feed suggests the presence of a *tracheo-oesophageal fistula*, This diagnosis should have been suspected earlier as there is almost always associated hydramnios and excessive nasopharyngeal secretions. The diagnosis is established by failure to pass a tube with a radio-opaque marker down into the stomach. If doubt remains, an X-ray should be taken to locate the tip. This condition is a surgical emergency. Oral feeds should be abandoned until after surgery. It is often possible to achieve a primary end-to-end anastomosis and close the fistula. If this is impossible the fistula must be closed, a gastrostomy created and continuous pharyngeal suction commenced.

CYANOSIS

The predominance of fetal haemoglobin in the immediate neonatal period ensures that cyanosis will not occur until the arterial oxygen tension is less than 4 kPa, as long as normal acid–base balance is maintained. A fall in pH from 7.3 to 7.1 produces a right shift of the dissociation curve so that cyanosis will occur when the arterial oxygen tension falls to 6 kPa, mimicking adult haemoglobin. Peripheral cyanosis is very common in healthy babies in the first few days of life and can be ignored provided the baby is otherwise healthy. Traumatic cyanosis due to massive petechial haemorrhages can be misleading to the casual observer but the mucous membranes of the mouth remain pink.

Cyanosis developing secondary to severe RDS does not as a rule present a diagnostic problem but there are occasions in which it is difficult to decide whether the cyanosis is due to cardiac, respiratory or even CNS causes. A *hyperoxia* test is helpful in distinguishing cardiac and respiratory causes. A preductal arterial blood sample is taken (e.g. from the right radial artery) and the Po_2 measured. The baby is then placed in a headbox with 100% oxygen for 15 minutes, and the sample repeated. In cyanotic congenital heart disease the Po_2 may rise by 1–2 kPa, but never above 14 kPa, while in respiratory disease there will be a significant rise, often above 20 kPa in all but the most severe lung involvement.

Problem
- Fetal distress or difficult delivery (usually, but not always).
- Central cyanosis usually present from birth.
- Loud pulmonary second sound.
- Chest X-ray showing well expanded oligaemic lungs.
- Blood gases show hypoxia with a relatively normal Pco_2.
- Often little improvement in saturation on breathing 100% oxygen.

Diagnosis — Persistent pulmonary hypertension
Nurse the baby in a high oxygen concentration, and ventilate if necessary, aiming to keep the Pco_2 in the low normal range. Give nitric oxide 5–20 ppm. Other cardiac causes include transposition of the great vessels, tricuspid atresia, pulmonary atresia, total anomalous pulmonary venous draining and severe heart failure complicating left heart syndrome, cardiomegaly or obstructive lesions such as coarctation of the aorta and pulmonary stenosis.

Problem

- History of severe fetal distress, birth trauma or excessive maternal sedation.
- Quiet, unresponsive baby who is breathing very shallowly.
- Blood gases revealing carbon dioxide retention affecting the baby to the same degree as the oxygen desaturation.

Diagnosis — Alveolar hypoventilation

These babies pick up dramatically on raising the inspired oxygen to 0.3. They require further investigation to identify the underlying neurological problems.

Problem

- Cyanosis usually present from birth.
- No significant rise in saturation on increasing inspired oxygen.
- Blood remains blue-brown on shaking in air and shows a high oxygen tension in the presence of a very low saturation.

Diagnosis — Methaemoglobinaemia

When cyanosis persists in an apparently healthy baby, consider the possibility of methaemoglobinaemia. Acquired methaemoglobinaemia is rare in the neonatal period, although it has been described secondary to absorption of aniline dyes from the nappy. This is also a complication of inhaled nitric oxide therapy. The congenital form can provide a diagnostic problem. Blood gases carried out while the baby is breathing oxygen enriched air will show a high Pa_{O_2} despite cyanosis. This is a dangerous situation and has on occasions lead to retinopathy of prematurity. Venous blood shaken in the tube with air will fail to turn pink. The diagnosis is confirmed by Hb electrophoresis. Rapid improvement results from giving large doses of reducing substance, e.g. ascorbic acid.

CHRONIC LUNG DISEASES

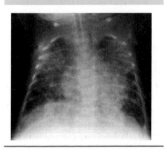

Bronchopulmonary dysplasia

Approximately 10% of preterm babies requiring respiratory support in the immediate neonatal period will require prolonged ventilation, be oxygen dependent and have respiratory problems and abnormal chest X-ray for many months, a condition diagnosed as bronchopulmonary dysplasia. This condition is due to the use of high inflation pressures, oxygen toxicity, aspiration, and infection. Approximately 30% will die. They require oxygen therapy for long periods and may be helped by physiotherapy. The role of bronchodilators is unclear. Systemic steroids, e.g. dexamethasone 0.2 mg/kg three times a day, reducing over 2–4 weeks, often assists weaning from respiratory support and may produce long term benefit. All episodes of infection must be treated with antibiotics.

Problem

There is a further but rare respiratory disease which can cause a diagnostic problem. These babies have:

- A history of severe prematurity usually with birth weight less than 1200 g.
- Onset of progressive tachypnoea, chest wall recession and oxygen dependency commencing at 2–3 weeks of age.
- X-ray showing hyperinflation and a lace-like pattern with small cystic areas.

Diagnosis — Wilson–Mikity syndrome

This poorly understood condition may be related to immaturity of the airways and tends to get progressively worse for 2–3 weeks followed by slow recovery. The baby is liable to have further respiratory problems later in infancy and the chest X-ray will usually not revert to normal for 1–2 years.

Other respiratory problems causing neonatal respiratory distress

Congenital diaphragmatic hernia occur approximately 1 in every 5000 deliveries and affect the left side in 85% of cases. Those presenting with difficulty in resuscitation at birth have a relatively high mortality due to associated *pulmonary hypoplasia*. The aim should be to stabilise the baby and achieve satisfactory blood gases before proceeding to surgery and repairing the diaphragmatic defect. Many have persisting pulmonary hypertension requiring pulmonary vasodilator drugs. A high pressure and high rate ventilation is often needed.

Thoracic dystrophy

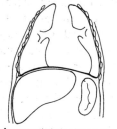

Apparently large heart: liver and spleen easily palpable in abdomen

Asphyxiating thoracic dystrophy can also produce respiratory distress in the immediate neonatal period. The defect lies in the poor development of the thoracic cage, producing a constriction of the lungs.

Bilateral choanal atresia presents with severe respiratory distress and cyanosis when the mouth is closed, but the infant turns pink on crying! This can be helped dramatically by inserting an oral airway which should be left in place until cannulae can be inserted through the atretic area.

APNOEA

Fetal respiratory movements commence by the end of the first trimester but are intermittent, probably only occurring in rapid eye movement sleep. They are thought to be important in stimulating lung growth and development. Most babies adapt to a regular pattern of respiration on delivery without difficulty, although subtle changes do occur over the next few days of life. Prematurity or illness can cause the baby to have recurrent apnoea. Apnoea occurs in three forms: central, i.e. cessation of all respiratory efforts (45%); obstructive, where the baby continues to make respiratory efforts against a closed upper airway (5%); and mixed attacks in which there are both central and obstructive components. Bradycardia (rate less than 90/min) regularly accompanies prolonged central apnoea but occurs earlier in obstructive or mixed apnoea. 'Apnoea' is defined here as cessation of air flow for 10 seconds or longer. Apnoea presents in two ways:

Problem (1)

- Commencing usually within 3 days of delivery in preterm babies.
- Baby otherwise well and vigorous between apnoeic episodes.

Diagnosis — Apnoea of prematurity

Problem (2)

- Onset usually after the first 3 days of life in a baby who has previously had regular respiration.
- Baby lethargic or irritable often feeding or tolerating feeds poorly.

Diagnosis — Apnoea secondary to infection, cerebral damage including IVH, ischaemia, brain trauma and metabolic disorders, including hypoglycaemia

Assess the baby's general appearance, recording pulse, respiration, core temperature and peripheral perfusion. Check the fontanelle tone, as raised intracranial pressure resulting from hydrocephalus, meningitis or intraventricular haemorrhage may present with apnoea. If the baby appears to have uncomplicated apnoea of prematurity, no additional investigations are required other than blood glucose and full blood picture. Those with secondary apnoea will, in addition, require an infection screen including throat, umbilical and rectal swab, blood culture, lumbar puncture, urinalysis, chest X-ray, serum calcium and blood gases to assess the metabolic state. All babies will require respiration monitoring. Unfortunately this will not detect obstructive or mixed episodes, so heart rate monitoring will also be required. The most effective method for identifying significant episodes of apnoea is to use a transcutaneous saturation monitor set to alarm at 88%.

Management. If systemic infection is suspected the baby will need to be commenced on intravenous antibiotics, e.g. penicillin and gentamicin, pending the results of the infections screen. Any hypoglycaemia (blood glucose below 2.5 mmol/l), is an indication for intravenous 20% dexrose giving 5 ml/kg stat. followed by 10% dextrose 75 ml/kg/day. If the baby has a metabolic acidosis the cause for this should be sought and where possible treated (see p. 103). Significant acidosis persisting can be counteracted by giving intravenous sodium bicarbonate over 30–60 minutes. Most attacks are either self-limiting or can be terminated by skin stimulation, flicking feet or blowing cold air/oxygen over the baby's face using a face mask. If this fails gentle aspiration of the pharynx using suction pressures of up to 100 mmHg may help. Failure to respond to this is an indication for bag and mask or mask and T-piece resuscitation. If the baby does not improve within 20–30 seconds proceed to endotracheal intubation and a brief period of IPPV.

Prevention

Added oxygen. Increasing the inspired oxygen fraction to 0.25 may reduce the incidence of apnoea; it is essential to monitor the baby's blood gases frequently, as this concentration may be sufficient to induce retinopathy of prematurity in the very immature baby.

Theophylline. 1–2.5 mg/kg body weight 8 hourly orally. This can be very effective but can sometimes lead to gastro-intestinal distension and vomiting. The half-life of theophylline is long and variable in the immediate neonatal period. Measure serum levels after 24 hours and weekly subsequently. Adjust dose to ensure blood levels of 5–12 μg/ml. Oral caffeine is also effective in reducing the incidence of apnoea given in a dose of 20 mg/kg/day. As this is considerably less toxic than theophylline it is not necessary to measure the blood levels. Those not tolerating any oral intake can be given aminophylline 5 mg/kg i.v. over 20 minutes followed by 4.4 mg/kg per day as a continuous infusion or i.v. caffeine.

Continuous distending pressures. Pressures of up to 5 cmH$_2$O are highly effective in reducing obstructive and mixed apnoea but have no influence on the frequency of central apnoea. On average this form of therapy will reduce the apnoeic attacks by 50%. This can be given by a single nasal catheter reaching back to the oropharynx.

Intravenous doxapram. This is a strong respiratory stimulant with a relatively short life. The recommended dose is 1–2 mg/kg body weight. Abnormal neurological signs do sometimes develop on this form of therapy.

IPPV. If frequent intubation is required or the baby is failing to respond rapidly to bag and mask ventilation, the baby should be commenced on ventilatory therapy and may need support for 1–2 weeks. It is necessary to measure blood gases initially, but if the baby is stable relatively infrequent sampling may be possible, particularly if a transcutaneous oxygen analyser or saturation monitor is available. The baby is unlikely to develop pneumothoraces or chronic lung disease providing low inflation pressures are used, however many babies produce considerable volumes of secretions in response to the ET tube and require frequent ET suction using scrupulously sterile techniques. Physiotherapy may also help to clear secretions. Nutrition can often be maintained via a nasogastric or nasojejunal tube as long as there are no contraindications such as sepsis. Secondary apnoeas are slightly less likely to respond to treatment other than IPPV.

Recommended initial ventilator settings

F$_{O_2}$ — 0.25
Inflation pressure — 15 cmH$_2$O
Respiratory rate — 20/min
I : E ratio — 1 : 2

BLEEDING

Bleeding in newborns can be very serious because a lot of blood can be lost in a few minutes from the umbilical stump and because intracranial haemorrhage may occur.

Problem

- An otherwise well baby bleeds on the 2nd to 4th day of life.
- Usually solely breast fed.

Diagnosis — Vitamin K deficiency bleeding

Certain essential clotting factors are synthesised in the liver by a mechanism for which vitamin K is an essential cofactor — principally prothrombin but also factors VII, IX and X. Transfer of vitamin K from the mother to the fetus is low so that newborn plasma levels are less than one-tenth of maternal levels. The baby's concentrations of vitamin K dependent clotting factors therefore fall in the first few days of life, and haemorrhage may occur. Bottle fed babies are unlikely to develop haemorrhagic disease as the milks are vitamin K supplemented. Solely breast fed babies have inadequate intake The disease can be prevented by giving all newborns 0.1–.0.5 mg of vitamin K i.m. soon after birth or 1 mg orally. Babies who are breast fed and given the oral formulation, will require additional oral doses at 7–10 days and at 6 weeks.

Problem

- A sick baby develops petechiae at any time from birth onwards.
- Often there is a severe infection, hypoxia, shock or acidosis.

Diagnosis — Disseminated intravascular coagulation

The insult to the baby results in thrombin formation and intravascular coagulation which consumes platelets and clotting factors. The prothrombin time, APPT and thrombin times are all prolonged and there are low levels of fibrinogen and platelets and elevated fibrin degradation products. The underlying problem must be treated vigorously and fresh frozen plasma given.

Problem

- Purpura, echymoses and perhaps cephalhaematoma soon after birth.
- A maternal history of idiopathic thrombocytopenic purpura.

Diagnosis — Immune neonatal thrombocytopenia

The low platelet count in the baby is due to transplacental transfer of anti-platelet antibodies. The thrombocytopenia persists for 2–3 months but the purpura clears more quickly. In severe cases, steroids and exchange transfusion are helpful.

OEDEMA

Oedema occurs in most newborns in small amounts with swelling of the eye-lids after birth, and in preterms oedema may be more generalised even in those who are well. However in a number of situations oedema may indicate serious disease.

Problem

- Gross oedema at birth with fluid in serous cavities.

Diagnosis — Hydrops fetalis

Efforts should be made to resuscitate all hydropic infants at birth since some have severe haemolytic disease, such as rhesus incompatibility (immune hydrops), which are compatible with normal survival, and in others it is important to keep the baby alive to establish a diagnosis, so that counselling can be given later. Non-immune causes include cardiac anomalies, including arrhythmias, chromosomal abnormalities and other recognisable syndromes, *alpha-thalassaemia,* and *twin-to-twin transfusions.* Up to 50% of all cases will be idiopathic.

Treatment consists of intubation and IPPV from birth to control pulmonary oedema, with aspiration of pleural and peritoneal effusions if the infant does not start to improve. Umbilical catheters enable CVP and BP to be monitored, and blood samples to be taken for the many tests needed to find a cause.

Problem

- Progressive oedema developing in the days after birth.
- Increasing respiratory distress or ventilator dependence.
- Sometimes the development of a ductus murmur.

Diagnosis — Acquired oedema

This will result if there has been fluid overload due to excessive fluids given intravenously for maintenance or to keep arterial catheters open, or due to untoward incidents with infusion pumps. Alternatively there may be fluid retention due to renal failure occurring in the sick neonate who has RDS or shock and hypotension, or due to CNS damage with inappropriate ADH secretion, or simply due to hypoalbuminaemia.

The underlying cause must be treated together with fluid restriction to 50–60 ml/kg/24 h. More severe restriction is needed, if inappropriate ADH secretion is present as shown by a low serum osmolality together with a urine osmolality greater than 200 mOsmol/kg. If there is no diuresis give frusemide 1–2 mg/kg. A salt-poor albumin infusion may be needed.

Problem

- Very firm shiny swelling of the limbs or abdominal wall.
- Poor capillary perfusion in association with any severe illness.

Diagnosis — Sclerema

In the past the appearance of sclerema in a baby with sepsis or any severe illness usually signalled death, but recently vigorous supportive treatment, including fresh frozen plasma or even exchange transfusion with fresh blood, has resulted in recoveries.

JITTERS, TWITCHES AND FITS

Tone and response to stimuli vary widely in the neonatal period. It is obviously most important to identify babies who lie at the extremes of the normal range from those who have underlying neurological abnormalities. Intermittent focal fits (twitching) in an otherwise healthy baby can be difficult to differentiate from the 'jitters'. Grand-mal convulsions are not seen at this age but generalised twitching commonly occurs often not associated with either apnoea or cyanosis. The type of convulsion is of little help in establishing the diagnosis. The following approach will identify the cause in approximately 50%.

Problem

- A baby who reacts to minor physical stimuli or even a loud noise with a Moro reflex.
- Hyper-reflexia often with bouts of clonus at the knee and ankle.
- Otherwise healthy and alert, feeding or tolerating feeds well.
- Normal blood sugar and serum calcium.

Diagnosis — Normal jittery baby

If the blood glucose is reduced, i.e. less than 2.5 mmol/l, the likely diagnosis is *symptomatic hypoglycaemia*. In this situation give 25% dextrose 1–2 ml/kg body weight over 2 minutes. This should lead to an improvement in the clinical condition if the diagnosis is correct. Continue with 10% dextrose i.v. at 4–6 mg/kg body weight/min for 12–24 hours while increasing milk feeds. The baby should be weaned off the dextrose infusion over a further 24 hours to prevent rebound hypoglycaemia.

Problem

- If there is severe, persistent or recurrent hypoglycaemia.
- And the 10% dextrose infusion rate to maintain normo-glycaemia is >5 ml/kg/h >8 mg/kg/min).

Diagnosis — Substrate or enzyme deficiency

Take blood samples for cortisol, growth hormone, TSH, electrolytes, 17-hydroxyprogesterone, lactate and pyruvate, amino acids and urine for metabolic screen. Continue adjusting the dextrose infusion appropriately to keep blood sugar normal and consider giving hydrocortisone 2.5–5.0 mg/kg i.v. 12 hourly.

Problem

- If there is severe, persistent or recurrent hypoglycaemia.
- And the 10% dextrose infusion rate to maintain normo-glycaemia is >6 ml/kg/h.

Diagnosis — Hyperinsulinism

Take two or more paired glucose and insulin measurements while hypoglycaemic. The cause may be nesidioblastosis or insulinoma which may be found on CT scanning and surgery indicated. Meanwhile treat with glucagon, diazoxide and chlorthiazide.

Problem

- If serum calcium is less than 1.5 mmol/l and phosphate greater than 3.5 mmol/l.

Diagnosis — Hypocalcaemic fits

These fits are relatively uncommon since the introduction of low phosphate containing milks but do still occur occasionally. They respond immediately to i.v. 10% calcium gluconate (up to 0.5 ml/kg slowly into drip). Subsequently the baby should be given clear fluids for 24 hours and then fed on either breast milk or a low phosphate containing milk. The hypocalcaemia which often accompanies hypoxic or traumatic brain damage, and occurs in the first few days of life, is probably worth treating, although clinical improvement is rarely seen. Maintenance therapy can be given as 10% calcium gluconate, 5 ml/kg/24 h either i.v. or orally. Neonatal serum calcium levels vary widely making interpretation difficult. It is important not to impede venous return during collection or to squeeze the extremity, as this will elevate the calcium content.

Problem

If the CSF contains:

- Increased numbers of leucocytes, i.e. greater than 10 and usually in excess of 100 mm³.
- Raised protein, i.e. greater than 1.5 g/l in term infants or 2.0 g/l in preterms.
- Reduced glucose, i.e. considerably lower than simultaneous blood glucose and often less than 1.0 mmol/l.
- Sometimes the presence of organisms on microscopy.

Diagnosis — Meningitis

In the absence of organisms the diagnosis can be difficult as intracranial haemorrhage, either in the form of an intraventricular or subarachnoid haemorrhage, will elevate the CSF protein, may produce a cellular response and often leads to a reduction in CSF sugar. However, if not treated, neonatal meningitis is nearly always fatal and even those identified early have a significant mortality. The child must be commenced immediately on i.v. antibiotic therapy with cefotaxime or chloramphenicol (or penicillin for streptococcal infection). Gentamicin may act synergistically with cefotaxime but is completely inadequate alone. If chloramphenicol is used, blood and CSF levels must be measured to ensure that the baby does not develop the 'grey baby syndrome' due to excessive levels. Treatment must be continued for a minimum of 3 weeks. Phenobarbitone may be needed to control irritability or fits, and the best nursing and supportive care are essential. On these regimens approximately 70% of babies will survive, and of these approximately 80% will subsequently have normal developmental progress. Some babies develop hydrocephalus and require shunts.

Intrauterine infections can also produce fits in the neonatal period. The IgM will always be elevated. Screen for rubella, CMV and toxoplasma. Viral culture and complement fixation tests against other viral infections are indicated if the previous investigations have been normal.

Problem

- Sometimes there is a history of a difficult delivery or perinatal asphyxia requiring prolonged resuscitation.

Diagnosis — Fits secondary to hypoxic brain damage or cerebral trauma (hypoxic ischaemic encephalopathy)

The fits can sometimes be controlled by giving anticonvulsants. If response is poor and the baby is not hypoxic as a result of the fitting, there is probably little point in pushing the anticonvulsant therapy until the baby is virtually unconscious.

The outlook in babies who have brief fits and do not have obvious cerebral damage or meningitis is good. At least 70% will show no long-term brain damage and although follow-up is important, it is entirely justified to be optimistic when discussing the likely outcome.

Drugs for neonatal fits

Phenobarbitone	i.v., i.m. or oral	
	Loading dose	20 mg/kg
	Maintenance	3–4 mg/kg/day
Phenytoin	i.v.	
	Loading	20 mg/kg over 30 min
	Maintenance	3–4 mg/kg/day
Diazepam	i.v.	0.25–0.5 mg/kg over 3–5 min
Paraldehyde	Rectally 2–4 hourly	0.3 ml/kg/dose mixed with equal volume of arachis oil
Clonazepam	i.v.	
	Loading	50–500 µg/kg
	Maintenance	10–60 µg/kg/h

Opisthotonus. Those babies who are hypertonic, lying in opisthotonous with legs and arms held in full extension, fitting continuously, are in an entirely different category. This is usually due to severe hypoxia or traumatic brain damage, to an overwhelming meningitis or intracranial haemorrhage. Initially the babies are often unable to swallow and sometimes have disseminated intravascular coagulation with bleeding from puncture sites. Even if the diagnosis of severe brain damage is strongly suspected, the following investigations are indicated: blood glucose, blood calcium and phosphate, blood culture, lumbar puncture, blood pH and acid–base balance, and skull X-ray.

In these babies the calcium is often low but response to intravenous calcium therapy is minimal or absent. Persistent acidosis raises the possibility of a congenital metabolic disorder. This is more likely in a baby who is hypotonic. The opisthotonus responds very poorly to anticonvulsants but they should still be given, as periods of apnoea and cyanosis often accompany convulsions in this age group. If cerebral oedema is suspected (a full fontanelle and a generalised echo-bright appearance on cranial ultrasound scan), give 20% mannitol, 7 ml/kg as an infusion over 20 minutes.

Many die in the next few days. Those surviving tend to show some improvement, often become hypotonic but require prolonged periods of nasogastric feeding. The occasional child does well but the majority have severe developmental delay and cerebral palsy. Babies who show signs of deterioration in the first few days of life, sliding into respiratory failure, probably should not be given ventilatory support unless there is reason to think that this is due to a temporary deterioration in cerebral function. This is, of course, a very difficult decision to make and if there is any doubt it is probably reasonable to provide support for a limited period of 1–2 days.

FLOPPY BABIES

As with jittery babies there are a group of healthy neonates who represent the hypotonic floppy end of the normal distribution and have a good long-term outlook, although they tend to be a little slow in walking and often bottom shuffle.

Problem

- Hypotonic.
- Feed poorly.
- Drowsy and respond badly to handling.
- Possibly also have fits.

Diagnosis — Hypotonia secondary to cerebral dysfunction

Some are unresponsive and drowsy from birth. The most likely cause is hypoxia or traumatic cerebral damage and this may be apparent from the baby's history. It can be closely mimicked by maternal drug sedation. The opiates produce hypotonia, shallow breathing and unresponsiveness but this usually passes off within 24–48 hours. If present, a dramatic improvement follows i.v. naloxone, 0.2 mg to a large baby, 0.1 mg to a small baby. This drug is safe given in this situation, unlike nalorphine, it does not produce respiratory depression if given inappropriately. Diazepam and other tranquillising drugs which are sometimes given in large doses to control maternal pre-eclamptic toxaemia are metabolised slowly by the baby and can produce a picture of hypotonia, lethargy and reluctance to feed lasting up to 1 week. Although the mechanism is obscure, there is evidence that intravenous naloxone helps. Other causes of cerebral dysfunction present from birth include intrauterine infections (rubella, CMV, toxoplasma), arrested brain development (microcephaly) and severe chromosomal abnormalities, for example trisomy 13, 15 and trisomy 17–18. These severe genetic abnormalities are not compatible with sustained life.

Problem

• Some babies show deterioration in responsiveness and develop hypotonia after having previously been alert. They become less active and reluctant to feed, sometimes developing abdominal distension. Those with orogastric feeding are unable to tolerate the volumes of milk that previously did not present any problem. Some develop attacks of apnoea. On examination the babies appear pale and lack the normal spontaneous activity.

Diagnosis — Systemic infection, particularly urinary tract, pneumonia, septicaemia and meningitis

This picture can also result from hypoglycaema, intracranial bleeds, particularly intraventricular haemorrhages in preterm babies, or a metabolic acidosis secondary to a congenital metabolic disorder or congenital renal disease. As they have potentially fatal but sometimes eminently treatable conditions, immediate investigation is imperative, including: chest X-ray to exclude aspiration or pneumonia; urine for cells and culture (bag urine may be satisfactory but if in doubt collect urine by suprapubic tap or clean catch); blood culture to exclude septicaemia and lumbar puncture for cells and organisms. A CSF which is uniformly blood stained suggests a subarachnoid haemorrhage or in the preterm baby an intraventricular haemorrhage, which has broken through into the CSF. Xanthochromia is a common finding in the first few days of life.

If an infection is suspected, antibiotic therapy must be commenced immediately after the infection screen has been completed, as a baby with *septicaemia* is unlikely to survive the 24–48 hours required for the result of the cultures. Likely organisms include streptococcus, staphylococcus, *E.coli* and other gram-negatives. To cover these organisms a combination of gentamicin 3 mg/kg/dose together with penicillin G 30 mg (50 000 units)/kg/dose or flucloxacillin 50 mg/kg/dose should be given intravenously every 12 hours to babies under 1 week of age, and every 8 hours to those above 1 week. This will be sufficient in a septicaemia, pneumonia or urinary tract infection. If the lumbar puncture reveals an excess of polymorphs then cefotaxime or chloramphenicol will be needed as already described. The large majority of babies with systemic infections will show an improvement within 1–2 days, and the length of treatment will depend on the site of the infection but should be at least 7 days for septicaemia.

Sometimes there may be special reasons to be worried that listeria may be the pathogen, for example the presence of meconium in a preterm delivery. Then ampicillin should be used. Anaerobic organisms are treated with metronidazole and pseudomonas with ceftazidine.

| Problem | • Sudden deterioration with hypotonia in the preterm baby. |

Diagnosis — Intraventricular haemorrhage

This is particularly likely to occur after hypoxia or asphyxia but may also affect babies who have thrived in the first few days of life. Often the haemorrhage breaks through into the ventricular system and tracks down into the spinal CSF producing uniform contamination of the fluid. Nothing can be done for this catastrophy other than attempts to maintain the baby's blood gas and base balance.

The extent of the haemorrhage can be seen on cranial ultrasound or CT scanning and is usually graded:

I   Germinal layer haemorrhage only.
II   Intraventricular haemorrhage (IVH) but not distending the ventricular system.
III   IVH with distension of the ventricular system.
IV   IVH with intracerebral extension into the brain parenchyma.

IVH almost always occurs in the first 3 days of life, and now that neonatal units carry out routine ultrasound scanning on babies under 1.5 kg or 33 weeks, we know that some degree of haemorrhage is very common, occurring in about 50% of the most immature babies. The prognosis for babies with asymptomatic Grades I and II haemorrhages is very good. Babies with Grade III have a 30–40% risk of a neurodevelopmental problem at follow-up, and those with Grade IV developing hydrocephalus and needing shunting have a 60–75% risk of abnormality later.

Ultrasound has also shown that some babies have another characteristic scan appearance called *periventricular leucomalacia* (PVL). This may occur in association with IVH or independently and there is usually a preceding history of asphyxia or hypoxia. This results in hypoxic-ischaemic damage to the region of the brain around the lateral ventricles, an area which is particularly vulnerable as it is in a watershed between arterial supplies. The early appearance is of an echodense 'flare', which later resolves and periventricular cystic areas may then develop. Follow-up studies have shown that these babies are at very high risk (up to 90%) of major handicap, i.e. spastic diplegia or other cerebral palsy, and often with other developmental delays. The appearance of Grade IV IVH or of PVL is therefore important information to include in the overall assessment of a seriously ill neonate on ventilation, helping to determine the appropriateness of continuing intensive care.

Problem

- Onset of hypotonia within a few days of birth, sometimes with drowsiness, loss of consciousness, fits and vomiting.
- Tachypnoea and tachycardia with a metabolic acidosis in the absence of respiratory or cardiac disease.
- Improvement on i.v. dextrose saline fluid. Relapse on reintroducing feeds.
- Sometimes history of previous infant or early neonatal death.

Diagnosis — Suspected inherited metabolic disorder

Babies with suspected metabolic disorders need urgent investigation if they are to have a chance of surviving. If the baby has been on clear fluids for more than 24 hours the results may be equivocal or even negative and it will then be necessary to repeat the investigation after milk has been reintroduced. If all the investigations cannot be carried out locally, arrangements should be made to send plasma and urine to a reference laboratory.

Management. This will obviously depend on the cause. If the tests have failed to establish a diagnosis, it is worth gradually introducing a low protein diet (<1 g protein/kg/day) accompanied by megavitamin therapy in an attempt to get the child to thrive. If the baby dies despite all efforts it is very important to obtain and store as much plasma as possible for future analysis and also if possible take a generous liver biopsy at the time of death on which histochemical tests can be performed at a later date for the sake of future children in the family.

Finally, there is a group of babies who are persistently hypotonic from birth but are neurologically alert. Conditions such as Down syndrome and Werdnig–Hoffmann disease should be considered.

Megavitamin therapy	
Thiamine	50 mg
Riboflavin	50 mg
Biotin	100 mg
Nicotinamide	600 mg
Pyridoxine	50 mg
Vitamin B$_{12}$	1 mg
Folic acid	15 mg
Ascorbic acid	3000 mg

VOMITING AND ABDOMINAL DISTENSION

Abdominal distension is a frequent occurrence in the immediate neonatal period. It is particularly common in the extremely preterm baby.

Problem

- Preterm baby in the first few days of life.
- Increasing gastric residue with abdominal distension.
- Bowel sounds present but diminished.
- Little or no meconium passed.

Diagnosis — Functional ileus secondary to immaturity

Ileus developing within the first few days is a frequent occurrence in preterm babies and often occurs at a time when the volume of feeds is increased, leading to gastric and gut distension. This tends to settle after 2–3 days on intravenous fluids followed by slow reintroduction of oral feeds. Ileus, however, also arises in association with systemic infection, particularly septicaemia. If the baby's general condition is in any way worrying a full infection screen (urine, blood culture, C-reactive protein, CSF and chest X-ray) must be performed and the baby commenced on intravenous antibiotics.

Problem

- A preterm or sometimes a full-term baby.
- Abdominal distension with or without bile-stained vomiting.
- Intermittent runny stools, often bile-stained.
- Abdominal X-ray showing bowel with fixed dilated loops with the appearance of gas in the gut wall.

Diagnosis — Necrotising enterocolitis

In spite of multi-centre studies this is still a poorly understood condition in which the final common pathway of damage is ischaemia of the bowel wall with the development of infection and septicaemia. The cause is probably multi-factorial and has been attributed to hypoxia, umbilical catheterisation, nasojejunal feeding and exchange transfusion. The prevalence varies widely between different neonatal units. Perforation is not uncommon and the baby may die or may survive with a considerable risk of bowel strictures.

Management is to stop all feeds, keeping the babies nil by mouth for 10–14 days, while starting broad spectrum antibiotics and metronidazole intravenously. Parenteral nutrition is used to maintain nutrition for the time that the bowel is rested. Surgical exploration is indicated if there is perforation or failure to improve on the medical management, and then resection of severely affected small bowel is often needed.

Necrotising enterocolitis

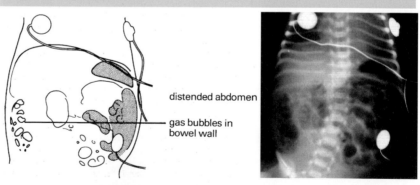

distended abdomen

gas bubbles in bowel wall

Problem

- Progressive abdominal distension from birth.
- Active bowel sounds.
- An increasing gastric residue with onset of vomiting.
- Little or no passage of meconium.
- Dilated gut with fluid levels on abdominal X-ray.

Diagnosis — Intestinal obstruction

The obstruction may occur at a number of different sites. It may be due to intraluminal lesions, for example meconium ileus, problems arising from abnormalities of the bowel wall, including *intestinal atresia*, stenosis and *Hirschsprung disease* or to external abnormalities such as malrotation, reduplication cysts and even obstructed hernias. Less commonly seen in association with Down syndrome is duodenal atresia. *Rectal agenesis* can often be diagnosed by inverting the baby and X-raying him!

Rectal atresia

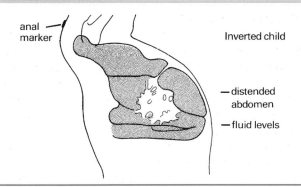

anal marker

Inverted child

— distended abdomen

— fluid levels

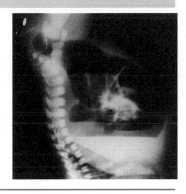

FURTHER READING

Anon 1993 Randomized study of high-frequency oscillatory ventilation in infants with severe respiratory distress syndrome. HiFO Study Group. Pediatrics 122. 609–619

Abman SH, Groothius JR 1994 Pathophysiology and treatment of bronchopulmonary dysplasia. Current issues. [Review] Pediatric Clinics of North America 41: 277–315

Archer N 1993 Patent ductus arteriosus in the newborn. [Review] Archives of Disease in Childhood 69(5 Spec No). 529–532

Brion LP, Goyal M, Suresh BR 1992 Sudden deterioration of intubated newborn: four steps to the differential diagnosis and initial management. Journal of Perinatology 12: 281–293

Coulthard MG, Vernon B 1995 Managing acute renal failure in very low birthweight infants. [Review] Archives of Disease in Childhood 73: F187–192

de Louvois J 1994 Acute bacterial meningitis in the newborn. [Review] Antimicrobial Agents and Chemotherapy 34 (Suppl A): 61–73

Field DJ, Pearson GA 1994 Neonatal extra corporeal membrane oxygenation (ECMO). [Review] Journal of Perinatal Medicine 22: 565–569

Emery EF, Greenough A, Gamsu HR 1992 Randomised controlled trial of colloid infusions in hypotensive preterm infants. Archives of Disease in Childhood 67(10 Spec No): 1185–1188

Gartner LM 1994 Neonatal jaundice. [Review] Pediatrics in Review 15: 422–432

Greenough A 1995 Patient-triggered ventilation. Pediatric Pulmonology (Suppl) 11: 98–99

Halliday HL 1995 Overview of clinical trials comparing natural and synthetic surfactants. Biology of the Neonate 67 (Suppl 1): 32–47

Holm BA 1993 Surfactant replacement therapy. New levels of understanding [editorial; comment]. [Review] American Review of Respiratory Diseases 148(4 Pt 1): 834–836

Kang JH, Shankaran S 1995 Double phototherapy with high irradiance compared with single phototherapy in neonates with hyperbilirubinemia. American Journal of Perinatology 12: 178–180

Kelsall AW 1993 Neonatal Unit, Rosie Maternity Hospital, Cambridge. Resuscitation with intraosseous lines in neonatal units Archives of Disease in Childhood 68(3 Spec No): 324–325

Klarr JM, Faix RG, Pryce CJ, Bhatt-Mehta V 1994 Randomized, blind trial of dopamine versus dobutamine for treatment of hypotension in preterm infants with respiratory distress syndrome [see comments] Journal of Pediatrics 125: 117–122

Kjartansson S, Arsan S, Hammarlund K, Sjors G, Sedin G 1995 Water loss from the skin of term and preterm infants nursed under aradiant heater. Pediatric Research 37: 233–238

Lagercrantz H 1995 Improved understanding of respiratory control—implications for the treatment of apnoea. European Journal of Pediatrics 154(8 Suppl 3): S10–12

Lemelle JL, Schmitt M, de Miscault G, Vert P, Hascoet JM 1994 Neonatal necrotizing enterocolitis: a retrospective and multicentric review of 331 cases Acta Paediatrica Scandinavica Supplement 396: 70–73

Ment LR, Oh W, Ehrenkranz RA, Philip AG, Duncan CC, Makuch RW 1995 Antenatal steroids, delivery mode, and intraventricular hemorrhage in preterm infants. American Journal of Obstetrics and Gynecology 172: 795–800

Mitton SG 1994 Amino acids and lipid in total parenteral nutrition for the newborn. [Review] Journal of Pediatric Gastroenterology and Nutrition 18: 25–31

Phibbs RH 1995 Erythropoietin therapy for extremely premature infants. [Review] Journal of Perinatal Medicine 23: 127–131

Poland RL 1995 Stabilization of the very-low-birthweight infant. Pediatrics in Review 16: 316–317

Raju TN, Langenberg P 1993 Pulmonary hemorrhage and exogenous surfactant therapy: a metaanalysis. Journal of Pediatrics 123: 603–610

Rosenfeld LE 1993 The diagnosis and management of cardiac arrhythmias in the neonatal period. [Review] Seminars in Perinatology. 17: 135–148

Roze JC, Tohier C, Maingueneau C, Lefevre M, Mouzard A 1993 Response to dobutamine and dopamine in the hypotensive very preterm infant. Archives of Disease in Childhood 69(1 Spec No): 59–63

Shaffer TH, Wolfson MR, Clark LC Jr 1992 Liquid ventilation. [Review] Pediatric Pulmonology 14: 102–109

Weindling M 1995 Periventricular haemorrhage and periventricular leukomalacia. [Review] British Journal of Obstetrics and Gynaecology 102: 278–281

White A, Marcucci G, Andrews E, Edwards K, Long W 1995 Antenatal steroids and neonatal outcomes in controlled clinical trials of surfactant replacement. The American Exosurf Neonatal Study Group I and The Canadian Exosurf Neonatal Study Group. American Journal of Obstetrics and Gynecology 173: 286–90

Ear, nose and throat

Traditionally diseases of the ears, nose and throat (ENT) are considered together. This is as it should be, for a symptom or sign suggesting a problem at one of the three sites is often due to a disease at another (e.g. ear-ache in children often occurs with tonsillitis). Certain symptoms obviously arise from the ears, nose or throat, for example sore throat, hoarseness, stridor, nasal obstruction, discharge or nose bleeds, ear-ache, aural discharge or deafness, but others, cough, pyrexia, and headache, are less specific. Whatever the presenting feature, the possibility of a systemic disorder should be considered and a proper clinical enquiry will extend well beyond the ears and upper respiratory tract.

SORE THROAT

One of the commoner ear, nose and throat complaints in children is a sore throat. It may be acute or chronic. Acute sore throats are relatively common in childhood but not all acute sore throats are due to tonsillitis.

Problem

- Sore throat of sudden onset often with pain radiating to the ears.
- Malaise, the child voluntarily goes to bed or to lie on a sofa.
- Fever, a raised temperature sometimes above 39°C.
- Upper deep cervical lymphadenopathy, the jugulo-digastric, tonsillar, nodes are enlarged, tender and painful.
- Tonsils are inflamed with or without pus in the tonsillar crypts.

Diagnosis — Acute tonsillitis

This is a systemic illness and prior to the availabilty of antibiotics was considered to be serious. It is a common complaint in children, particularly in the early school years. Investigation rarely adds to the clinical picture. Bacteriology swabs for culture and sensitivity may be taken and these will usually show haemolytic streptococcus if they show anything. The preferred form of treatment is one of the penicillin antibiotics with analgesics.

Tonsillar infection

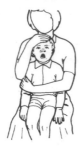

TONSILLITIS

 acute
parenchymatous

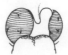 asymmetrical—
suspect quinsy

 acute—
follicular

 very rarely
causes
obstruction

Complications. Rarely the illness may be unresponsive to treatment or sufficiently severe to justify admission. If there is asymmetry of the clinical signs then the possibility that a quinsy has developed should be considered. There may be trismus and more rarely stridor. A poor response to parenteral antibiotic therapy suggests that pus has formed and drainage is required. In these circumstances giving a general anaesthetic can be technically difficult and should only be attempted by a highly skilled anaesthetist experienced in dealing with children. There is a real possibility of rupture of the quinsy with the associated danger of aspiration of the pus. As an alternative, mild sedation and local analgesia may be used to facilitate incision and drainage of the abscess. The diagnosis of quinsy is rarely made in children; it is more often suspected retrospectively when peri-tonsillar fibrosis is found at tonsillectomy.

Prognosis. Following an acute attack of tonsillitis a full recovery is to be expected. A few children fail to show full recovery and subsequently develop a state of chronic tonsillitis.

Problem

- Recurrent episodes of tonsillitis (perhaps more correctly called relapsing tonsillitis).
- The child is never 100% well in between (this chronic malaise often only becomes apparent in retrospect after tonsillectomy when the improvement in the child's general health and appetite becomes manifest).

Diagnosis — Chronic tonsillitis

A persistent sore throat may be ascribed to chronic tonsillar infection, even in the absence of a history of repeated acute attacks. In addition to the complaint of a sore throat there may be a history of poor general health, lack of energy, bad breath and occasional ear-ache. Examination will often reveal the presence of enlarged upper deep cervical lymph glands and, as in cases of recurrent acute tonsillitis, a variable picture on pharyngeal inspection. Again a reliable sign is the presence of a marked flush on the anterior faucial pillars. Whilst bacteriological culture of a pharyngeal swab will probably disclose the infecting organism, usually streptococcus, it is unlikely to alter the management. A long course (2–3 weeks) of a broad spectrum antibiotic may be tried; if this fails then tonsillectomy is indicated.

Tonsillectomy

Age is an important factor when considering the need for the operation. Children are most prone to repeated tonsillitis between the ages of 4 and 8 years and spontaneous resolution of the symptoms is likely as the child grows older, so that children do 'tend to grow out of it'. The severity of the symptoms in the individual child must be taken into account in assessing the need for tonsillectomy, but it is not usually recommended that the tonsils should be removed unless:

— The child suffers from at least four attacks of tonsillitis per year, these attacks occurring during the winter months, and requiring several weeks' absence from school each year.
— Children under the age of 4 years who develop recurrent tonsillitis are likely to continue having recurrences of infection for many years and tonsillectomy might be considered with as few as 2 or 3 attacks per year.
— In children over the age of 8 years spontaneous resolution of the attacks is also less likely and tonsillectomy is advised if attacks persist at a rate of 2 to 3 each year.

Rarely does tonsillar appearance affect the decision of whether or not to operate. The appearance may vary from very small and deeply buried tonsils to massive fleshy and pitted structures. It is only in the extreme case that the tonsils are sufficiently large to interfere with swallowing food. Very rarely tonsillar enlargement may cause respiratory obstruction with carbon dioxide retention and hypoxia at night leading to pulmonary hypertension. This is more likely in dysmorphic children, e.g. Down syndrome. A common sign in cases of recurrent tonsillitis is the presence of a marked flush on the medial border of the anterior faucial pillars. A history of nephritis, cardiac disease or other systemic disease such as diabetes mellitus will of course influence the decision to operate. Frequently after tonsillectomy for recurrent acute tonsillitis the parent will make the observation that the child's general health is better, the child appears considerably brighter, healthier and happier and frequently that his or her appetite has improved dramatically. This has been attributed to the removal of a source of chronic sepsis.

Problem

• Generalised sore throat in a miserable child.
• Nasal congestion.
• Diffuse inflammation of the oropharynx.

Diagnosis — Acute pharyngitis
This is very common, usually presenting as part of the clinical picture of a coryzal attack. The infecting organism is usually a virus, either an adenovirus or an influenza virus, and a throat swab will add little information. Hospital admission is not required and treatment is

symptomatic, requiring rest at home, frequent hot drinks and analgesics. Throat pastilles will help soothe the sore throat.

Acute pharyngitis is a precursor of measles; Koplik's spots will usually be seen as discrete white nodules with a surrounding area of erythema on the mucosa of the inside of the cheek. The possibility of infectious mononucleosis should be considered if the child fails to show the early recovery expected in coryzal and influenzal infections or if he or she develops a membrane on the tonsils and pharynx. Often these children have a line of petechial spots where the hard palate joins the soft. In these cases, a Paul Bunnell or Monospot test and a full blood count should be carried out. If glandular fever is suspected the use of ampicillin should be avoided as there is a high risk of producing a rash.

Acute pharyngitis occurs in scarlet fever, typhoid and diphtheria. The clinical picture in the two former is that of the underlying disease; diphtheria is now rare in the UK, as is Vincents angina — acute membranous pharyngitis — in which there is a mild sore throat accompanied by a high temperature. Examination in this latter condition shows a membrane over the tonsil which is readily stripped. Culture shows the two infecting organisms, the spirochaete and *Bacillus fusiformis*. Response to penicillin is usually rapid.

Acute pharyngitis may also be the presenting symptom of several haematological disorders, including acute lymphatic leukaemia, agranulocytosis and Hodgkin disease. Examination of a blood film is therefore indicated if one of these conditions is suspected.

Some children may present with a persistent sore throat and a history of nasal airway obstruction; in these children the cause of the sore throat and associated symptoms is a chronic adenoiditis and sinusitis and this will be discussed under nasal diseases.

Immunocompromised children, including those with HIV, may present with a sore throat due to oral candidiasis. HIV should also be included in the differential diagnosis of children with persistent cervical lymphadenopathy.

If a child complains of a sore throat and there is a history suggesting a foreign body, pharyngeal inspection is required. If it is not possible to obtain the child's co-operation then examination under anaesthetic will be necessary. Radio-opaque foreign bodies can be excluded by a lateral soft tissue radiograph.

Problem

- Persistent nasal obstruction with snoring but no rhinorrhoea.
- Often mild chronic pharyngitis, enlarged cervical lymph nodes and history of recurrent or persistent night-time cough.

Diagnosis — Nasal obstruction secondary to enlarged adenoids

Other than the common cold, the commonest cause of nasal obstruction is the presence of enlarged adenoids. This may occur in children at any age and the diagnosis needs also to be considered in infancy, although typically it is a much more common problem in children between the ages of 4 and 8 years of age. The symptoms of sore throat and night-time cough are usually due to a combination of mouth breathing and mucopurulent postnasal discharge. Sometimes this discharge may be so severe as to cause relative anorexia and if ingested, as is not uncommon, may cause vomiting and failure to thrive, especially in the younger child.

Examination of the postnasal space is frequently unrewarding in children. The child with enlarged adenoids presents as a mouth breather with dry lips and a 'nasal' voice (rhinolalia clausa). The child may sniff frequently due to the presence of a persistent postnasal discharge. Enlarged cervical glands are often palpable and on occasions even visible.

Treatment with topical nasal decongestants in the form of drops or sprays has no place in the management except in the very short term, and effective treatment is by adenoidectomy and attention to any associated sinus infection.

Adenoids (the child is wearing an ear ring!)

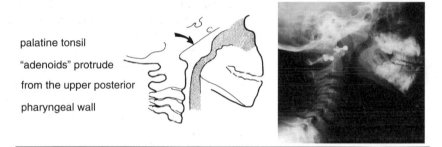

palatine tonsil

"adenoids" protrude

from the upper posterior

pharyngeal wall

NASAL DISCHARGE

Problem

- A history of persistent nasal airway obstruction associated with clear rhinorrhoea, which at times becomes purulent.
- Sneezing.
- Examination of the nasal mucosa shows rather pale congested mucosa especially over the turbinates and the presence of a thin film of clear mucus.

Diagnosis — Allergic rhinitis or vasomotor rhinitis

These can be considered together as many of their symptoms are identical. The main difference is that in nasal allergy the symptoms are related to some specific event or environment in which an allergen is to be found. There may be a seasonal variation as with hay fever. Close questioning of the parent is essential and it is helpful to go through a list of common allergens on several consultations as it is not uncommon for a parent to return on a subsequent visit and give a rather more detailed account, having had time to reflect on possible relevant factors.

Sneezing is common and the child may have an itchy nose, frequently rubbing it. This may result in a horizontal linear crease just above the tip of the nose and the child may typically be seen to rub the palm of his hand vertically over the tip of the nose — the so called allergic salute. There may be an associated history of bronchospasm. In many children there is a positive family history of allergy or other atopic disorder, and there may be other stigmata of allergic disease such as eczema.

Sinuses

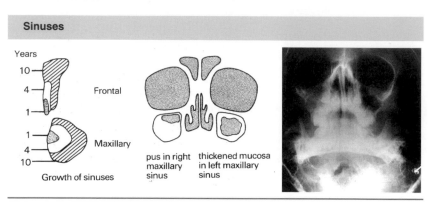

First attempt to establish the nature of the allergen(s). They are not necessarily inhalants but they may be ingested. Confirmation of the allergen can be demonstrated by showing an improvement in the symptoms after removal of the offending agent from the child's environment. Skin testing is rarely carried out now; nasal provocation testing is also rarely used. Full blood count and microscopic examination and nasal smears may show the presence of numerous eosinophils. Serum IgE levels and RAST tests (radioallergosorbent test) help to confirm the allergic basis of the rhinitis. If allergens cannot be incriminated a diagnosis of vasomotor rhinitis is assumed.

Assessment of the part played by a deflected septum is not always easy and the other conditions should be treated first. Septal surgery is unwise in young children and should be left whenever possible until the growth of the facial and nasal skeleton has finished, usually by the age of 17 years. However, severe septal deformity will be seen from time to time and will require correction to prevent frequent recurrent or persistent sinusitis. In these cases the correct surgery is septoplasty rather than submucous resection.

Problem

• Nasal congestion with a persistent purulent discharge.

Diagnosis — Chronic sinusitis

As a general truism the child who has nasal obstruction has enlarged adenoids; the child with nasal congestion and a purulent discharge has sinusitis, often coupled with adenoiditis. These symptoms may occur secondary to other nasal pathology, including septal deviations. Nasal polypi are rare in childhood, other than in cases of cystic fibrosis.

| Problem | • Unilateral clear rhinorrhoea with a previous history of a head injury. |

Diagnosis — CSF rhinorrhoea due to a skull fracture of the anterior cranial fossa

This requires treatment with prophylactic antibiotics until it dries up; failure to do so merits referral to a neurosurgical unit for formal repair of the dural defect.

| Problem | • Purulent unilateral rhinorrhoea, often offensive or blood stained. |

Diagnosis — Probably a foreign body

Unilateral purulent nasal discharge should always suggest the possibility of a foreign body in the nose and anterior rhinoscopy will usually reveal its presence. The discharge is frequently offensive. If it is not possible to remove the offending object in the out-patient department, the child may require admission for the removal of the foreign body under a short general anaesthetic.

NASAL OBSTRUCTION AT BIRTH

Choanal atresia

Associated abnormalities include:
    mental deficiency
    short stature
    deafness
    coloboma

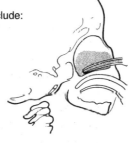
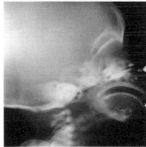

| Problem | • A newborn infant is unable to respire despite strenuous attempts and becomes cyanosed.
• The obstruction can be relieved by inserting an oral airway and fixing this in place. |

Diagnosis — Bilateral posterior choanal atresia

If suspected, the diagnosis can readily be confirmed by passing a catheter into the nose and demonstrating that it cannot be passed into the nasopharynx. Surgical treatment can then be carried out in the next few days when the atresia segment is either broken down or bored through and polythene tubes inserted to maintain the lumen. Unilateral atresia is often overlooked until the child is 4 or 5 years old, when he or she may present with unilateral nasal obstruction and a runny nose. The diagnosis can be confirmed by probing the nose with a soft rubber catheter after the use of topical anaesthesia. CT scanning has become the accepted radiological investigation; it may show whether the atresia plate is bony or fibrous. Tumours of the nose are rare in children. They may be congenital — nasal glioma or encephalocoele, dermoid tumour, or develop later — usually sarcoma, the commonest being rhabdomyosarcoma.

NOSE BLEEDS

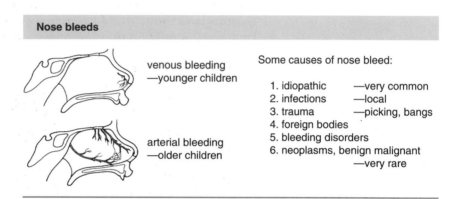

Nose bleeds

venous bleeding
—younger children

arterial bleeding
—older children

Some causes of nose bleed:

1. idiopathic   —very common
2. infections   —local
3. trauma   —picking, bangs
4. foreign bodies
5. bleeding disorders
6. neoplasms, benign malignant
                   —very rare

Management

In accident and emergency department. This is a common problem in children of all ages but particularly between the ages of 4 and 8 years. Hospital admission is rarely required. Bleeding is almost invariably from Little's area and in most epistaxes, pressure on the soft part of the nose is sufficient to arrest the bleeding. Pressure should be maintained for 15 minutes by the clock.

In-patient. Very rarely, if the simple measures outlined above fail, the child may need admission and even more rarely insertion of a small nasal pack. Any history of any tendency to bleed or bruise readily in the child or any family is sought. A full blood count and film and assessment of bleeding and clotting characteristics should be carried out.

Outpatient. Children are frequently seen as outpatients with a history of repeated nose bleeds but who are not bleeding at the time. In all these children a blood count should be taken. Examination of the nose will show dilated vessels in one or both Little's areas. These become particularly prominent after application of a small cotton wool pledget soaked in 10% cocaine solution. Once local anaesthesia is achieved chemical cautery agents (e.g. silver nitrate in solid form, chromic acid bead or trichloracetic acid) are applied to the vessels feeding the plexus. If a small scab is seen over a site of recent bleeding, care should be taken not to disturb this as fresh bleeding may be provoked.

Surgery. Should the use of chemical cautery not prove successful, it will be necessary to admit the child for a short general anaesthesic in order to cauterise the bleeding area using electrocautery. It should always be stressed that nose picking is a common cause of nose bleeds, especially after nasal cautery. Any haematological abnormality must be followed up as appropriate.

EAR-ACHE

Ear-ache is a common symptom in childhood. It is frequently an accompaniment of acute tonsillitis, the pain being referred to the ears, although it should always be remembered that otitis media can occur in association with tonsillitis and therefore the ears must be examined even in the presence of obvious tonsillar infection. Similarly in the post-tonsillectomy period ear-ache is common. Mild or moderate ear-ache is a frequent symptom in otitis media with effusion.

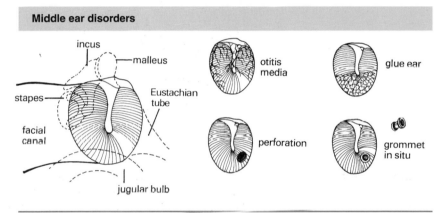

Middle ear disorders

Otitis externa is uncommon in childhood and the finding of an oede-matous infected external auditory canal must always prompt the search for an underlying otitis media. Clinically one of the pointers in the history which distinguishes acute otitis media and externa is the relative timing of the pain to any discharge. Typically the pain precedes the discharge in acute otitis media. The reverse occurs in otitis externa.

Problem

- Ear-ache which may be sufficiently severe for the child to wake up from sleep.
- High temperature in an unwell child.
- Often evidence of upper respiratory tract infection.
- Inflammatory changes involving the tympanic membrane.

Diagnosis — Acute otitis media

In early cases the eardrum will appear injected, even slightly indrawn due to negative intratympanic pressure resulting from the acute salpin-gitis; subsequently there is bulging and marked reddening of the tympanic membrane followed by rupture and discharge of a purulent, often blood-stained, matter. Assessment includes examination of the nose and pharynx when the origin of the ear infection may be found. In many cases the drum does not perforate and assessment is confined to the clinical appearance of the ear and the general well being of the child.

Medicines. Treatment is started empirically with antibiotics, preferably with one of the penicillin group, the organism being one of the following: *Haemolytic streptococcus*, *Staphylococcus pyogenes*, pneumococcus or *Haemophilus influenzae*. Start the treatment parenterally and change this to oral agents as soon as the temperature drops and the child can more readily take drugs by mouth. Analgesics are necessary, and it is desirable to prescribe also a suitable nasal decongestant, both systemically and topically.

Ear toilet. If the ear is already discharging the pain will have been largely relieved; a swab can be taken for bacteriological examination and the ear gently dry mopped providing the child can co-operate sufficiently. It is pointless to persist if the child is restless and agitated as more harm, both physical and psychological, may be caused.

Surgery. Hospital admission is rarely required for cases of acute otitis media. The main indication is failure to respond to out-patient treatment. In these cases large doses of intramuscular antibiotics will often settle the infection. Occasionally a myringotomy will be needed requiring a short general anaesthetic. By this means the abscess is drained and pus can also be sent for culture and sensitivity, so that treatment can be amended accordingly. Very rarely a child may present with a facial palsy in association with acute otitis media. Then it is necessary to carry out a myringotomy at a very early stage in order to obtain pus for culture and sensitivity. Large doses of antibiotics should be administered; as the acute otitis media settles the facial palsy is likely to resolve.

Problem

• Rarely a child may present with swelling or marked tenderness in the post-auricular region associated with other symptoms of acute suppurative otitis media.

Diagnosis — Acute mastoiditis

Urgent admission is required. X-rays usually show marked clouding of a well pneumatised mastoid air cell system with coalescence or

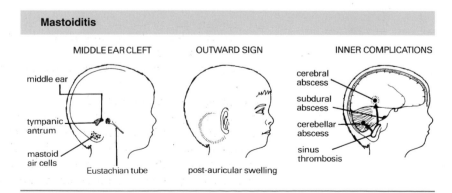

Mastoiditis

MIDDLE EAR CLEFT — middle ear, tympanic antrum, mastoid air cells, Eustachian tube

OUTWARD SIGN — post-auricular swelling

INNER COMPLICATIONS — cerebral abscess, subdural abscess, cerebellar abscess, sinus thrombosis

necrosis of the bony septa between the air cells; this helps to differentiate mastoiditis from furunculosis of the ear canal. Treatment is with analgesics, large doses of antibiotics by injection, preferably one of the penicillins, followed by surgical exploration of the mastoid and cortical mastoidectomy, at the earliest opportunity.

EAR DISCHARGE

It is necessary to distinguish between the common waxy discharge and a purulent discharge. Wax may vary from a thin light brown material to a dark brown, hard impacted substance. Its differing appearance and quantity have no clinical significance. The discharge of acute suppurative otitis media is often blood stained and there is usually a clear history of the acute infection. In chronic suppurative otitis media (CSOM) the discharge may be either profuse and mucopurulent or thin, offensive and scanty. This provides an important indication to the aetiology, pathology and hence management of the underlying disorder.

Problem

- A profuse mucoid or mucopurulent discharge.
- Central tympanic perforation revealing oedematous and congested middle ear mucosa.
- Little tenderness.

Diagnosis — Tubotympanic disease

This type occurs more commonly in children from poorer social backgrounds where personal hygiene is less and where there is a greater prevalence of upper respiratory tract disorder. It is associated with signs of upper respiratory tract infection and is often unilateral. There is usually a concomitant deafness, but rarely any serious complications. Bacterial examination of the discharge usually reveals upper respiratory tract pathogens. The management is directed towards the underlying upper respiratory tract infection.

Problem

- Offensive, thin, scanty aural discharge.
- Defect in the pars flaccida or Schrapnell's membrane which may be difficult to see.
- Sometimes a cholesteatoma which is visible through the defect.

Diagnosis — Attico-antral disease

In this there is a real danger of complications such as facial palsy, labyrinthine fistula or intracranial problems, hence the terminology of so-called 'safe' and 'unsafe' ears. If examination of the ear by direct vision, even with the assistance of the Siegle or pneumatic, proves unsatisfactory, then examination under the operating microscope

Cholesteatoma

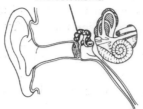

cholesteatoma

Surgery:

approached from mastoid
—peeled free then sucked
out

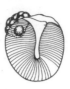

becomes essential, with or without the benefit of general anaesthesia. In both types of disease aural polypi may be found either deep in the meatus or, if sufficiently large, presenting at the introitus of the auditory canal. These must be removed and the ear closely inspected.

Whilst X-rays may show signs of chronic ear disease, they seldom influence management and therefore do not need to be taken routinely. Gram-negative organisms such as proteus species and pseudomonas may be cultured from the discharge. In attico-antral disease conservative management includes the use of topical antiseptics or antibiotics with the intention of controlling any secondary infection and suction toilet of the defect under anaesthetic. Early surgical exploration of the mastoid is required. Cholesteatoma may occur in the presence of a moderately well pneumatised mastoid in children and may, therefore, be very extensive.

A history of a clear aural discharge after a head injury should always alert the doctor to the possibility of skull fracture, with escape of cerebrospinal fluid which is initially blood stained. Even if X-rays do not show any fracture the patient should be treated as if one is present and penicillin and one of the sulphonamides prescribed, the ear covered with a sterile dressing and head injury observations instituted. Usually CSF otorrhoea settles spontaneously. However, the possibility of either a conductive or sensorineural hearing loss secondary to the head injury must not be forgotten.

DEAFNESS

Deafness may present in children in a variety of ways. It may present purely and simply by the parent or perhaps the school teacher noticing the child having difficulty in hearing. Should a parent bring a child with such a history it is imperative that the child is regarded as having a hearing loss until and unless it can be clearly shown on testing that this is not so. Whilst a positive history of a child having difficulty in hearing is of immense value, it should be stressed that lack of parental awareness of a hearing loss does not necessarily mean the child hears normally. Children may, however, present with a variety of other complaints related to and directly or indirectly caused by the hearing loss.

In the case of the very young child a history of late talking or failure to develop normal speech and language may be of great significance. Clearly this history must be taken in conjunction with the child's general developmental history. The older child who is already at school may present with learning difficulties and in particular may show slowness in learning to read compared with other educational skills. A history of underachievement may be of great significance.

Children of all ages may present with behaviour disturbance, such disturbance may take the form of disobedience, either as an attention-seeking device or simply because the child does not hear what is said. Other forms of behaviour disturbance occur such as tantrums or becoming enuretic. Withdrawal is not an uncommon finding in children who develop a hearing loss.

Assessment

The methods of assessment and management of deafness are determined by the age of the child as well as the degree and nature of the hearing loss. All children should receive a screening test of hearing initially between the ages of 6 and 9 months when the child is able to respond to simple distraction methods of testing, later at the age of 2 or 3 years and subsequently on school entry. It is important that any child who fails this test of screening should be followed up by an otologist and further more definitive testing of the child's hearing carried out. Pre-term babies requiring intensive care in special care baby units are particularly at risk of deafness and may be screened using one of several techniques including oto-acoustic emissions and brainstem electric response audiometry. In almost all children it is possible to carry out some form of subjective audiometry, determined by the age of the child, and of course by the child's general development. Clearly a child with multiple handicaps, and in particular one with mental retardation, may require other methods of testing such as evoked response audiometry.

Whilst distraction testing is suitable for children between approximately 6 and 18 months, older children may be encouraged to carry out play audiometry and the child may be conditioned to respond to sound, for example by placing a toy in a container. Above the age of 3–4 years, it is usually possible in an otherwise healthy child to construct conventional pure tone audiograms using audiometry.

Problem

- A child with a mild to moderate hearing loss, noticed by parents or school teachers or picked up on routine screening testing. A history of recurrent mild or moderate ear-ache. Recurrent acute suppurative otitis media.
- A history of upper respiratory tract infection with nasal obstruction.
- The ear drum may be abnormal in appearance, but often it is difficult to distinguish the appearance of the ear drum from normal.

Diagnosis — Otitis media with effusion (OME)

The commonest cause of deafness is glue ear or otitis media with effusion. This condition has received a variety of synonyms and is common throughout childhood, even in children under 1 year of age. Suspicion of the hearing loss is all important in the diagnosis and management of a child with OME. The hearing loss varies from child to child and, even more importantly, an individual child's loss may fluctuate. Although many clues suggest the presence of OME, the final diagnosis rests on a combination of examination, audiometry and tympanometry. Examination of the child's ear reveals a range of appearances. At one extreme the ear drum may appear almost completely normal unless the Siegle (pneumatic) speculum is used to assess drum mobility. Other appearances include loss of the normal light reflex, a completely dull and featureless drum head, a yellow sheen to the tympanic membrane and a deep slate blue discoloration. The drum may be quite retracted with the handle of the malleus directed almost horizontally. Fluid levels and air bubbles may be seen but these are less common findings. By the age of 5 years it may be possible to elicit a Rinne test using the C2–512 Hz tuning fork. A negative result indicates bone conduction to be better than air conduction and suggests a conductive element of approximately 20 dB or greater. Pure tone audiometry may demonstrate the conductive loss but tympanometry is diagnostic

Management

The initial stage in the management of all children with a conductive hearing loss (and indeed a sensorineural one) is parental advice and guidance. In many children this may be all that is required to help the child and the parents or teachers cope with the deafness. Parental smoking is an important risk factor for OME.

Surgery. Insertion of ventilating tubes or grommets will result in improvement in the hearing and the United States Department of Health has drawn up guidelines for their use. Adenoidectomy, particularly in children between the ages of 4 and 8 years, has been shown to promote resolution of OME. Tonsillectomy is not an operation to be considered in the management of OME, although other indications for tonsillectomy may co-exist with OME.

Two groups of children are prone to secretory otitis. First, almost all children with Down syndrome have OME and in the majority surgery is not applicable, in part at least due to the very narrow auditory meati found in these children. Treatment with a hearing aid is the most appropriate method of providing adequate hearing. Second, children with cleft palate also invariably have OME; for them long term middle ear ventilation is often the best method of managing deafness and is preferable to hearing only with the help of a hearing aid.

Problem

- Failed neonatal hearing screen, or screen at 6/9 months.
- Parental concern about hearing.
- Poor or absent language development.

Diagnosis — Sensorineural hearing loss

Many children with these symptoms will have a conductive hearing loss but a few will have a severe or profound sensorineural hearing deficit. Wherever there is concern about the hearing in infants, adequate tests must be carried out to be sure that their hearing is normal. Failure to pick up a severe hearing loss early will lead to a lost opportunity to help the child and can be very frustrating to parents. About one in a 1000 children has a congenital, severe or profound hearing loss. This may be hereditary (dominant, autosomal recessive or X-linked), associated with severe neonatal problems, congenital infections (e.g. Rubella), part of a syndrome or of unknown cause. It is especially common in low birthweight preterm babies.

Hearing aids. Treatment with hearing aids can start at a few months of age. The earlier hearing aids are fitted, the better chance the child has of developing normal speech and language. With early hearing aids and input from specialist teachers of the deaf, normal or near normal speech and language can be achieved by many deaf children.

Sensorineural hearing loss can also be acquired at any time in childhood. Meningitis is the commonest reason for this and can lead to profound deafness. All children should have their hearing tested after bacterial meningitis. Children who appear to hear normally but have poor language development may have a high-tone hearing loss. Even a quiet voice will be heard but the high frequency components (the consonants of speech) will be lost, so that words do not make sense. This leads to much frustration until the correct diagnosis is made and appropriate hearing aids are fitted. A small number of children with severe or profound sensorineural deafness will fail to show benefit with even the most powerful hearing aids; in these children cochlear implantation may be considered. It is estimated that in the UK about 250–300 children per year will require this method of (re)habilitation.

HOARSENESS

This may be caused by acute laryngitis, chronic laryngitis or Singer's nodes. Hoarseness is a relatively common complaint in children, usually short lived and associated with acute upper respiratory tract infection. Occasionally, however, it may persist and come to the attention of the laryngologist. It is rarely possible to visualise the larynx in a child, partly due to lack of co-operation on the part of the child. However, even when the child is able and willing to allow indirect laryngoscopy, the normal anatomy of the child's larynx precludes a view of the vocal cords due to the omega-shaped epiglottis which obscures vision. Thus it may become necessary to carry out direct laryngoscopy under a general anaesthesia for a firm diagnosis to be made. Whether chronic diffuse laryngitis or Singer's nodes are found, it is not necessary to remove any tissue.

The child should be instructed in the presence of the parents on the need to rest the voice; in a child this essentially means avoiding shouting, as complete voice rest is a forlorn hope. Speech therapy may help. Attention is paid to any sepsis in the upper respiratory tract, and the child kept under review until the condition settles.

FURTHER READING

Chalmers D, Stewart I, Silva P, Mulvena A 1989 Otitis media with effusion — The Dunedin Study. McKeith Press, London

Crombie IK, Barr G 1990 An investigation into factors that may influence tonsil morphology. Journal of the Royal Society of Medicine 83: 20–21

Davis A, Wood S, Healy R, Webb H, Rowe S 1995 Risk factors for hearing disorders: epidemiologic evidence of change over time in the UK. Journal of the American Academy of Audiology 6: 365–370

Gibbin KP 1993 Otological considerations in the first five years of life. In: McCormick B (ed) Paediatric audiology 0–5 years. Whurr Publishers, London

Hadfield PJ, Birchall MA, Novelli V, Bakley CM 1996 The ENT manifestations of HIV infection in children. Clinical Otolaryngology 21: 30–36

Haggard MP, Hughes E 1991 Screening children's hearing A review of the literature and the implications of otitis media. HMSO, London

McCormick B, Archbold S, Sheppard S 1994 Cochlear implants for young children. Whurr Publishers, London

Mills R 1996 The management of childhood otitis media with effusion. Journal of the Royal Society of Medicine 89: 132–134

Nelson JD (ed) 1990 Update on otitis media. International Congress and Symposium Series Number 164. Royal Society of Medicine Services Limited, London

Parson DS (ed) 1996 Pediatric Sinusitis. Otolaryngologic Clinics of North America. Vol 29

Sell D 1987 Disorders of speech. In: Evans JNG (ed) Scott-Brown's Otolaryngology, vol 6, 5th edn. Paediatric Otolaryngology Butterworth, London

9 Airways and lungs

The respiratory tract responds to a wide variety of pathological processes with a limited number of symptoms and signs. Nevertheless it is usually possible to define the part of the airway or lung most affected and to guess at the aetiology from the history, age and clinical findings. The most helpful diagnostic symptoms and signs are acute stridor, chronic stridor, coughing and wheezing attacks often with breathlessness, recurrent coughing without wheezing, and chronic coughing with persistent or progressive breathlessness.

ACUTE STRIDOR

Stridor is a harsh sound caused by obstruction in the larynx or trachea and is predominantly inspiratory, although a quieter expiratory component may be present, especially in lesions involving the trachea.

Problem (common)

- Coryzal symptoms for 1–2 days with cough and hoarseness.
- Often commences at night, worse on crying or when disturbed.
- Sternal retraction and use of accessory muscles.
- Little constitutional disturbance with mild or absent pyrexia.

Diagnosis — Acute laryngo-tracheo-bronchitis (croup)

This condition, which is always viral (usually the para-influenza, RSV or rhino-virus), is produced by airway narrowing as a result of mucosal oedema and secretions in the upper airway. The following should be assessed and documented; severity of stridor and whether or not it is present at rest, degree of recession, heart and respiratory rate, presence of cyanosis or pallor and level of consciousness. Indications for admission to hospital include cyanosis, exhaustion or drowsiness, stridor present at rest, parental anxiety or poor social conditions. Lateral X-ray of the neck may be helpful if a foreign body or epiglottitis is suspected but is usually unnecessary.

Management

As acute upper airway obstructions are potentially fatal and yet eminently treatable, it is crucial that the children should be monitored carefully for signs of increasing obstruction so that appropriate measures can be taken before irreversible changes have occurred. The features that need monitoring are heart rate, respiratory rate, severity of stridor, degree of recession, colour and level of consciousness.

Croup

1. Consider possibility of foreign body or acute epiglottitis

2. Do not attempt to visualise epiglottitis unless you are prepared for immediate intubation/tracheostomy

3. Do not leave the child unattended at any time—even in the X-ray Dept.

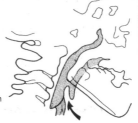 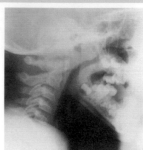

Reassurance. The normal tendency for the larynx to collapse on inspiration is grossly exaggerated in croup. All efforts should therefore be made to reassure and calm the child in order to lessen these dynamic changes.

Mist therapy. Warm mist or steam may be useful at home, but there is no evidence that cold mist in hospital is of any value. Jet nebulisers are most unlikely to have any effect on the relative humidity in the airways. Ultrasonic nebulisers will raise the water content, but at the expense of hiding the child in a dense mist, making careful observation and nursing care difficult. Such a mist may also induce lower airways obstruction in susceptible children.

Medicines. Antibiotics are not indicated unless acute epiglottitis is suspected. Systemic steroids are useful, particularly in children requiring intubation. Intravenous hydrocortisone (100 mg 6 hourly) or oral prednisolone (1–2 mg/kg body weight/24 h) can be given. There are now several studies which have shown that high dose inhaled topical steroids, e.g. nebulised budesonide 1–2 mg, shortens the episode, and if given in domiciliary practice, reduces the need for hospital admission. Inhalation of adrenalin (1 ml of 1/1000) from a nebuliser and face mask device will often produce relief. This, however, will only last for 20–30 minutes and is sometimes followed by rebound deterioration. It is therefore not suitable for out-patient treatment, but can be used to buy time and may avoid the need for intubation in some children.

Intubation. Approximately 1% of children with croup requiring admission to hospital undergo intubation. Indications for intubation are drowsiness or restlessness due to hypoxia and rising heart and respiratory rate. If time permits, intubation should be carried out by a highly skilled anaesthetist as this is a difficult procedure. If the child is deteriorating rapidly then emergency intubation may be necessary but this should only be carried out when facilities for an immediate tracheostomy are to hand. Extubation is usually possible after 2–3 days.

The majority of children have a single isolated attack. Some children have recurrent attacks of croup and a small number undoubtedly go on to develop asthma in later childhood.

Problem (rare)

- Acute illness with high temperature (often 39.5°C+) and associated toxic state, unwell for less than 2 days.
- Acute onset of severe inspiratory and expiratory stridor which is rapidly progressive.
- Child appears anxious, still, swallowing is painful and so there often is drooling of saliva.

Diagnosis — Acute epiglottitis

This is a severe bacterial infection caused by *Haemophilus influenzae*, Type B. The incidence has fallen following the introduction of Hib immunisation. The peak-age incidence is 2–3 years, unlike croup which is seen most in the second year of life. Document in the same way as in acute viral croup. Carefully assess the severity of the child's condition, as it may be necessary to bypass the obstruction immediately to prevent death. Whenever this condition is suspected the child must be admitted to hospital. Lateral X-ray of the neck will usually visualise the epiglottis, but the trip to the X-ray department may be hazardous. Direct inspection of the epiglottis by an experienced paediatric anaesthetist, under general anaesthetic and intubation if necessary, is the ideal course of action. Blood culture often confirms infection with *H. influenzae*.

Epiglottitis

pharyngeal ballooning

pea-like epiglottis

no apparent foreign body

Swollen epiglottis

It is of paramount importance to observe very carefully as the obstruction can progress rapidly.

Medicines. As some strains of *H. influenzae* are resistant to amoxycillin it is usual to give a third generation cephalosporin, e.g. cephotaxime. Intravenous hydrocortisone or oral prednisolone are sometimes given, but it is not known whether either contribute to the child's recovery. Any child who shows signs of cyanosis or hypoxia requires intubation.

Intubation. Many units now electively intubate all children with acute epiglottitis, others are more conservative but even so some 60% of all children admitted require intubation. The tube will need to be left in place for 12–24 hours to allow time for the inflammation to settle.

Problem

- Moderate pyrexia for 2–3 days.
- Croupy cough with increasing upper airway obstruction.
- Extensive tracheal inflammation and copious secretions with no gross epiglottic changes on laryngoscopy.

Diagnosis — Acute bacterial tracheitis (pseudomembranous croup)
This condition is relatively rare and can mimic both acute laryngo-tracheo-bronchitis and acute epiglottitis. It is important that it is recognised because it is usually but not always due to *Staphylococcus aureus* or *H. influenzae*. Virtually all the children will require intubation and both anti-staphylococcal and broad spectrum anti-biotics, e.g. flucloxacillin and ampicillin. Frequent tracheal toilet is required and the children often require intubation for several days.

Problem

- No history of previous upper respiratory tract infection.
- A history of sudden onset of coughing and stridor whilst running around or playing with small objects.

Diagnosis — Foreign body
This should always be considered in any child with acute stridor, par-ticularly if there are any atypical features. Lateral X-ray of the larynx will show up radio-opaque objects clearly, for example tin soldiers. Often, however, other objects can also be visualised by contrast with the laryngeal and trachea air. If the child's condition permits, the for-eign body can be removed in theatre under direct vision under general anaesthesia. If the child is cyanosed and/or unconscious try to visu-alise the object with a laryngoscope. If this is impossible proceed with emergency tracheostomy.

Problem

- Very occasionally children have onset of painless swelling involving various parts of the body, e.g. hands, feet, genitals, joints, face and lips, often with areas of urticaria. Rarely these children develop stridor.

Diagnosis — Angioneurotic oedema
Give i.v. hydrocortisone (100–200 mg) and i.v. antihistamines (e.g. chlorpheniramine 2–5 mg). If the stridor is severe and the response is slow, inject subcutaneous adrenaline 0.5–1 mg (1/1000) over 5 minutes.

Problem

- Very rarely in the UK a child presents with toxaemia, oedema of the neck with ulcerating lesions of the tonsillar bed forming a membrane which tends to bleed.

Diagnosis — Diphtheria

Send a throat swab for gram stain and microscopy. All will require intubation/tracheostomy, i.v. fluids for maintenance requirements with benzyl penicillin 300–600 mg 6 hourly for 7–10 days, and anti-toxin 20 000 u i.m. plus 20 000 u i.v. Beware sensitivity reactions. Give either 0.1 ml of 1/1000 intradermally or 0.2 ml of 1/10 subcutaneously and observe for 1–2 hours before. Complications include acute heart failure (10%) which must be treated with digoxin, cardiac arrhythmias (10%) and peripheral and bulbar neuritis (5–10%). Treat these symptomatically.

Problem

- Children who have been in fires and exposed to hot gases, e.g. steam from a teapot, sometimes develop acute stridor even though there are no burns to the skin.

Diagnosis — Laryngeal burns

These children are difficult to manage particularly if they also have extensive skin burns. However, i.v. hydrocortisone, 100–200 mg 6 hourly may be helpful. Mist therapy using ultrasonic nebulisers may relieve some of the obstruction. Often intubation for 2–3 days is required to maintain an airway until the oedema has settled.

Problem

- The occasional child presents with a history of lethargy and possibly anaemia over the previous weeks or months. Sometimes the superficial lymph glands, liver and spleen are enlarged. A chest X-ray and lateral X-ray of the thoracic inlet shows a large tumour.

Diagnosis — Stridor secondary to mediastinal tumour, usually lymphosarcoma

The mass usually shrinks rapidly on treatment with DXT and cytotoxic drugs. Intubation may be necessary initially, as the treatment may cause a transient increase in the size of the mass lasting 2–3 days. The subsequent management is that of the underlying pathology.

Problem

- Children with a malabsorption problem, or on a low vitamin D-containing diet, or more rarely hypoparathyroid disorders, may present with a sudden onset of inspiratory stridor, sometimes, but not always, with clinically obvious rickets. Trousseau's and Kvostek's signs are positive.

Diagnosis — Tetany

Give calcium gluconate i.v. slowly (5–10 ml of 10%). If the diagnosis is correct this will relieve the stridor within 1–2 minutes. The subsequent management is that of the underlying disorder.

PERSISTENT STRIDOR

Congenital web

Rt. recurrent nerve palsy

Bilateral nerve palsy

Juvenile papillomatosis

Persistent stridor is almost always a disease of infancy and early childhood. Most present at or soon after birth and cause a great deal of parental anxiety. The main problem is to decide which children require investigations. In the large majority the stridor begins within the first 4 weeks of life.

Diagnosis – Persisting stridor? Cause
Any infant with a persistent stridor and *recession* requires laryngoscopy. In the newborn period an anaesthetic is often not needed. This investigation may reveal several different abnormalities apart from the above.

Unilateral or bilateral cord palsy. One of the cords may cross the midline when the larynx is closed and fail to move normally. Alternatively, both cords may remain adducted. The unilateral form sometimes occurs in association with congenital heart disease, the bilateral form more usually with neurological abnormalities, i.e. the Arnold–Chiari abnormality. Children with unilateral cord palsies do not require treatment and often improve in subsequent months. Those with bilateral palsies are more likely to get into trouble and may require prolonged nasotracheal intubation. Occasionally tracheostomy is required.

Sub-glottic haemangioma. A mass is seen projecting into the lumen of the larynx with loose and wrinkled mucosa. The lesion is soft and readily compressible by a probe. The sub-glottic haemangiomas follow a similar time course to the cavernous haemangiomas appearing in the skin. The symptoms develop in the first 1–3 months of life, with progressive inspiratory stridor. The symptoms then stabilise and improvement is seen in the second year of life. Surgical excision or X-ray treatment can almost always be avoided.

Laryngeal papilloma. Very occasionally multiple papilloma can be observed, particularly in the region of the vocal cords. Laryngeal papilloma or warts occur in infancy and early childhood. These lesions can produce major problems with severe airways obstruction. Surgical clearance is rarely possible. In some children the papillomas disappear spontaneously in later childhood. Permanent tracheostomy is often required.

Subglottic stenosis, narrowing below the glottis. This can be congenital but more frequently arises secondary to prolonged

Subglottic stenosis

intubation in the neonatal period or early infancy. These are difficult conditions to treat when severe, repeated dilatation sometimes produces long term benefit, but on occasions surgical correction will be required; this is a major procedure with poor long-term results. Tracheal transplants may have a place in those with the most severe obstruction but most children will show improvement with time.

Congenital floppy larynx. In the majority of children investigated, the larynx will appear to be normal except for a tendency to collapse in inspiration, sometimes with an abnormally large epiglottis which tends to fall back occluding the larynx.

Problem

- The symptom is only present when the child cries, is excited, or has an upper respiratory tract infection.
- The infant has no respiratory distress when at rest and the stridor is not getting worse.

Diagnosis — Infantile larynx (floppy larynx — presumed)

Laryngomalacia

By far the commonest cause of persistent stridor in infancy is the infantile or floppy larynx. There appears to be no anatomical abnormality, except that the normal tendency for the trachea to collapse on inspiration is exaggerated. Mild chest cage deformity is common and a degree of intercostal recession provides an indication of the severity of the obstruction. No invasive investigations are required.

Management. Stridor is a very worrying symptom to the child's parents. Time must be spent explaining the nature of the lesion. If the child does not have stridor at rest no further investigations are required, but the child will need to be assessed every 2–3 months so that the initial diagnosis can be reviewed. Symptoms gradually subside in the first and second years of life. Parents should be warned that symptoms are likely to get worse when the child has a cold. If the child has stridor at rest, has respiratory distress or indeed if the stridor is not apparent until after the first 6 weeks of life, further investigations are required. Chest X-ray and lateral X-ray of the neck and thoracic inlet will identify any large mass or cyst compressing the airway from without.

Problem

- Occasionally the barium swallow will show a persistent, obliquely running, filling defect in the mid-thoracic region.

Diagnosis — Vascular ring

External compression of the trachea usually caused by vascular abnormalities can produce persistent stridor. This is again predominantly inspiratory and there may be associated difficulty in swallowing as the oesophagus is also enclosed in the tight ring. The vascular ring is

Aortic ring

trachea
vascular ring
oesophagus
Ao
PV
RA
RV

usually due to a double aortic arch enclosing the oesophagus and trachea or to an anomalous origin to the left subclavian artery. Angiography is required to demonstrate the anatomy and surgery to release the oesophagus and the trachea.

COUGHING AND WHEEZING ATTACKS: AGE 0–2 YEARS

With the exception of the immediate neonatal period, wheezing and coughing attacks occur throughout the childhood. The pattern of disease is age dependent. The most common diagnostic problem is between acute bronchiolitis and early asthma.

Problem

- The baby, usually between the ages of 1 and 9 months, has a 2–5 day history of coryzal symptoms with progressive tachypnoea (up to 130/min), difficulty with feeding and gross hyperinflation. Fine crepitations are heard all over the chest, sometimes accompanied by rhonchi.

Diagnosis — Acute bronchiolitis

Record heart and respiratory rate, and assess the degree of hyperinflation, recession, cyanosis and distress. Measure oxygen saturation

Bronchiolitis

depressed diaphragm

horizontal ribs

streaky hilar shadows

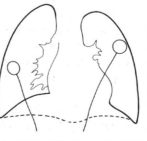
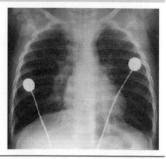

using a cutaneous probe if possible. Chest X-ray shows overinflation, sometimes with patchy areas of collapse/consolidation, but a chest X-ray is not required unless the signs are atypical or the child is very ill. Nasopharyngeal secretions should be aspirated and sent for immunofluorescence. This is usually positive for respiratory syncytial virus (RSV) in winter epidemics. Occasionally bronchiolitis is due to adenoviral infection, especially types 3, 7 and 21, and identification will require viral culture and paired antibody titres.

Management

Heart and respiratory rates should be monitored with transcutaneous oxygen saturation in addition if available. Apnoea and bradycardias are common. The baby may become severely hypoxic and carbon dioxide retention is common. Oxygen should be given, using a headbox, if the baby is blue, pale or restless, if the respiratory rate is above 60/min or oxygen saturation below 90%. The baby should be nursed in a comfortable position and handled as little as possible. Nasogastric tube feeding or i.v. fluids are often required.

Medicines. Ribavirin is now available for RSV infection. It is extremely expensive, and has to be given as a mist using a special form of nebuliser for prolonged periods each day. At present its use, which remains controversial, is confined to infants at particular risk, especially those with bronchopulmonary dysplasia, severe congenital heart disease, cystic fibrosis, suffering from immunodeficiency or less than 6 weeks old. Bronchodilators and steroids are ineffective in bronchiolitis. Antibiotics are not indicated unless the child is very ill and there is evidence of pneumonia. Staphylococcal infection should then be considered and an antibiotic combination such as flucloxacillin and ampicillin or gentamicin prescribed. Physiotherapy does not improve the symptoms or shorten the duration of the illness.

Ventilation therapy should be commenced on clinical grounds rather than on the results of blood gases and then only for persistent apnoea, deterioration in level of consciousness or exhaustion. Ventilatory support is difficult in these babies as high pressures are required often for prolonged periods. Those with such severe disease may then be left with lung pathology similar to bronchopulmonary dysplasia seen in preterm babies. The most suitable pattern of ventilation has yet to be defined but I:E ratios greater than 1:1 are unlikely to be helpful in this situation. Pressures in excess of 30 cmH$_2$O are often needed. There is now some evidence that continuous positive airway pressure given using a face mask, nasal catheters or endotracheal tube may obviate the need for IPPV and should be considered before the child is exhausted. Ribavirin can be given to children receiving ventilatory support. Those not responding to IPPV may be helped by ECMO.

Complications

Many babies with bronchiolitis develop episodes of apnoea or periodic breathing. Careful observation and prompt stimulation will often prevent severe hypoxic episodes requiring intubation. Cardiac failure is overdiagnosed, because of the apparent enlargement of the liver due to overinflation of the lungs. It rarely occurs in the absence of any underlying cardiac defect. Occasional babies are left with severe persistent airways damage (obliterative bronchiolitis), especially after adenovirus infection, which tends to improve slowly if the baby survives. Over-distension of one lung (Macleod syndrome) sometimes occurs.

Macleod syndrome

Unilateral overinflation:
  bronchiolitis

Differential diagnosis:
partial obstruction of main bronchus
  tuberculous glands
  foreign body
  tumour
  aberrant vessels

Congenital anomalies:
  lobar emphysema
  cysts

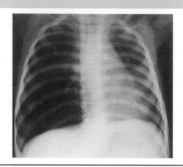

Most babies make a complete recovery in 10–14 days. There is a high risk of recurrent bouts of coughing and wheezing in the next few years.

Problem

- Older children, particularly those who are in the latter part of the first year and who are overweight, show a similar but milder disorder with wheezing a prominent feature.

Diagnosis — Early asthma

Although the plump, wheezy 9-month-old baby who is not particularly distressed is very different from the acutely distressed, grossly hyperinflated 6-week-old baby with acute bronchiolitis, the two conditions merge and the differentiation will become a matter of personal clinical opinion. Chest X-ray will show less hyperinflation than during an attack of acute bronchiolitis but may be otherwise indistinguishable. Nasal secretions for viral immunofluorescence will help identify the current viral population, but will be unlikely to alter the management.

Management

Four-hourly recording of heart and respiratory rate are usually adequate. Oxygen saturation should be measured in sick babies and oxygen given if necessary.

Drugs. Most of these babies will settle in a few days, irrespective of treatment. Beta 2 stimulants are often ineffective in the first 12–15 months of life but it is worth trying a nebulised solution, for example, salbutamol or terbutaline, to assess any response. This should be discontinued if the child does not appear to benefit. There is no evidence that xanthine drugs, e.g. i.v. aminophylline or oral theophylline, are effective but these are given in some units. At least one-third will improve rapidly on receiving nebulised or aerosol/coffee cup ipratropium bromide (125–250 μg) at 6-hourly intervals. Systemic steroids appear to work in the second year of life and can be used to terminate a prolonged attack, e.g. prednisolone 1–2 mg/kg body weight/24 h). Inhaled topical steroids given either via a spacer and face mask system or as a nebulised solution (budesonide) are helpful in the management of infants with troublesome and persistent symptoms.

Physiotherapy may help if symptoms are prolonged.

Episodes of bronchitis with wheeze in infancy are part of the spectrum of asthma. Many children will have recurrent episodes with viral infection but often lose this tendency by school age.

Problem	• Acute onset of coughing and wheezing not associated with coryzal symptoms.
	• Often a history of vomiting or regurgitation.
	• A tendency to cough during feeds.
	• Sometimes features suggesting hypotonia or developmental delay.

Diagnosis — Aspiration (presumptive)

There may be repeated episodes of lower respiratory tract problems with areas of patchy consolidation on X-ray. The episodes of aspiration may be due to impaired pharyngeal co-ordination, either as an isolated defect or as part of generalised delay, gastro-oesophageal reflux, rarely due to an H-type tracheo-oesophageal fistula (TOF), but not infrequently after repair of oesophageal atresia. Cine/video barium swallow may show inco-ordination and identify some of the children with TOF. A small H-type fistula can best be excluded by high intubation, injecting lipiodol into the tract and manually inflating the child. The positive pressure will open and delineate the fistula.

Acute aspiration

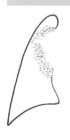 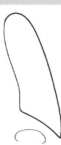

collapse
consolidation
Rt. upper lobe

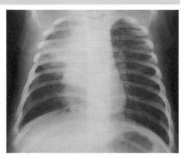

Examine tracheal aspirate for fat-laden macrophages which are likely to be present if significant milk aspiration has occurred. Recurrent aspiration can also be identified by giving the infant a radioactive technetium labelled milk feed and screening with a gamma camera immediately and 4 and 12 hours later looking for radioactivity in the lung fields.

Management. The acute attack is an indication for systemic antibiotic therapy and for physiotherapy.

Problem	• Occasionally children with acute wheezy attacks in the first 2 years of life have a history of frequent offensive stools, failure to gain weight adequately and previous attacks of lower respiratory tract infection.

Diagnosis — Cystic fibrosis (presumptive) (see p. 164)

COUGHING AND WHEEZING ATTACKS: CHILDREN OVER 2 YEARS

Problem (common)	• A history of attacks of wheeze and cough, often with upper respiratory infection. • A personal or family history of eczema or hay fever. • Dyspnoea and wheeze which is mainly expiratory. • Hyperinflation, recession, use of accessory muscles.

Diagnosis — Asthma

Assess how well the child is able to talk, walk, eat and sleep. Record the heart and respiratory rates, blood pressure (pulsus paradoxus of greater than 20 mmHg indicates severe asthma) and assess colour, severity of dyspnoea, wheeze, recession and overinflation. Record the treatment already given and the past history, especially of severe attacks. Measure oxygen saturation, and peak flow if this is possible.

Initial treatment

Give salbutamol (2.5–5 mg) or terbutaline by nebuliser, using either a face mask or mouth tube. In the absence of a nebuliser, 5–10 puffs from an inhaler can be given slowly, using a spacer device or a paper cup as a face mask. If the child responds well (measure peak flow), and maintains this improvement for at least 2 hours, he or she may go home to continue on an increased dose of inhaled bronchodilator for a few days. If the response is poor, the child is severely ill or having a prolonged attack, admission to hospital is required, especially if the child has a past history of severe attacks or is taking inhaled steroids.

In-patient management

Frequent careful observation is required, including measurements of oxygen saturation and peak flow.

Drugs. Nebulised bronchodilators may be repeated at 1–2 hour intervals and then continued 4–6 hourly. Prednisolone (2 mg/kg/day) should be started. If the child is vomiting, give i.v. hydrocortisone (100 mg 4–6 hourly). If the response to salbutamol is poor it may be helpful to give nebulised ipratropium (100–500 mg) 6–8 hourly in addition.

Overinflated lungs

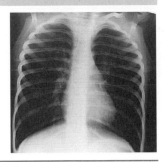

Poorly responding children may be given an i.v. aminophylline loading dose (4 mg/kg) but only if no oral theophylline preparations have been given in the last 24 hours, then 0.7 mg/kg/h. Oxygen should be given to all children with severe acute asthma, but blood gases are required only if the attack is severe and the child deteriorating.

Intermittent positive pressure ventilation is rarely needed if effective early treatment is given. It may be required for exhaustion, or following cardiorespiratory arrest. It should not be started on blood gas measurements alone, though a rising $PaCO_2$ is an indication that IPPV may be needed.

Treatment should be reduced as the child improves. A single dose of oral steroid may be adequate for some but many will need a few days' course, the dose and duration being judged by the child's response. Before discharge the child's regular treatment should be reviewed and altered if necessary and his or her inhaler technique checked. Regular bronchodilator therapy and an increased dose of prophylactic therapy should be given for a week or two. The need for compliance with regular therapy should be emphasised.

Out-patient management

It is important to assess the severity of the asthma and the main trigger factors. Diary records including regular peak flow measurements at home are very helpful.

Bronchodilator drugs used in the treatment of asthma

Drug	Delivery system	Unit dose	Dose/frequency
Salbutamol	Oral (Tabs)	2,4 mg	1/4–6 hourly
	(Syrup)	2 mg/5 ml	2.5–5 ml/4–6 hourly
	Oral slow release (Volmax)	4,8 mg	1/12/24 hourly
	Dry powder (Rotahaler)	200,400 µg	1/4 hourly
	(Diskhaler)	200,400 µg	1/4 hourly
	(Accuhaler)	200,400 µg	1/4 hourly
	MDI	100 µg	1–2/3–4 hourly
	MDI (Autohaler)	100 µg	1–2/3–4 hourly
	Nebules	2.5,5 mg	2 ml/3–4 hourly
Terbutaline	Oral (Tabs)	5 mg	Half tab/4 hourly
	(Syrup)	1.5 mg/5 ml	5 ml/3–4 hourly
	Dry powder (Turbohaler)	500 µg	1/3–4 hourly
	MDI	250 µg	1–2/3–4 hourly
	Respules	5 mg/2 ml	2 ml/3–4 hourly
Salmeterol	Dry powder (Diskhaler)	50 µg	1/12–24 hourly
	(Accuhaler)	50 µg	1/12–24 hourly
	MDI	25 µg	1–2/12–24 hourly
Ipratropium bromide	MDI	20/40 µg	1–2/4–6 hourly
	MDI (Autohaler)	20 µg	1–2/4–6 hourly
	Neb. solution	250 µg/ml	0.5–1 ml/4–6 hourly

Inhaled drugs used in the prophylaxis against asthma

Drug	Delivery system	Unit dose	Dose/times daily
Sodium cromoglucate	Powder (Spinhaler)	20 mg	1/3–4 times
	MDI (with Fisonair)	5 mg	2/3–4 times
	Neb. Solution	20 mg	1/3–4 times
Beclomethasone	Dry powder (Rotacaps)	100,200 mg	1–2/twice
	(Accuhaler)	100,200,400 mg	1–2/twice
	MDI	50,100,200 mg	1–3/twice
Budesonide	Dry powder (Turbohaler)	100,200,400 mg	1–2/twice
	MDI	50,200 mg	1–3/twice
	Neb. Solution (Respules)	0.5,1.0 mg	1/2–3 times
Fluticasone	Dry powder (Diskhaler)	50,100,200 mg	1–2/twice
	(Accuhaler)	50,100,200 mg	1–2/twice
	MDI	50,125,250 mg	1–2/twice

Side effects of asthma therapy

Group	Examples	Side effects
Beta agonists	Salbutamol, terbutaline salmeterol (long acting)	Tremor; tachycardia, hyperactivity Mild oxygen desaturation
Anticholinergic	Ipratropium bromide	Tachycardia, dry mouth, constipation, urinary retention
Xanthines	Theophylline, aminophylline	Tachycardia and arrhythmias Nausea and vomiting Hyperactivity, convulsions Bed wetting
1 Antiinflammatory	Sodium cromoglycate	Mild throat irritation
2 Antiinflammatory (inhaled topical steroids)	Beclomethasone Budesonide Fluticasone	Oral thrush, dysphonia Temporary growth suppression and adrenal suppression at high doses
3 Antiinflammatory (Systemic steroids)	Prednisolone Dexamethasone Prednisone	Fluid retention, growth and adrenal suppression Hypertension, diabetes, immune suppression

Asthma therapy guidelines

Level	Indication	Relief therapy	Prophylaxis
1	Occasional wheezing	Inhaled beta agonist	None
2	Needs relief therapy at least thrice weekly	Inhaled beta agonist	Sodium cromoglycate
3a	Poor control on sodium cromoglycate	Inhaled beta agonist	Low-dose inhaled steroids
3b	Persisting nocturnal and exercise symptoms	Inhaled beta agonist and long-acting agonist	Low-dose inhaled steroids
4	Control still poor	Inhaled beta agonist and long-acting agonist	High-dose inhaled steroids
5	Control still poor, repeated hospital admissions, poor school attendance	Inhaled beta agonist and long-acting agonist	High-dose inhaled steroids and daily or alternate-day systemic steroids

Triggers			
Infection	Allergens	Irritants	Exercise
Viral, e.g. rhinovirus, RSV, parainfluenzavirus, adenovirus	House dust mite	Mist	
	Animals, especially cat and horse	Cigarette smoke	Excitement
		Aerosol sprays	
	Grass pollen		Fizzy drinks
	Feathers		

Medicines. Children with only occasional mild attacks can be treated satisfactorily with intermittent bronchodilator therapy, preferably by inhalation. A spacer device or dry powder inhaler should be prescribed and the child and parent instructed in its use. The bronchodilator can be given as required and before exercise. Prophylactic therapy should be started if the child is having frequent attacks or persistent symptoms which affect daily life. Sodium cromoglycate should be tried first, as it is entirely free of side effects. It also has the advantage of blocking exercise-induced asthma. If 4–6 weeks' treatment, given regularly, does not bring about improvement the child should be changed to an inhaled steroid, given in the smallest dose that controls the symptoms, which may vary from time to time. If despite inhaled doses of 400 mg per day (200 mg of fluticasone) frequent bronchodilators are still required, add in long acting beta agonists (salmeterol) morning and night. This often dramatically reduces nocturnal and exercise symptoms. The next step is to increase the dose of inhaled steroids. Very high doses of inhaled steroid may produce side effects, especially adrenal suppression and fluid retention.

Short courses of topical steroids (3–5 days) can safely be given for acute deterioration whatever the level of regular therapy. Occasionally children with severe chronic asthma require prolonged courses of oral prednisolone. Alternate day prednisolone results in fewer side effects (growth suppresssion, facial change) than daily treatment, but may not control the asthma.

Information. Parents and children need a thorough explanation on asthma and its management. Acute attacks may cause much anxiety, and a plan of action needs to be discussed. Direct access to the hospital ward saves time in a bad attack and helps relieve anxiety. Written instructions about treatment are helpful. Home peak flow meters are useful in those with severe or brittle asthma. Parents should be encouraged to allow children to take part in all activities, with appropriate premedication, and to avoid school absence. Known allergens should be avoided as far as possible.

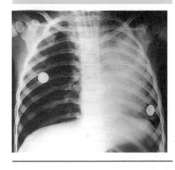

Lung collapse in an asthmatic child

Prognosis

Wheezing attacks are most common in the pre-school years, and many children lose their tendency to wheeze with colds by school age. Others with more troublesome asthma improve later in childhood, but may have a recurrence of symptoms in adult life. Boys are more likely to lose their asthma.

Problem

- Very occasionally the story is that of sudden onset of coughing, wheezing and retching in a child who was previously well.
- Not infrequently, the attack starts while the child is running with either toys, nuts or other objects in the mouth.
- Often there are localised rhonchi rather than generalised wheezing.

Diagnosis — Inhaled foreign body

Inhalation of foreign bodies occur most frequently at this age. These children are in a very precarious situation as total obstruction can result from movement of the article in the trachea. If possible get films on inspiration and expiration as mediastinal shift and localised areas of hyperinflation may only be apparent on expiration.

Management. Urgent bronchoscopy is required so that the foreign body can be removed. This can be a difficult procedure and should only be undertaken by someone with considerable experience. Occasionally a transbronchial approach at thoracotomy will be needed.

Non-opaque foreign body in the right main bronchus

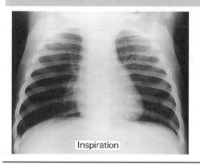
Inspiration

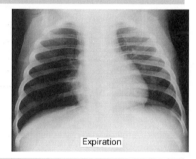
Expiration

ACUTE COUGHING EPISODES

Attacks of coughing without wheezing are seen throughout childhood.

Problem (common)

- 2–3 day period of coryzal symptoms leading to coughing attacks.
- Little or no pyrexia.
- No respiratory distress.
- No hyperinflation.
- Chest X-ray which may show bronchial wall thickening but is otherwise clear.

Diagnosis — Acute bronchitis

This condition occurs at all ages but rarely leads to admission to hospital unless social conditions are very poor. These attacks are almost all viral and so antibiotics are not indicated unless sputum culture reveals a secondary bacterial infection. Expectorants are of no proven value. Use of cough suppressants, e.g. linctus codeine 5 ml, may help to provide a good night's sleep.

Problem

Sometimes, particularly in children over the age of 3 years, a more dramatic history emerges:

- Coryzal symptoms increasing to irritant cough within a few days.
- Onset of paroxysmal cough within 2–3 weeks often with an inspiratory whoop and terminating in vomiting.
- Chest X-ray showing little other than bronchial wall thickening although there are on occasions areas of atelectasis.
- A relative and absolute lymphocytosis.

Diagnosis — Probably whooping cough

This condition tends to occur in epidemics and is not always prevented by previous immunisation. Symptoms are likely to be particularly severe and dangerous in the first year of life. Occasionally an identical clinical picture can be caused by adenovirus infection. Chest X-ray will show some bronchial wall thickening with small local areas of collapse-consolidation. The lungs are not over-inflated. Pharyngeal swab should be taken and cultured for *Bordatella pertussis*. It is unusual to be able to culture this organism if the child has had symptoms for more than 2 weeks. Viral culture and paired viral antibody titres should be measured if the picture is in any way atypical or occurring outside the epidemic as other viruses, particularly the adenovirus, can produce an identical picture.

Management. Little can be done to alter the course of the disease. If the child is seen within the first 2–3 weeks of the onset of symptoms it is worth prescribing oral amoxycillin or erythromycin. Cough suppressants rarely have any effect, although some would prescribe phenobarbitone 15–30 mg tds in the hope that this will reduce the incidence of paroxysms. Exposure to cold air undoubtedly triggers coughing and should be avoided. It may also be worth giving Beta-2 adrenergic stimulants as there is some evidence that they help.

Complications include failure to thrive due to excess vomiting, secondary bacterial infection of the respiratory tract (broncho-pneumonia, segmental collapse, otitis media), intracranial haemorrhages, peripheral neuritis, encephalitis and frenula ulcers. A large number of babies recover virtually unscathed after symptoms persisting for weeks or months. A few babies are left with lung damage in the form of bronchiectasis. Mortality is restricted to babies within the first few months of life. It is probably justifiable to treat infant siblings with erythromycin in the hope of aborting the illness.

Problem

- Acute onset of illness with coughing sometimes following an upper respiratory tract infection.

- Pyrexia often with tachypnoea, respiratory distress and grunting respiration.
- Evidence of an area or areas of consolidation on chest X-ray usually, but not always, with areas of relative dullness to percussion and crepitations.

Diagnosis — Pneumonia

This can be patchy and diffuse — bronchopneumonia — or with local areas of dense consolidation — lobar pneumonia. It is sometimes possible to guess at the lobe involved from the symptoms, e.g. pain referred into the abdomen is usually from the right or left lower lobe, and associated neck stiffness occurs with right upper lobe pneumonia. The diagnosis can be difficult as pneumonia can produce a very varied picture in childhood ranging from a mild pyrexial illness with no respiratory symptoms through to peripheral circulatory shock and severe respiratory failure. Often the diagnosis is only made on X-ray as even quite large areas of consolidation can be very difficult to pick up on clinical examination.

Pneumonias easily missed without lateral radiographs

Upper segment RUL   Lower segment RLL   Rt. Middle Lobe   Lt. Lower Lobe

Investigations

Take lateral radiographs as well, as the standard PA views for collapse/consolidation of a left lower or right upper lobe are easy to miss on the standard films alone. Right upper lobe pneumonias occur frequently in the first year of life, presumably due to aspiration when lying down. A very high polymorph count on blood film indicates a bacterial aetiology, although in viral infections there may be a significantly raised polymorph count persisting for 1–2 days. Blood culture will often be positive and identify the organism. Throat swab is often misleading with the exception of pneumococcal infections. Sputum results are more useful than throat swabs. This can best be collected by gentle oropharyngeal suction. There is now an increasing number of viruses which can be identified by immunofluorescence within a few hours. Viral culture is a slow process and is unlikely to be of much help during the acute phase of management.

Lung tap. Aspirating secretions from the affected lung using a 21 needle attached to a 10-ml syringe provides the most reliable way of identifying the infecting organism. As this is an invasive procedure and may induce a pneumothorax or haemoptysis, it should not be used unless unusual organisms are suspected, for example in patients with immuno-suppression or in those in whom recovery is slow.

Blood gases. These are not indicated unless the child is very ill. Carbon dioxide retention is rare except in severe staphylococcal infections but desaturation occurs early due to shunting of blood through unventilated areas. Those with peripheral shock will have a metabolic acidosis.

Management

If the child is not critically ill it is satisfactory to record pulse, respiration, temperature, colour and clinical condition every 4 hours. Those with peripheral collapse will require intensive monitoring. Most children are more comfortable if nursed in a semi-recumbent position. Infants can best be nursed in a Derbyshire chair. Many are able to take drinks satisfactorily. Those who cannot will require i.v. lines to provide maintenance fluids.

Oxygen. Oxygen saturation should be monitored if possible, and oxygen given as required to keep Sao_2 above 90%. Signs of hypoxia include restlessness, pallor and cyanosis with a rising heart rate. Oxygen can be given to infants using a head box or older children by face mask and nasal cannula. It should be humidified, but mist is not helpful.

Physiotherapy. The place of physiotherapy has yet to be defined, but it is probably useful in those in whom the pneumonia is secondary to aspiration. Gentle oropharyngeal suction appears to give young infants with excessive secretions some relief.

Antibiotics. The antibiotic to be selected depends on the age and the suspected organism. Even though the majority of attacks of pneumonia are viral in origin, it is extremely difficult to exclude a bacterial aetiology. All except those with trivial symptoms and minimal chest X-ray changes should therefore be given antibiotics.

In the first year of life, as throughout childhood, streptococcus pneumoniae is the commonest cause of bacterial pneumonia. However, staphylococcal infections occur more frequently at this age and gram-negative bacilli, like *E. coli* are not uncommon. *Chlamydia trachomatis* can also cause pneumonia in early infancy, an infection producing quite dramatic chest X-ray changes in infants who are not that ill. For this reason anti-staphylococcal agents should be considered with a broad spectrum antibiotic, for example flucloxacillin and gentamicin systemically. Chlamydial infections respond best to erythromycin.

Over 1 year of age the antibiotic of choice is probably penicillin, as over 90% of infections will be due to the pneumococcus. If the child is very ill it is wise to adopt the policy used for infants. If mycoplasma is identified the child should be given erythromycin. The possibility of tuberculosis should always be considered.

Prognosis

Most children respond within a few days. The main complications are pleural effusions particularly those with pneumococcal infections, and empyemas and pneumothoraces in those with staphylococcal infections. Tension pneumothoraces will require immediate drainage. Some empyemas settle on adequate i.v. antibiotic therapy. If the child remains sick and the empyema shows no sign of resolving, surgical drainage will be required. Occasionally, affected lobes are slow to reinflate. These children need vigorous physiotherapy. If the lung fails to respond, consider bronchoscopy to exclude a foreign body and to clear the airway.

Problem

- Very occasionally children present with coughing who have poor peripheral perfusion with a pulse rate and high respiratory rate, clinical and radiological evidence of cardiomegaly, hepatomegaly and sometimes splenomegaly.

Diagnosis — Heart failure (see Ch. 8)

RECURRENT OR CHRONIC COUGH

Children with persistent or recurrent episodes of cough may cause a great deal of anxiety to their parents and can be difficult diagnostic problems. A chest X-ray is indicated and may reveal areas of persistent collapse/consolidation following infection which will respond to physiotherapy. If the chest X-ray is normal, asthma is a likely cause of frequent, especially nocturnal cough in young children and a therapeutic trial may resolve the problem. Other diagnoses include cystic fibrosis, recurrent aspiration, foreign body, ciliary dysfunction, immune deficiency states and congenital abnormalities of the lung.

Problem

- History of recurrent chest infections, often starting in infancy.
- Loose, offensive stools, usually, but not always, with failure to thrive.
- Overinflated lungs, often with chest deformity.
- Clubbing may be present by 3 years of age.

Diagnosis — Cystic fibrosis

This is an inherited disorder of salt and water transport which affects about one in 2500 births in the UK. With neonatal screening the majority are identified soon after birth. If there is no screening 10–20% present with meconium ileus, others present in infancy with offensive stools and failure to thrive or with persistent or recurrent cough and/or wheeze. The degree of pancreatic insufficiency is variable and in the absence of newborn screening, only 60% of cystic fibrosis (CF) patients are diagnosed in the first year of life. A large appetite may ensure a reasonable weight gain until respiratory infection occurs. The severity and rate of progression of the disease are very variable.

Neonatal screening. In Trent UK, immunoreactive trypsin (IRT) is measured on the 5th day Guthrie specimen. If raised, the blood spot is tested for deltaF508, the common CF mutation. Children who are homozygous for this mutation — about half of CF cases — are diagnosed immediately. Heterozygotes have a repeat IRT at 4 weeks, and other CF mutations are sought. If the second IRT is raised, the child is referred for a sweat test. Occasional children are missed on screening, especially if they do not carry deltaF508.

Meconium ileus presents with a low small bowel obstruction in the newborn period due to viscid meconium. About one-third can be treated by a contrast enema under X-ray control, but the majority require surgery. Atresia, perforation and volvulus may be present and some gut may need resection. The thick meconium is cleared and a temporary ileostomy often made. Post-operatively there may be delay before the micro-colon functions, requiring a period of total parental nutrition. Temporary food intolerances are common, but for most infants the longer term outlook is good. The diagnosis of CF must always be confirmed.

Diagnosis rests on two positive sweat tests (Na and Cl > 60 mmol/l) based on 100 mg of sweat obtained using the pilocarpine iontophoresis method. The diagnosis can also be made and confirmed by genotype. Examination of stool for fat content, fat globules and chymotrypsin will indicate the degree of pancreatic deficiency.

Management

There is no curative treatment. The aim is to control the malabsorption with pancreatic enzyme supplements, ensure good nutrition and delay progression of lung disease.

— Pancreatic enzyme supplements (Creon, Pancrease) should be given with each meal and snack. The dose is adjusted to get the stools reasonably normal and the child gaining weight well. In view of recent cases of fibrosing colonopathy associated with high enzyme dosage, the dose should not exceed 10 000 u lipase/kg/day. Some children benefit from the addition of an H_2 blocker which prevents gastric acid delaying the release of the enzyme from the pH dependent coating when pancreatic bicarbonate secretion is inadequate.
— Diet should be of high energy and protein content. Fat does not need to be restricted. Dietary supplements are only needed for periods of ill health or if intake is poor.
— Vitamins A, D and E are given routinely.
— Salt is needed in hot weather and for babies.
— Physiotherapy is advised twice daily from diagnosis and exercise encouraged.
— Smoking should be forbidden in the house, and contact with infection avoided if possible.

— Antibiotic treatment is advised for all respiratory infections and may be given on a long term basis.
— Give full immunisation, including influenza.
— The child and parents should be seen regularly preferably in a special CF clinic by an experienced team. Sputum cultures, lung function and growth should be monitored to guide treatment. Ongoing family education and support, including genetic counselling, is essential.

Hospital admissions are usually for exacerbations of lung disease, sometimes for abdominal pain.

Exacerbations

Increased symptoms may be due to intercurrent viral infection, which may permit bacterial invasion, or to lack of home treatment. Ask how cough, sputum, wheeze and activity compare with the child's usual level, and look for objective evidence of deterioration such as a fall in lung function, Sao_2 or weight. Unless there is wheezing or advanced disease, the lungs are usually clear on examination. A chest X-ray is usually unnecessary unless pneumothorax is suspected. Early treatment of children with mild and moderate disease is very important to prevent deterioration.

Antibiotic therapy. This should be based on recent sputum cultures. In the absence of positive cultures, treat for staphylococcus and *H. Influenzae*, and aim to eradicate these pathogens if isolated, irrespective of symptoms. Oral antibiotics should be given in high dosage for a prolonged period. Once pseudomonas is established it will not be eradicated for any length of time by antibiotic therapy. Treatment of initial isolates with oral ciprofloxacin and nebulised colistin for 3 weeks delays establishment. Once established, pseudomonas should in general only be treated when the child's conditions warrants it and

Antibiotic therapy in cystic fibrosis

Pathogen	Antibiotic	Dose	Duration
Staph.aureus	Flucloxacillin	100 mg/kg/day in 4 doses (oral)	4 weeks
	Erythromycin	50 mg/kg/day in 4 doses (oral)	4 weeks
	Clindamycin	30 mg/kg/day in 4 doses (oral)	4 weeks
Haemophilus influenzae	Amoxycillin	50–100 mg/kg/day in 3 doses (oral)	10–14 days
	•Co-amoxiclav	50–100 mg/kg/day in 3 doses (oral)	10–14 days
	Trimethoprim	92 mg/kg/day in 2 doses	10–14 days
	•Cefachlor	40 mg/kg/day in 3 doses	10–14 days
	(• = also covers Staph.)		
Pseudomonas aeruginosa	Ciprofloxacin	125–500 mg b.d. (oral)	10–14 days
	Ceftazidime	150–200 mg/kg/day i.v. in 3 doses (to 2 g t.d.s.)	14 days
	Azlocillin	300 mg/kg/day in 4 doses i.v.	14 days
	Gentamicin	9–10 mg/kg/day in 3 doses	14 days
	Tobramycin	(adjust according to blood levels)	
	Colistin	75 000 u/kg/day i.v. in 3 doses 0.5–2 megaunit b.d. by nebuliser	
	Gentamicin	20–80 mg b.d.	

Advanced CF

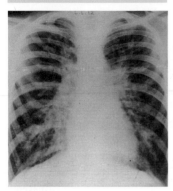

Bilateral:
  cystic shadows
  linear shadows
  overinflation
  patchy collapse
  and consolidation

oral antibiotic therapy for other pathogens has failed, though some children benefit from semi-elective treatment at intervals. Intravenous antibiotic therapy is then usually required and should be given for at least 10–14 days. A neonatal long line, or an implanted device such as the Portacath, should be used and great care taken to preserve the veins. High doses of aminoglycosides are required and blood levels should be measured. Apart from skin rashes, side effects are uncommon and i.v. antibiotic therapy can be given safely at home after training, with nursing supervision. When in hospital, children with multi-resistant pseudomonas or *Burkholderia cepacia* should be nursed separately from other CF children to prevent cross infection.

Ribavirin therapy — consider for infants with RSV bronchiolitis.

Oxygen may be needed, especially at night. Aim to keep SaO_2 90–95%, using low flow nasal cannulae or a Ventimask to avoid CO_2 narcosis.

Bronchodilator therapy (usually nebulised salbutamol) may be helpful given before physiotherapy. Assess peak flow response.

DNase (alfa dornase, Pulmozyme) should be continued in hospital if the child is having it long term. DNA in sputum is broken down, making sputum easier to clear and improving lung function. It is not yet clear if intermittent treatment in exacerbations is useful and there may be considerable problems about prescribing this expensive drug.

Nebulised antibiotics (usually colistin or gentamicin) are rarely helpful in the acute situation but have a modest long term benefit when given regularly.

Lung complications

Pneumothorax, allergic aspergillosis, lobar collapse and haemoptysis may occur.

Advanced disease

The rate of progression of the lung disease to respiratory failure — the main cause of death in CF — is very variable. The response to treatment decreases with repeated courses and transplantation becomes the only option. Assessment at a referral centre is required before the end stage is reached, but the lack of donors means that few patients will achieve a successful transplant. Care should be taken not to prolong the process of dying, and there should be no hesitation in giving opiates to relieve breathlessness and anxiety. Cardiopulmonary resuscitation and IPPV should not be attempted, and arrangements made for the child to spend his or her last days at home, if the family wish.

Abdominal pain

Acute abdominal pain may be due to:
— Constipation — treat with increased fibre and laxatives rather than by reducing pancreatic enzyme dose (unless this is excessive).
— Distal intestinal obstruction syndrome (meconium ileus equivalent). There is usually a palpable mass in the right iliac fossa. Oral lactulose and n-acetyl cysteine (Fabrol) may be effective. If not, give oral gastrografin and/or rectal cisapride. Sub-acute bowel obstruction may occur and is best treated by oral lavage with Klean Prep or a gastrografin enema, which must be

performed under X-ray control and will also serve to confirm the diagnosis.

— Intussusception.
— Fibrosing colonopathy.
— Adhesions from previous surgery.
— Gall stones.

Other complications

Liver disease. An enlarged firm liver, especially the left lobe, indicates biliary cirrhosis. Patients with an enlarged spleen have portal hypertension and haematemesis may occur requiring urgent treatment. Hepatocellular failure is uncommon.

Diabetes. Glucose intolerance is common, and diabetes requiring insulin treatment occurs in about 10% of teenage and adult CF patients. Ketoacidosis is rare, the patient presenting with weight loss, polydipsia and polyuria.

Infertility is almost invariable in males, due to obstruction or absence of the vas. Females are fertile but pregnancy may impair the mother's health.

The prognosis for CF patients has improved greatly, especially in the first year of life. The median life expectancy is currently 25–30 years.

Problem

- In the first 2 years of life.
- History of recurrent lower respiratory tract infections.
- Sometimes but not always a tendency to vomit.
- X-rays suggestive of repeated aspiration.
- A history of coughing on feedings, sometimes with other signs of developmental delay.

Diagnosis — Recurrent aspiration

Inhalation of milk and solids produce recurrent episodes of coughing due to lung collapse and consolidation. There are many possible underlying causes, from oesophageal inco-ordination to the Riley–Day syndrome.

Radiological features of chronic aspiration

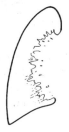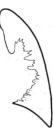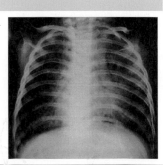

hyperinflation

hilar shadowing

Problem

- Recurrent or persistent cough, sometimes with evidence of bronchiectasis on the chest X-ray.
- Persistent nasal discharge with opaque antra on chest X-ray.

Diagnosis — Chronic sinusitis with lower respiratory tract infections

Whether the sinusitis is itself responsible for the infections or (and perhaps this is more likely) purely denotes an altered susceptibility of the respiratory tract resistance to infection, has yet to be determined. However, aggressive management of the sinusitis with antibiotics, decongestants and, if necessary, antral washouts seem appropriate. In some children the sinusitis and bronchiectasis are associated with non-functional respiratory cilia which on electron microscopy have abnormalities or absence of the dynein arms, the so-called *immotile cilia syndrome*. Of these at least 50% have dextrocardia (*Kartagener syndrome*). Prophylactic physiotherapy will help keep the lungs clear of secretions but frequent courses of antibiotics will also be required for intercurrent bacterial infections.

Problem

- There is a further group of children who have repeated recurrence of pneumonia in the same lobe of the lung which responds only briefly to antibiotic therapy.

Diagnosis — Probable foreign body

There is not always a history of inhalation. X-rays in inspiration and expiration may help, but bronchoscopy will usually be necessary. A longstanding foreign body may result in an area of bronchiectasis.

Foreign body!

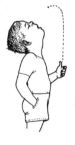

a flicked peanut if not caught in the mouth may go to the right middle lobe

peanuts are not radio-opaque wire springs are!

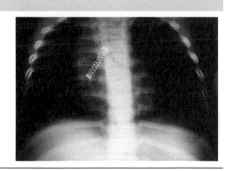

Problem

- Recurrent lower respiratory tract infections.
- Chronic cough and sputum production, which is often green.
- Sometimes a history of haemoptysis.
- Ring shadows on chest X-ray usually involving lower lobes.

Diagnosis — Bronchiectasis

The commonest cause of bronchiectasis is cystic fibrosis and this condition will obviously have to be excluded with a sweat test. Other conditions which need to be considered are immunological disorders, including agammaglobulinaemia (*Burton disease*) which is inherited as a sex-linked recessive and the *immotile cilia syndrome*. In some children the bronchiectasis is localised and arises from a previous insult, including prolonged collapse of a lobe in an asthmatic child, foreign body which was not removed for weeks, or even months, or a pneumonia which was either bacterial, e.g. staphylococcal, or viral, e.g. adenovirus type 7. These children will require a full immunological work up in addition to sweat test. It is also justified to carry out a bronchoscopy if necessary, progressing to bronchography.

Management. This consists of treating intercurrent infections vigorously with antibiotics and ensuring that the child leads as active a life as possible and has physiotherapy twice daily to aid clearance of secretions. Surgery is now rarely indicated unless a lobe or segment of the lung is persistently collapsed and acting as an infection source. Those with hypo- or agammaglobulinaemia can often be radically improved by weekly and then monthly gammaglobulin injections. Those with bronchiectasis secondary to the immotile cilia syndrome or to lung injury often show considerable improvement in later childhood. There is a tendency for the sputum production and cough to disappear.

Problem

- Fairly progressive breathlessness.
- Irritant dry cough, occasionally, but atypically with wheezing.
- Poor appetite and failure to thrive.

Diagnosis — Atypical pneumonia or fibrosing alveolitis

Pneumonia developing in the first weeks of life in babies born small for dates sometimes with congenital abnormalities, suggests pneumonia due to inter-uterine infection. Both congenitally acquired rubella and cytomegalovirus infection can produce pneumonia persisting for several months. Symptoms are not always present from birth but can develop in the first few months with cough, tachypnoea and breathlessness. Both produce widespread streaky opacities, similar to those seen after aspiration of bronchial pneumonia. Both can be diagnosed by isolating the virus from secretions and urine and finding high antibody titres. Gancyclovir may be useful in the treatment of cytomegalovirus pneumonia, but mortality remains high.

Children with immunological deficiency states, e.g. combined immunological deficiency, HIV, those with malignant disease, e.g. leukaemia, and those on cytotoxic drugs are particularly likely to develop *Pneumocystis carinii* infection. This protozoal organism produces a slowly progressive tachypnoea, dry cough and dyspnoea with little constitutional reaction. Little can be heard on auscultation and the chest X-ray tends to show hazy opacities stretching out from the hilar regions, which later becomes more widespread with a generalised regularity. This condition can usually be diagnosed by bronchial lavage but sometimes it is necessary to resort to lung biopsy or transbronchial biopsy. Treatment of choice is high dose co-trimoxazole, which appears to be as effective as pentamidine isothyonate, but does not have the associated toxic reactions.

Fibrosing alveolitis is a poorly understood condition in which there are inflammatory changes involving the alveolar lining and terminal airways, associated with proliferation of the alveolar lining cells and exudation of fluid. In some of these children there is progressive lung fibrosis. This condition is difficult to diagnose without an open lung biopsy, although it is probably preferable to first give a prolonged course of steroids (prednisolone 1 mg/kg body weight tds for 4–6 weeks) after having excluded an infectious aetiology. If the child shows further deterioration or fails to respond, then a lung biopsy is required to establish a diagnosis. The majority will survive but prolonged steroid therapy will be required.

Fibrosing alveolitis

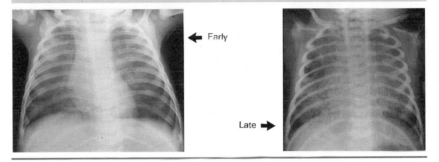

Early

Late

FURTHER READING

Anderson HR, Butland BK, Strachan DP 1994 Trends in prevalence and severity of childhood asthma. British Medical Journal 308: 1600–1606

Bokulic RE, Hilman BC 1994 Interstitial lung diseases in childhood. Pediatric Clinics of North America 1: 543–567

de Lorimier AA 1994 Congenital tracheal stenosis. Seminars in Thoracic and Cervical Surgery 6: 206–211

Doull I 1995 Corticosteroids in the management of croup. British Medical Journal 311: 1244

Green CP, Price JF 1992 Prevention of exercise-induced asthma by salmeterol Xinafoate. Archives of Disease in Childhood 67: 1014–1017

Guidelines in the management of asthma 1993 Thorax 48: S2–S24

Kravitz RM 1994 Congenital malformations of the lung. Pediatric Clinics of North America 41: 453–472

Kristjansson S, Berg-Kelly K, Winso E 1994 Inhalation of racemic adrenaline in the treatment of mild and moderate croup. Acta Paediatrica 83: 1156–1160

Milner AD, Murray M 1989 Acute bronchiolitis in infancy: treatment and prognosis. Thorax 44: 1–5

Parks DP, Ahrens RC, Humpries T, Weinberger MM 1989 Chronic cough in childhood: approach to diagnosis and treatment. Journal of Pediatrics 115: 856–862

Priftis K, Milner AD, Conway E, Honour JW 1990 Adrenal function in asthma. Archives of Disease in Childhood 65: 838–840

Tibballs J, Shann FA, Landou LI 1992 Placebo-controlled trial of prednisolone in children intubated for croup. Lancet 340: 745–748

Vogt-Moykopf I, Rau B, Bramscheid 1993 Surgery for congenital malformations of the lung. Annales de Radiologie (Paris) 36: 145–160

Cystic fibrosis

Hodson ME, Geddes DM (eds) 1995 Cystic fibrosis. Chapman & Hall Medical, London

Hodson ME, Warner JO 1992 Respiratory problems and their treatment. British Medical Bulletin 48: 931–948

Hoiby N 1993 Pseudomonas infection in cystic fibrosis. In: Dodge JA, Brock DJH (eds) Cystic fibrosis: current topics. Wiley, Chichester, p 251–268

MacDonald A 1996 Nutritional management in cystic fibrosis. Archives of Disease in Childhood 74: 81–87

Children with heart disorders are usually healthy and only occasionally require hospital admission. There are many cardiac abnormalities, mainly congenital, but the ways in which they present are limited. A knowledge of the usual age and mode of presentation of the more common lesions, a careful examination, a chest X-ray and an electrocardiogram (ECG) will narrow the diagnostic possibilities — an echocardiogram will usually make the diagnosis. The main concern of the hospital paediatrician is the immediate management of the child. Does the child, for example, need to be referred to a cardiac centre or the next cardiac clinic? If referral is necessary, how urgent is it? A complete anatomical diagnosis and decisions about surgery require a specialist cardiology opinion. Heart disease in children shows itself in one of four ways — heart failure, central cyanosis, a heart murmur and funny turns.

HEART FAILURE

The symptoms and signs of heart failure in a child are essentially the same as those in an adult. In infants it may be confused with septic shock, a metabolic disorder or acute respiratory disease.

Symptoms

— Breathlessness, especially on exertion — the infant pants for breath during a feed or after crying.
— Feeds take longer to complete.
— Failure to thrive.
— Sweating, especially on exertion.
— Abdominal pain, due to rapid enlargement of the liver.
— Collapse and shock, particularly in the neonatal period.
— Metabolic acidosis.

The last three are associated with the rapid onset of severe failure caused by an obstructive lesion or by myocardial disease. The examination of an infant with suspected heart failure should be carried out with care.

Signs

— Dyspnoea, an increased rate and difficulty in breathing, is always present, even during sleep. Chronic dyspnoea leads to deformity of the lower ribs (Harrison's sulci).

— Central cyanosis relieved by oxygen, and grunting respiration occur if there is pulmonary oedema.

— Tachycardia is usual, even at rest. If the heart rate exceeds 220 per minute, the tachycardia is likely to be the cause of the failure.

— Hypotension with weak pulses, cold peripheries and poor capillary filling occur in severe acute failure. If there is raised blood pressure this may be the cause of the heart failure.

— Cardiac enlargement is usual. The apex beat is seen or felt outside the normal position of the 5th intercostal space and the mid-clavicular line. The sternum may bulge forward and the cardiac impulse is usually prominent.

— Auscultation is rarely normal. The heart sounds are loud or muffled, and there is often a murmur or gallop rhythm.

— Hepatomegaly indicates a rise in right atrial pressure and it is easier to detect than a raised jugular venous pressure. The liver may be tender.

Peripheral oedema is a poor sign of heart failure in young children. Auscultation of the lungs is usually remarkably normal, a useful distinguishing feature from lung disease. A chest X-ray separates heart failure from lung disease since there is almost always marked cardiac enlargement with prominent pulmonary vascular markings. Total anomalous pulmonary venous drainage of the infra-diaphragmatic type is the only important exception. The chest X-ray here may show a heart of normal size and the pulmonary venous congestion may be mistaken for lung disease.

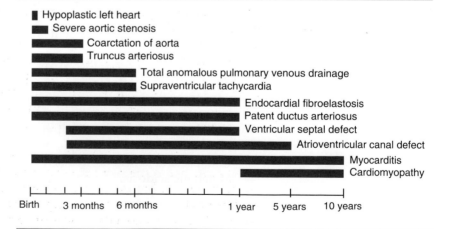

Usual age of presentation of disorders causing heart failure

- Hypoplastic left heart
- Severe aortic stenosis
- Coarctation of aorta
- Truncus arteriosus
- Total anomalous pulmonary venous drainage
- Supraventricular tachycardia
- Endocardial fibroelastosis
- Patent ductus arteriosus
- Ventricular septal defect
- Atrioventricular canal defect
- Myocarditis
- Cardiomyopathy

Birth   3 months   6 months   1 year   5 years   10 years

Diagnosing the cause

Consider the child's age. For example, babies with the hypoplastic left heart syndrome only present in the first 2 weeks of life, whilst babies with uncomplicated ventricular septal defects rarely develop heart failure before 2 months of age. Analyse the heart sounds and murmurs but remember a heart murmur may be absent in hypoplastic left heart syndrome, coarctation, total anomalous pulmonary venous drainage, myocarditis and endocardial fibroelastosis.

Hypoplastic left heart syndrome. The baby collapses in the first few days with severe heart failure, the shocked appearance simulating septicaemia. There is acute renal failure and a metabolic acidosis. Diagnosis is made by echocardiography which shows a tiny left ventricle with atresia or hypoplasia of the mitral and aortic valves and ascending aorta. Surgical correction is not possible and the baby usually dies within a few days. A continous infusion of diamorphine relieves the pain of a congested liver and the distress of breathlessness.

Hypoplastic left heart syndrome

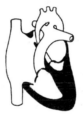

Clinical findings
  absent or weak pulses
  pallor and poor capillary filling
  prominent RV impulse
  gallop rhythm +/- systolic murmur
  large liver

CXR
  cardiomegaly
  pulmonary venous congestion

ECG
  unhelpful

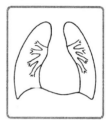

Coarctation of the aorta. Severe coarctation, often with an associated ventricular septal defect, presents in a very similar way to the hypoplastic left heart syndrome although the baby may be older. The poor cardiac output again leads to acute renal failure and metabolic acidosis, with hypotension in the arms, weak brachial pulses and absent femoral pulses. With effective resuscitation (frusemide, dopamine, sodium bicarbonate, oxygen and mechanical ventilation) and use of prostaglandin E to open the ductus arteriosus, the brachial pulses become easily palpable, urine output increases and the acidosis improves. The baby is then fit for transport to a cardiac unit for surgical repair of the coarctation. Echocardiography shows a normal sized left ventricle, a dilated right heart and pulmonary artery, and a narrowing in the distal part of the aortic arch.

Aortic stenosis. Severe ('critical') aortic valve stenosis presents in a similar manner to the two previous conditions. All peripheral pulses are very weak. Echocardiography shows a normal sized left ventricle, a dilated right heart and pulmonary artery, and a thickened immobile aortic valve. The resuscitation measures are the same as used for coarctation of the aorta but valvotomy (by surgery or balloon dilatation) is less successful.

Truncus arteriosus. The baby usually develops heart failure after the first week of life and the onset is more insidious. Echocardiography shows a large common artery arising from both ventricles with a high ventricular septal defect. The pulmonary arteries arise, separately or together, from the posterior wall of the truncus which then continues as the aorta. Mild desaturation is measurable by pulse oximetry but not usually observed clinically. The baby is treated with diuretics in the hope that surgery can be postponed. A synthetic conduit containing a homograft valve is attached to the right ventricle and connected to the pulmonary arteries, whilst the ventricular defect is closed so that the truncus becomes the ascending aorta (Rastelli procedure).

Truncus arteriosus

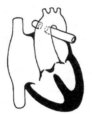

Clinical findings
collapsing pulses
ejection click
systolic murmur

CXR
cardiomegaly
pulmonary plethora

ECG
unhelpful in early infancy
RVH or RVH + LVH present in
older children

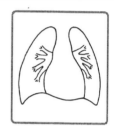

Patent ductus arteriosus (PDA). This usually presents as a heart murmur without symptoms although it is a common cause of increasing respiratory difficulty and ventilator dependence in preterm infants recovering from hyaline membrane disease. Occasionally it gives rise to heart failure in infancy. The symptoms are insidious and failure to thrive is a prominent feature.

Ventricular septal defect (VSD). Large or complicated defects may cause heart failure in infancy. The peak age of presentation is around 3 months when pulmonary vascular resistance reaches its lowest level and the resultant left to right shunt is at a maximum. The heart failure is treated medically in the usual way in the hope that the defect will get smaller. Surgery is necessary if medical treatment fails. The defect is usually closed unless it is complex. If this is the case, a palliative pulmonary banding is performed.

Atrioventricular septal defect. This is the severest form of endocardial cushion defect and a relatively common abnormality in infants with Down syndrome. Heart failure develops insidiously in the first few weeks and failure to thrive is prominent. Intensive medical treatment with high calorie feeds is often successful at first but surgical correction is necessary if this fails. Early development of pulmonary vascular disease makes some patients inoperable but gives rise to an improvement in symptoms as the left to right shunt diminishes.

Atrioventricular defect

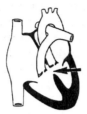

Clinical findings
  normal pulses
  enlarged forceful heart
  systolic murmur
    large liver

CXR
  cardiomegaly
  pulmonary plethora

ECG
  superior QRS axis (S wave>R wave in aVF)
  incomplete right bundle branch block

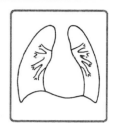

Total anomalous pulmonary venous drainage. In the cardiac and supracardiac type, the presentation is usually with heart failure and failure to thrive in infancy. Mild cyanosis detectable by pulse oximetry is a common feature. The diagnosis is made on echocardiography and early surgical correction is very successful.

Endocardial fibroelastosis. Scarring of the endocardium of the left ventricle results in dilatation and hypertrophy. Symptoms of heart failure develop in infancy. Echocardiography shows a dilated, poorly contracting left ventricle with bright endocardial echos: the heart is anatomically normal. Digoxin and diuretic therapy is often effective and should be continued in the long term. The disease may regress.

Endocardial fibroelastosis

Clinical findings
  reduced pulses
  no cyanosis
  enlarged heart
  gallop rhythm
  no murmur
    (sometimes an apical pansystolic murmur)
  enlarged liver

CXR
  enlarged heart
  pulmonary venous congestion

ECG
  LVH
  T wave inversion in I, aVL and V4-6

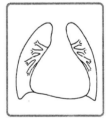

Myocarditis. This presents in infancy or childhood with heart failure, often precipitated by or associated with a respiratory infection. The pulses are weak, the heart sounds are muffled, a gallop rhythm is usually present and there is no murmur. Hepatomegaly may be present but is not marked. A chest X-ray taken because of respiratory symptoms is often the first clue to the diagnosis and shows an unexpectedly large heart with pulmonary venous congestion. An ECG shows widespread ST and T wave changes in the chest leads. An echocardiogram shows a dilated, poorly contracting heart with no structural abnormality. Cardiac enzymes may be elevated at the beginning of the illness and Coxsackie B virus may be isolated from the stool. The treatment is digoxin (at half the usual dose to avoid toxicity) and diuretics. Some recover fully, some develop a permanent cardiomyopathy and others, particularly young infants, deteriorate rapidly and die.

Cardiomyopathy. This non-specific disorder of heart muscle may be isolated, familial, associated with a disorder of voluntary muscle or follow irradiation and chemotherapy. Presentation and findings are similar to those of myocarditis but usually more gradual in onset. Treatment is the same but recovery is rare.

Supraventricular tachycardia (SVT). Infants in heart failure are likely to have SVT if their heart rate exceeds 220 per minute. Diagnosis and management are discussed later.

MANAGEMENT OF HEART FAILURE

Medicines

Inotropic agents. In severe acute heart failure, an i.v. infusion of dopamine (5 µg/kg/min) will improve cardiac output. In less severe cases digoxin can be used. Digoxin is particularly effective in infants and children with poor myocardial function (endocardial fibroelastosis, myocarditis, cardiomyopathy or obstructive lesions like coarctation). It is much less effective when there is volume overload (VSD, PDA, AV canal, truncus arteriosus) and often not used in such lesions. It should not be used in the preterm infant with a PDA.

Diuretics. Frusemide (2 mg/kg/day in 2 divided doses) is the most

Digoxin dosage	
Digitalization	40 µg/kg/day in 3 × 8-hourly doses over the first 24 hours, by mouth. If the oral route cannot be used, the intravenous dose is 30 µg/kg/day in 3 × 8-hourly i.v. injections, each given over 15 minutes, over the first 24 hours
Maintenance	10 µg/kg/day in 2 × 12-hourly doses, by mouth
Therapeutic level	1–3 µg/ml

effective. If used in the long term a potassium supplement (KCl 2 mmol/kg/day in 2 divided doses) or a potassium sparing diuretic such as spironolactone (2 mg/kg/day in 2 divided doses) is necessary.

Vasodilators. These are used in children with valvular lesions or myocardial disease to supplement diuretic therapy. They should be used with caution to avoid hypotension and should be started in hospital. Captropril (Capoten) and hydralazine (Aprescline) are alternatives.

Supportive therapy

Infants in heart failure feel better when semi-recumbent, children prefer to sit up. The need for calories is often neglected but urgent. Feeding by nasogastric tube may be necessary and if given continuously it may be better tolerated in a sick infant. Continuous overnight tube feeding may help an older child to thrive. Energy requirements are high, and calorie supplements may be needed. Effective treatment of heart failure results in a reduction in respiratory rate, heart rate and liver size, a small weight loss initially, improved feeding and then weight gain. When heart failure is due to structural abnormalities any improvement is likely to be short lived and surgery is the only effective therapy. The younger the patient, the more urgent the need for referral to a cardiac centre.

CENTRAL CYANOSIS

Peripheral cyanosis is very common, especially in newborn babies, and is of no significance. Perioral cyanosis is particularly common in older children who are cold, especially after swimming and, again, is of no importance. Central cyanosis is recognised as a purple or blue tinge to the lips and tongue. It is clinically detectable when the amount of reduced haemoglobin in capillary blood exceeds 3 g/100 ml. It is therefore readily recognised in a newborn baby with a high haemoglobin but less noticeable in an anaemic child. Pulse oximetry is very useful if there is doubt about the presence of cyanosis.

There are other causes of central cyanosis besides heart disease. In the newborn period, the following should be considered:

Problem

- The baby looks ill and has obvious respiratory difficulty.
- Arterial blood gases show a low Po_2 and a Pco_2 which may be normal or raised. A nitrogen washout test produces a rise in Po_2 to a level usually above 100 mgHg (14 kPa).
- The chest X-ray shows a normal heart size and abnormal lung fields.

Diagnosis — Lung disease
Hyaline membrane disease, pneumonia and meconium aspiration may all result in central cyanosis.

Problem

- There is a history of a cerebral insult such as birth trauma.
- It may be apparent from inspection that the baby is underventilating, with slow, shallow breathing.
- Arterial blood gases show a low Po_2 and a high Pco_2. A nitrogen wash-out test produces a rise in Po_2.
- The baby may exhibit other neurological abnormalities, e.g. fits.

Diagnosis — Cerebral disorder

Control of respiration may be affected by drugs, immaturity, trauma or asphyxia. Hypoventilation may occur, with resulting cyanosis.

Problem

- The baby looks well.
- Arterial blood gases show a normal P_{O_2}. This increases markedly when the baby is given 100% oxygen to breathe, even though cyanosis is still present.
- A sample of blood turns brown when shaken with air.
- Spectrophotometry of blood shows the presence of methaemoglobin.

Diagnosis — Methaemoglobinaemia

In this rare condition, the baby is centrally cyanosed but has a normal heart and lungs. Response to intravenous reducing agents, e.g. ascorbic acid or methylene blue, is usually dramatic.

Problem

- Clinical examination reveals a baby with central cyanosis.
- Arterial blood gases show a low P_{O_2} and a normal P_{CO_2}. The P_{O_2} of preductal blood is frequently more than 5 mmHg higher than that of postductal blood. Simultaneous transcutaneous P_{O_2} measurements from the right chest and the lower abdomen may show this. Arterial P_{O_2} changes little with 100% O_2.
- Auscultation reveals a loud pulmonary second sound.

Diagnosis — Persistent pulmonary hypertension (also called persistent transitional or fetal circulation)

This is the most difficult condition to distinguish from cyanotic congenital heart disease and referral to a cardiac centre may be necessary. After birth, the pulmonary vascular resistance remains high so that the right-sided pressures (in the right atrium, right ventricle and pulmonary artery) are high. Blood shunts from right to left through the normal fetal channels of the foramen ovale and the ductus arteriosus, resulting in central cyanosis. The phenomenon is seen in babies with severe lung disease, especially hyaline membrane disease and meconium aspiration, and group B haemolytic streptococcal pneumonia. It is also seen in the absence of lung disease in babies who are small for dates, asphyxiated at birth or polycythaemic. Echocardiography is useful because it demonstrates an anatomically normal heart with a right to left shunt at atrial level after peripheral contrast injection or on Doppler assessment.

Problem

- The baby looks well, with no respiratory difficulty.
- There may or may not be a heart murmur.
- The second heart sound is usually single.
- Arterial blood gases show low P_{O_2} and normal P_{CO_2}. After the

infant has been breathing oxygen (90% or more) for 10 minutes the arterial O_2 is unchanged or has slightly increased (not above 100 mgHg, 14 kPa).

• A chest X-ray shows no lung disease.

Diagnosis — Cyanotic congenital heart disease

The underlying lesion responsible for the cyanosis can often be deduced from the age at presentation, the chest X-ray and the ECG. The echocardiogram is diagnostic in all cases.

CYANOTIC HEART DISEASES PRESENTING IN THE FIRST WEEK OF LIFE

The important lesions are transposition of the great arteries, tricuspid atresia, pulmonary atresia, total anomalous pulmonary venous drainage with obstruction to the common pulmonary vein and Ebstein's anomaly.

Transposition of the great arteries. Cyanosis develops when the foramen ovale and ductus arteriosus start to close. In the absence of a ventricular septal defect, this often occurs within the first 24 hours. Although the infant is usually well initially, the increasing cyanosis leads to acidosis and death if no treatment is given.

Transposition of the great arteries

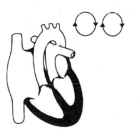

Clinical findings
  central cyanosis
  mild tachycardia
  loud single second heart sound
  no murmur

CXR
  'egg on side' appearance
  develops outside neonatal period
  pulmonary vascular markings are
  normal or increased

ECG
  RVH — normal in newborn

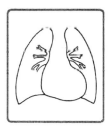

Affected infants may show some improvement in arterial Po_2 with prostaglandin E but urgent balloon septostomy may be needed to allow mixing of atrial blood. Transfer to a cardiac centre should take place at once. The operation of choice is now the arterial switch procedure which is usually carried out at a few days of age. For complicated cases and with late presentation, diversion of systemic and pulmonary venous returns using a baffle is carried out in older infants (Mustard operation).

Tricuspid atresia. There are a number of variants of this condition but the presentation is usually with central cyanosis in the early newborn period. The diagnosis is made on echocardiography although cardiac catheterisation is carried out later in childhood before definitive surgery. Prostaglandin E will reverse the cyanosis and allow unhurried transfer to a children's cardiac centre at a convenient time. A systemic to pulmonary anastomosis — an artificial patent ductus — is then created. The definitive operation is the creation of a right atrial to pulmonary artery anastomosis with a valved conduit (Fontan procedure)

Tricuspid atresia

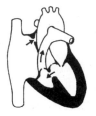

Clinical findings
  central cyanosis
  no tachycardia
  single second heart sound
  +/- soft systolic murmur

CXR
  small heart
  oligaemic lung fields

ECG
  superior QRS axis (S wave > R wave in aVF)
  reduce RV forces

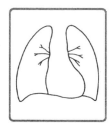

Pulmonary atresia (without a ventricular septal defect). This represents the severest form of pulmonary valve stenosis. Fetal echocardiography suggests that it develops in utero from progressive pulmonary stenosis. The right ventricle is thick walled but the cavity and the tricuspid valve are often small. Affected infants develop severe central cyanosis in the early neonatal period which can be reversed by infusion of prostaglandin E. An open pulmonary valvotomy or creation of a systemic to pulmonary anastomosis are the surgical options but the results are often disappointing.

Pulmonary atresia

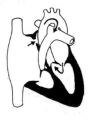

Clinical findings
  central cyanosis
  single second heart sound
  no murmur

CXR
  prominent right atrium
  mild cardiomegaly
  oligaemic lung fields

ECG
  right atrial hypertrophy
  normal axis
  reduced RV and increased LV forces

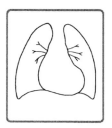

Total anomalous pulmonary venous drainage (TAPVD). The supracardiac and cardiac types present with heart failure, failure to thrive and minimal or no cyanosis. In the infracardiac type where the common pulmonary vein passes below the diaphragm and drains into the portal or systemic venous system, the pulmonary venous return is obstructed. The pulmonary veins are congested, there is pulmonary hypertension and pulmonary oedema. Symptoms develop in early infancy, often in the newborn period, with a combination of central cyanosis and respiratory distress. Always consider the diagnosis in any cyanosed infant with respiratory difficulty — without surgery death is inevitable, but operative correction is relatively straightforward and curative. Echocardiography will make the diagnosis in expert hands.

Total anomalous pulmonary venous drainage

Clinical findings
  central cyanosis
  tachypnoea and recession
  no murmur
  hepatomegaly

CXR
  small heart
  streaky hilar shadows
  hazy lung fields (oedema)

ECG
  often normal

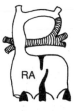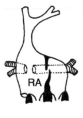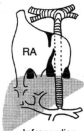

Supracardiac   Cardiac   Infracardiac

Ebstein anomaly. The leaflets of the tricuspid valve are deformed and are displaced distally towards the apex of the right ventricle. Thus the right atrium is large, the right ventricle is small and there may be tricuspid regurgitation. There is usually an associated atrial septal defect and there may be an accessory atrio-ventricular conduction pathway (Wolff–Parkinson–White syndrome). The severest form results in intra-uterine death, the milder forms are asymptomatic and compatible with normal life expectancy, but those in between present with symptoms. Central cyanosis may result from right heart dysfunction and a right to left atrial shunt and can develop in the newborn period, infancy or childhood. Failure to thrive and a reduced exercise tolerance are common. Diagnosis is suspected from the clinical findings, chest X-ray and ECG — it is confirmed by echocardiogram. Repair or replacement of the tricuspid valve is the surgical treatment.

Ebstein anomaly

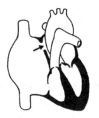

Clinical findings
  central cyanosis
  soft systolic and diastolic murmurs
  added sounds

CXR
  cardiomegaly
  large RA shadow
  oligaemic lung fields

ECG
  tall P waves
  prolonged PR interval
  right bundle branch block

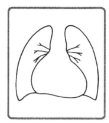

CYANOTIC HEART DISEASE PRESENTING AFTER THE FIRST WEEK OF LIFE

Fallot tetralogy. This is the commonest cyanotic congenital heart lesion presenting outside the immediate newborn period. Its severest form, pulmonary atresia with a ventricular septal defect, will result in central cyanosis at a very early age. There is a large sub-aortic ventricular septal defect with the aorta overriding both ventricles, pulmonary valve and infundibular stenosis and right ventricular hypertrophy. Infants or young children develop cyanosis insidiously, with tiredness and breathlessness on exertion. Occasionally cyanotic spells occur. Diagnosis is made by echocardiogram. Treatment is surgical — either total correction of the defects or (if symptoms occur in early infancy) a palliative systemic to pulmonary anastomosis. The latter, the modified Blalock procedure, is the creation of an artificial ductus arteriosus which improves pulmonary blood flow until a total correction is performed.

Fallot tetralogy

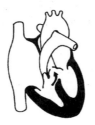

Clinical findings
  central cyanosis
  clubbing (after infancy)
  single second heart sound
  pulmonary systolic murmur

CXR
  boot shaped heart
  (RVH and small pulmonary artery)

ECG
  right axis deviation
  RVH

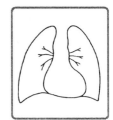

COMPLICATIONS OF CYANOTIC HEART DISEASE

Polycythaemia. An increased haemoglobin is a normal reaction to chronic hypoxaemia and is important to the child with cyanotic heart disease. Relative iron deficiency may result in a haemoglobin within the normal range but a low mean corpuscular volume and haemoglobin concentration, and causes marked exercise intolerance. When treated with iron the haemoglobin rises to polycythaemic levels and the child feels better. When the haematocrit exceeds 70%, however, there is a marked increase in blood viscosity with a tendency to thrombosis.

Infection. Children with any form of cyanotic heart disease are prone to endocarditis. This in turn may lead to a cerebral abscess (fever, headache, drowsiness and focal neurological signs).

Cyanotic spells. Children with Fallot tetralogy or tricuspid atresia may have severe bouts of cyanosis with hyperventilation and loss of consciousness. The attacks are more common in infancy and are usually preceded by bouts of persistent crying. Examination during an attack shows an unconscious child, deeply cyanosed with a brady-cardia and no heart murmur. On recovery the pulmonary systolic mur-mur reappears. These spells are thought to be caused by infundibular spasm. The treatment is to place the child in the knee-elbow position, give oxygen by mask and inject morphine intravenously (0.1 mg/kg). Urgent surgery is then necessary.

TRANSPORT OF BABIES TO A CARDIAC CENTRE

Babies with symptomatic heart disease need to be referred to a cardiac centre with facilities for surgery — the younger the baby the greater the urgency, since early presentation reflects a more serious abnormal-ity. Proper assessment and stabilisation is important, and heart failure should be vigorously treated. The use of prostaglandin therapy should be discussed with the cardiac centre.

Check List
1. Treatment of heart failure *before* transport.
2. Administration of prostaglandin (discuss).
3. Correction of metabolic acidosis.
4. Correction of hypoglycaemia.
5. A warm thermal environment, especially for cyanosed babies.
6. Consent for catheterisation and surgery.
7. A sample of maternal blood.

Prostaglandin (PGE). PGE maintains patency of the duct in fetal life. If administered as an intravenous infusion in the neonatal period it will often re-open a duct that has closed and therefore relieve cyanosis in infants with duct dependent pulmonary blood flow (tricuspid or pul-monary atresia) and improve perfusion in infants with duct dependent systemic blood flow (coarctation of the aorta). Cyanosis in transposition of the great arteries may be improved but not in persistent fetal circula-tion or total anomalous pulmonary venous drainage.

Prostaglandin (PGE$_1$ (alprostedil))

Administration	Side effects
Start i.v. infusion at a rate 0.005 µg/kg/min Increase in multiples of dose to a maximum of 0.05 µg/kg/min until the cyanosis improves or heart failure is controlled	Cutaneous vasodilatation Hypotension Jitteriness Fever Apnoea (occurs in 12% of babies — it is dose related and unusual at the quoted doses)

THE CHILD WITH A HEART MURMUR

Most children with congenital heart disease present with a murmur heard on routine or coincidental examination. The first task of a doctor who hears a heart murmur in a child is to decide whether a murmur is innocent or significant. The following scheme is useful for diagnosing a child with a significant murmur, based on its nature and its site. The older the child, the easier it is to make a diagnosis.

Distinguishing features of innocent and significant heart murmur

Innocent murmur	Significant murmurs
A healthy child	May be cardiac symptoms
Normal pulses	May be normal in volume or collapsing
No thrill	Thrill may be present
A mid-systolic murmur Musical, buzzing quality	May be pansystolic or diastolic
Usually soft	May be loud
Often variable	Consistent
Normal heart sounds	May be abnormal heart sounds
Normal CXR, ECG	CXR or ECG may show abnormality

Finding

- Pansystolic murmur, loudest at lower left sternal border. The murmur runs into the second heart sound, obscuring it. It is often loud and associated with a thrill.

Diagnosis — Ventricular septal defect (VSD)

Presents usually as a heart murmur which appears outside the immediate newborn period (when pulmonary artery and right ventricular pressures fall). If the left to right shunt is large heart failure may occur. The chest X-ray shows cardiomegaly, prominent pulmonary artery, pulmonary plethora and the ECG biventricular hypertrophy. The hole can usually be demonstrated by 2D imaging or Doppler and right ventricular pressure can be estimated.

Management. Heart failure is treated medically, with surgical closure reserved for infants where this is not successful. A VSD may get smaller or close spontaneously with time. If it persists and there are symptoms, or an appreciable shunt on investigation, or evidence of increasing pulmonary artery pressure, the defect should be closed by surgery. Complications include pulmonary vascular disease (increasing RVH clinically and on ECG, a shorter and softer murmur, a louder pulmonary second sound), and subacute bacterial endocarditis.

Finding

- Systolic ejection murmur in the pulmonary area with fixed splitting of the second heart sound. There is no thrill but there may be a mid-diastolic murmur in the tricuspid area.

Diagnosis — Atrial septal defect (ASD)

Presents with a heart·murmur, often not noted until school age. There may be reduced exercise tolerance, chestiness and underweight. Chest X-ray is the same as for VSD, depending on the size of the left to right shunt. An ECG shows right axis deviation and right bundle branch block. The defect can be seen on the echocardiagram.

Management. Surgical closure to prevent the development of heart failure, pulmonary vascular disease and atrial arrhythmias in later life.

Finding

- Systolic ejection murmur in the pulmonary area, often loud and with a thrill and preceded by an ejection click.

Diagnosis — Pulmonary stenosis

Presents with a heart murmur, often first heard in the neonatal period. In the severest form (critical pulmonary stenosis) the features are similar to pulmonary atresia. Chest X-ray shows post-stenotic dilatation of the main pulmonary artery, the ECG right ventricular hypertrophy (RVH). The narrowed valve is seen on the echocardiogram and the gradient estimated by Doppler.

Management. If the gradient exceeds 50 mmHg or there is RVH, the child should be routinely catheterised and the valve dilated with a balloon catheter (pulmonary valvuloplasty). Open valvotomy is rarely necessary.

Finding

- Absent femoral pulses (or weak, delayed femorals), variable systolic murmur over the precordium and hypertension in the arms.

Diagnosis — Coarctation of the aorta

Presents with heart failure in early infancy or as the chance finding of a murmur or hypertension in a healthy child. Chest X-ray shows a normal heart size, prominent descending aorta, rib notching in older children only; the ECG, left ventricular hypertrophy. Echocardiogram will reveal the narrowed aorta, usually just beyond the origin of the left subclavian artery. In well children a gradient across the narrowing can be measured by Doppler. Associated cardiac abnormalities (VSD, PDA or aortic valve lesions) are common.

Management. Unless the coarctation is mild, surgical correction is advised. Balloon dilatation is useful if coarctation reappears after surgery.

Finding

- Loud murmur under the left clavicle which extends through systole and the second heart sound into diastole, collapsing pulses and a very prominent precordial impulse.

Diagnosis — Patent ductus arteriosus

Presents with heart failure in infancy or a murmur on routine examination. Chest X-ray appearances as for VSD and ASD (signs of a left to right shunt) and the ECG shows left ventricular hypertrophy. The echocardiogram demonstrates the ductus, with turbulent flow throughout the cardiac cycle detected on Doppler.

Management. Catheter occlusion or surgical ligation in all cases, to prevent heart failure, pulmonary vascular disease and bacterial endocarditis.

Finding

- Systolic ejection murmur loudest at right upper sternal border radiating to the neck, often with a thrill (particularly in the suprasternal notch) and an ejection click.

Diagnosis — Aortic stenosis

Presents with a heart murmur as a chance finding. Symptoms are unusual and suggest severe stenosis. Chest X-ray shows post-stenotic dilatation of the ascending aorta. The ECG is normal or shows left ventricular hypertrophy. The thickened, narrowed aortic valve which opens poorly can be demonstrated on the echocardiogram and the aortic valve gradient measured by Doppler.

Management. In severe cases there is a risk of sudden death on exertion. If examination and the investigations suggest more than mild stenosis, cardiac catheterisation should be undertaken. Balloon valvuloplasty is often effective although open valvotomy may be necessary. If there is aortic regurgitation as well as stenosis, valve replacement will be needed. Antibiotic prophylaxis with dental treatment is vital.

Finding

- Late systolic murmur at the apex, variable and sometimes with a peculiar crowing or honking quality, often preceded by a systolic click.

Diagnosis — Floppy mitral valve

Chest X-ray is normal, ECG is normal, the echocardiogram shows long slender mitral valve leaflets which prolapse posteriorly into the left atrium during systole.

Management. Antibiotic prophylaxis with dental treatment is the only precaution.

'FUNNY TURNS'

Children often have sudden episodes in which there may be alteration of consciousness — these are sometimes caused by a cardiac arrhythmia. Features which suggest a cardiac origin are palpitations in the chest (the child is aware of a rapid, slow or irregular heart beat), extreme pallor before loss of consciousness, and a relationship to physical exertion or emotion. Most 'funny turns' are not cardiac but cerebral in origin but if they are caused by a cardiac arrhythmia they may be life-threatening. A child can be asked to describe his or her heart rate and rhythm and the mother can be asked to count the rate during an episode. 24 hour tape recordings of heart rate, brief event recorders and trans-telephone ECGs have made the diagnosis of significant arrhythmias easier.

Vasovagal faints are common in older school children, especially girls. The child feels weak, nauseated and has a 'swimming' feeling. Voices sound far away and the room appears to be moving. She looks pale, grey and clammy, and may lose consciousness briefly. The heart rate is slow and regular. If the child is allowed to lie down with her legs raised, she quickly comes round. Similar but more alarming episodes occur in toddlers following unexpected minor injury (reflex anoxic spells).

Diagnosis (1)

Supraventricular tachycardia (SVT)
This is an uncommon but important cardiac arrhythmia which can present in the fetus, newborn, infant or child. The younger the patient the less well the SVT is tolerated. This is partly because the heart rate is higher, diastolic filling is impaired and heart failure therefore develops sooner. The heart is usually structurally normal although a proportion (10–25%) have the Wolff–Parkinson–White (WPW) syndrome. Underlying cardiac abnormalities include Ebstein's anomaly, post-cardiac surgery, especially involving the atria, cardiac tumour and myocarditis.

Fetal SVT. This presents as a tachycardia on fetal heart monitoring or as fetal hydrops (heart failure) often with hydramnios.

SVT in the newborn and infant. Symptoms occur earlier and are most marked in the newborn. In the infant, SVT may be triggered by a febrile illness. The symptoms are those of cardiac decompensation: poor feeding, pallor, cold peripheries, increasing breathlessness with an expiratory grunt and vomiting.

The child with SVT complains of an unpleasant sensation in the chest, feels weak and looks pale. Palpitations can often be described.

The ECG permits the rate to be measured and ranges between 180 and 340/min. In the newborn and infant it exceeds 220/min. It is absolutely regular, with no beat to beat variation; the QRS complexes are narrow but normal; if P waves are seen, the axis is often abnormal.

Management

Admit to a high dependency area for close monitoring and observation. Treatment depends on the severity of symptoms (an effect of heart rate, duration of tachycardia and presence of underlying cardiac disease).

Diving reflex. This is the most effective method of vagal stimulation in the infant or child. Do not use eyeball pressure or carotid sinus massage. There are two techniques:

Treatment according to state

Well or mildly unwell
  Diving reflex
  Drugs
  DC cardioversion

III
  Drugs
  DC cardioversion

Extremely III
  DC cardioversion

1. *Facial cooling* — fill a polythene bag with cold water and ice cubes, place it on the face so that the forehead, eyes, nose, mouth and cheeks are covered; leave for 15 seconds and monitor ECG.
2. *Immersion (infants)* — wrap the trunk and limbs in a towel and immerse head and face completely in a washbasin full of iced water — leave for 5 seconds — do not cover the nose or mouth — the baby becomes temporarily apnoeic. Return to sinus rhythm usually occurs at once.

Adenosine. This has a very short half-life (15 seconds) and no important side effects. It is given as a rapid i.v. bolus followed by flushing the line with saline. The starting dose is 0.05 mg/kg increasing by increments of 0.05 mg/kg to a maximum dose of 0.3 mg/kg. It works instantly but SVT often recurs unless a regular anti-arrhythmic is given.

Verapamil. Hypotension, bradycardia and even death are described in infants given verapamil. It is *only* to be used after the age of 1 year and never in conjunction with a beta blocker. It is given as an i.v. bolus over 20 seconds in a dose of 0.15 mg/kg — return to sinus rhythm occurs in most children shortly after the injection. Calcium chloride for i.v. use should be available in case of severe hypotension.

Flecainide. Given as a *slow* i.v. injection (over 15 minutes) in a dose of 2 mg/kg. Return to sinus rhythm usually occurs within 10 minutes of the injection and side effects are mild and uncommon.

Digoxin. This is too slow acting to be useful in ill patients but may be used if the child is well. Digitalisation is by the oral or i.v. route as previously described.

DC cardioversion. Anaesthetise the child or sedate with i.v. midazolam in an emergency, giving oxygen by face mask. Apply the infant or child paddles to the chest (one at apex of the heart, the other at the right sternal border) through conducting pads. Ensure that the intervening skin is dry and free from electrode gel. Administer a shock of 1 joule/kg, synchronised if possible to the R wave of the ECG. Because it is always successful in converting SVT to sinus rhythm it is the first line treatment in a desperately ill infant or child, and the back up treatment in others if the diving reflex and drugs have failed.

If the episodes of SVT occur in infancy, prophylaxis with regular digoxin is usually effective. Outside infancy, a beta blocker such as propranolol (0.5 mg tds orally) can be used, except in children with asthma, to reduce the frequency of troublesome episodes. Amiodarone (350 mg/m² surface area/day for 10 days followed by 200 mg/m²/day) is useful for resistant cases and in the presence of the WPW syndrome. The choice of drug is an area for the specialist.

Diagnosis (2)

Complete heart block
This is usually congenital although it may follow cardiac surgery. In some cases there is an underlying structural heart defect. In the congenital form without a heart defect there is a high incidence of maternal collagen disease. Some children tolerate heart block well. Others develop Stokes–Adams attacks with sudden loss of consciousness,

extreme pallor and loss of peripheral pulses, often related to exertion. They may be mistaken for epileptic fits. Indications for a pacemaker are extreme bradycardia, escape beats and the development of heart failure in the young infants, or the appearance of Stokes–Adams attacks. If the complete heart block is intermittent the diagnosis may not be apparent on examination or ECG but 24-hour ECG recordings are useful.

Diagnosis (3)

Sick sinus syndrome

Some children with funny turns, dizzy spells, loss of consciousness, particularly on exertion, have a slow heart beat on examination — an ECG shows a sinus bradycardia, but 24-hour heart rate recordings show both rapid and slow arrhythmias. The former are treated with drugs and the latter with a pacemaker.

INFORMATION FOR PARENTS ON CONGENITAL HEART DISEASE

Antibiotic prophylaxis with dental treatment. There is a small risk of subacute bacterial endocarditis when children with congenital heart lesions have invasive dental procedures (extractions, fillings, scaling and polishing). The importance of antibiotic prophylaxis should be stressed to the parents and it is useful if they have written information to give to their dentist. Oral prophylaxis is satisfactory and amoxycillin is the antibiotic of choice (amoxycillin 1.5–3 g orally 1 hour before dental treatment).

Immunisation. Congenital heart disease is no contraindication to full immunisation — indeed it could be argued that immunisation is more important still.

Exercise restriction. Children with moderate or severe aortic stenosis should not be allowed to undertake strenuous exercise because of the small risk of sudden death. All other children with congenital heart disease should be allowed to exert themselves as much as they wish. They will stop if the exertion is too much for them.

Non-cardiac surgery in children with congenital heart disease. The only contraindications to surgery are frank cardiac failure or severe pulmonary hypertension. A general anaesthetic and an operation involve a considerable risk in these cases. Otherwise there is no reason why surgery should not be undertaken, regardless of the type of lesion or the type of operation contemplated. There are three provisos however:

1. Antibiotic prophylaxis is necessary for ENT or bowel surgery.
2. In children with aortic stenosis, hypotension must be avoided because this will result in poor coronary artery perfusion and myocardial damage.
3. In children with cyanotic heart disease and polycythaemia, thrombosis may occur if dehydration develops. The children must be well hydrated before, during and immediately after operation, if necessary by the i.v. route.

FURTHER READING

Anderson RH, Macartney FJ, Shinebourne MA, Tynan M 1987 Paediatric cardiology (2 volumes). Churchill Livingstone, Edinburgh

Jordan SC, Scott O 1989 Heart disease in paediatrics. Butterworths, London

Kugler JD, Danford DA 1996 Management of infants, children and adolescents with paroxysmal supraventricular tachycardia. Journal of Pediatrics 129: 324–338

11

Bowel

VOMITING
DIARRHOEA
ABDOMINAL PAIN
CONSTIPATION
GASTRO-INTESTINAL BLEEDING

Problems arising in the gastrointestinal system can produce a wide range of symptoms and are responsible for a high proportion of attendances at A&E departments and admissions to hospital. Many of the symptoms, for example vomiting and pain, are non-specific and so it is important to keep an open mind on the cause until a firm diagnosis is reached. The presenting symptoms of gut disorders considered in this chapter are vomiting, acute and chronic diarrhoea, acute and recurrent abdominal pain, constipation and gastrointestinal bleeding.

PERSISTENT VOMITING

Persistent vomiting in a newborn infant is a serious symptom; intestinal obstruction, systemic infection and a metabolic or renal disorder must all be considered. After the first week of life the priority is to distinguish innocent regurgitation and feeding problems from pathological disorders. The following are important in reaching a differential diagnosis: a record of recent weight gain; feeding regimen with details of the type of feed, volume, frequency and duration; the nature of the vomit and its time in relation to feeds, in particular it is important to

---

Causes of persistent vomiting

Innocent	**Cerebral disorders**
Possetting	Hydrocephalus
	Subdural bleed
Intestinal	
Gastro-oesophageal reflux	**Renal disorders**
Pyloric stenosis	Renal failure
Malrotation and partial obstruction	Renal tubular acidosis
Food intolerance	
	Metabolic-endocrine disorders
Infection	Adrenal failure
Urinary tract	Amino-acid disorders
	Hypercalcaemia

document the presence of either blood, coffee grounds or bile stains; careful examination looking for signs of thrush, dehydration, evidence of intestinal obstruction and raised intracranial pressure; and a test feed.

Problem(s)

- Excessive feeding with a daily milk intake well in excess of 150 ml/kg/day.
- Inadequate intake which can occur either in breast or bottle fed infants (it may be due to thrush or air swallowing).
- Problems due to teat hole size and the rate of milk flow.
- Inexpert handling during and after feed times or simply at napkin changing.
- The mother may be inexperienced, anxious or depressed.

Diagnosis — A feeding problem

The difficulty may be recognised on admission to hospital and supervision under experienced nursing staff. Information and guidance may be provided by sympathetic nurses or health visitors who have sufficient time to assist the mother and restore her confidence. Often inappropriate changes in milk formulae have delayed recognition and exacerbated the true problem.

Problem

- A normal, thriving infant.
- Appropriate feeding.
- Small volume milk vomits between feeds.

Diagnosis — Innocent regurgitation, possetting

The lower oesophageal sphincter is less established in early infancy. The mother may be concerned about the cause but usually regards the vomits as a nuisance rather than having any sinister implication. Management is by reassurance and possibly using a non-digestible thickener (such as Carobel or Nestargel). The problem resolves spontaneously with weaning and the adoption of a more upright posture.

Problem

- Frequent large volume vomits.
- Failure to thrive.
- Iron deficiency anaemia.
- Episodes of aspiration pneumonia.
- Irritability and neck posturing during feeds.

Diagnosis — Gastro-oesophageal reflux with or without a hiatus hernia (partial thoracic stomach)

Gastro-oesophageal reflux (GOR) is the involuntary passage of gastric contents into the oesophagus more than normal (on 24 hour oesophageal pH monitoring >4% of time at pH <4). When of greater duration it

Position of pH electrode and section of 24-hour recording of pH

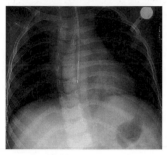

X-ray showing position
of electrode

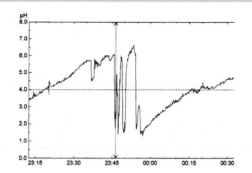

part of 24-hour recording showing
an event at 23.46 h

% time when pH below 4
Normal up to 4%
Moderate 4–15%
Severe more than 15%

may cause oesophagitis or respiratory complications. Factors such as thoracic stomach or hiatus hernia, lack of intra-abdominal oesophagus and loss of the cardia-oesophageal angle result in incompetence of the gastro-oesophageal sphincter mechanisms. The investigation to establish the diagnosis and severity of GOR is 18–24-hour oesophageal monitoring of the % time the pH is less than 4: 5–10% then it is mild, 10–15% moderate and more than 15% severe. Other investigations are to determine complications (haemoglobin, ferritin, faecal occult blood and chest X-ray) or secondary causes (e.g. anti-gliadin antibodies). Barium studies are indicated when an anatomical abnormality is suspected — hiatus hernia, oesophageal stricture, malrotation or gastric outflow obstruction. Endoscopy with a flexible fibre-optic instrument will detect oesophagitis and potential stricture formation as well as excluding a cause such as an enteropathy.

Sliding hiatus hernia

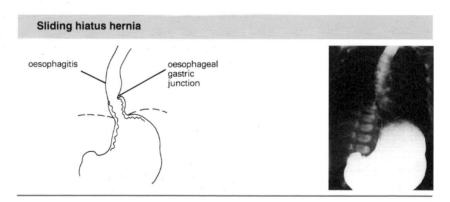

oesophagitis

oesophageal
gastric
junction

Management

Positioning. Reflux may be reduced in babies by nursing on the side with the head raised 30% from the horizontal.

Thickening and antacid. A non-digestible starch food thickener (e.g. Carobel or Nestargel) may reduce the number of vomits and an antacid such as Gaviscon may help symptoms.

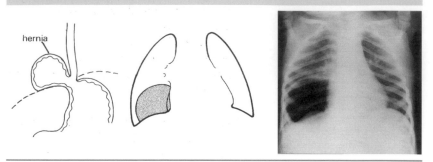

Para-oesophageal hernia

hernia

Acid suppression. More severe cases will require histamine-2 antagonist therapy (e.g. ranitidine) or a proton pump inhibitor (e.g. omeprazole).

Check sufficient therapy or compliance by measuring gastric pH. Acid suppression may help heal peptic oesophagitis but will not decrease reflux. Bile and food reflux may continue damage and symptoms.

Prokinetic agent. Cisapride improves lower oesophageal clearance, increases sphincter pressure and increases gastric emptying thus decreasing reflux episodes.

Surgery. Medical measures have failed when symptoms persist after 3 months' therapy or if there is refractory iron deficiency anaemia, further episodes of aspiration pneumonia or stricture formation. The conventional procedure is a Nissen fundoplication via the abdominal approach. There is a 20% relapse when the repair becomes undone. Medical measures often fail in children with neurodevelopmental problems and these patients will need assessment of the safety of oral feeding as a gastrostomy may be indicated at the same time as the fundoplication.

Summary of the treatment

Uncomplicated GOR
— No treatment await natural resolution.
— Or interventions to reduce vomiting (positioning, food thickening and reduced liquid intake, pro-kinetic agent).

Arrange for 24 hour pH monitoring if the above fails or if there are complications or if suspicion of silent reflux (no vomiting but symptoms suggesting reflux, e.g. repeated aspiration).

Moderate GOR (pH<4–15% of time).
— Add antacids or H-2 antagonists.
— Increase prokinetic agent and continue for up to 3 months.

Severe GOR (pH<4 more than 15% of time or evidence of oesophagitis)
— Proton pump inhibitor in place of antacids or H-2 antagonist.

Surgery if still failing to thrive or other complications after full medical treatment for 3-month period.

Problem

- Projectile non-bile stained vomiting.
- Weight loss and dehydration.
- Constipation.
- Persistent jaundice.
- A test feed revealing a hungry infant, a pyloric tumour, visible peristalsis, a projectile vomit sometimes containing blood or 'coffee grounds'.

Diagnosis — Infantile pyloric stenosis

Occurrence is partially determined by polygenic inheritance but the exact aetiology remains a mystery. For the test feed the infant is fed with head nursed on the right arm and examining with the left hand, feeling for the hypertrophied pyloric muscle just beyond the rectus sheath. Look out also for ravenous feeding, stomach peristalsis and projectile feeding. Plasma sodium, potassium and bicarbonate measurement reveals a hypokalaemic alkalosis which supports the diagnosis and indicates the necessity of fluid and electrolyte replacement. Imaging by radiology or ultrasound is needed in those few infants whose pyloric tumour cannot be definitely palpated on repeat test feeding. Typical features on barium swallow and/or ultrasound include a dilated stomach with delayed emptying, a narrowed pyloric canal, pouting of the pylorus into the antral cavity and 'doughnut appearance'. Gastro-oesophageal reflux is also a common finding.

Management. It is essential to correct the fluid and electrolyte deficit before general anaesthesia and surgery. Half normal saline in 5% glucose with added potassium chloride is an appropriate solution to correct the deficit and the alkalosis. Oral feeding should be stopped while awaiting surgery and the stomach emptied via a nasogastric tube. Following a Ramstedt procedure most infants tolerate rapid reintroduction of oral feeds. There is sometimes a problem with oesophageal reflux which usually settles spontaneously.

For infants whose vomiting does not follow the above patterns or is accompanied by fever, or other signs of systemic upset, the following investigations must be considered:

Urine, blood and CSF microscopy and culture — *urinary and other systemic infections.*

Plasma glucose, sodium, potassium, bicarbonate, urea and creatinine measurement; and urine reducing substances — *metabolic disorders — renal failure — renal tubular acidosis.*

Plasma calcium — *hypercalcaemia.*

Food intolerance such as cows' milk protein intolerance or gluten enteropathy may present with persistent vomiting without diarrhoea. Some infants with undiagnosed asthma present with vomiting precipitated with coughing. The older infant can develop behavioural vomiting in association with excessive liquid intake and faddy eating.

ACUTE DIARRHOEA AND VOMITING

Acute diarrhoea and vomiting may result from toxic or infective insult to the gut or be part of a systemic illness. Infective gastroenteritis results from several mechanisms by viral, bacterial and protozoal agents. In about 60% of admitted cases the agent is viral, 15% bacterial (*E. coli*, campylobacter, shigella and salmonella in decreasing order of frequency), 1% giardia or cryptosporidium and 24% no pathogen identified. The mechanisms include the production of enterotoxins which activate intestinal adenyl cyclase and stimulate fluid secretions, invasion of the mucosa and adherence to the mucosa with disruption of the microvillus brush border.

Problem

In winter months, the majority of children with infective diarrhoea present with:

- An acute onset of vomiting or diarrhoea. The vomiting may precede the diarrhoea by many hours.
- Colicky abdominal pain and abdominal distension.
- Watery stools.
- Mild pyrexia.
- Prodromal upper respiratory tract symptoms.

Diagnosis — Probably viral gastroenteritis (commonly rotavirus)

Problem

Other children present with a more systemic illness involving:

- High fever, irritability and convulsions.
- Bloody, mucoid stool.
- Occasionally erythema nodosum and arthritis.

Diagnosis — Invasive diarrhoea as caused by certain *E. coli*, campylobacter or shigella

In most cases the infecting agent cannot be accurately defined on clinical features. The first priority is to confirm the diagnosis of infective gastroenteritis, and to exclude other systemic or surgical disorders manifesting with fever and gastrointestinal symptoms. The differential diagnosis includes meningitis, diabetic ketoacidosis, acute appendicitis and intussusception. Also consider haemolytic uraemic syndrome, a rare complication of entero-invasive gastroenteritis (*E. coli* type 0157).

Management

The priorities in gastroenteritis are assessment of the dehydration and starting rehydration therapy at home or hospital depending on severity and social circumstances. In the assessment remember that the typical signs may be absent in hypernatraemic dehydration, especially in obese infants. In moderate to severe dehydration appropriate laboratory investigations may include blood count and haematocrit, plasma electrolytes and urea, stool microscopy and culture.

Assessment of i.v. fluid therapy in dehydration

	Clinical assessment	Laboratory aids
1. Volume losses	Signs of dehydration Signs of shock	PCV Blood urea
2. Osmolar changes	(a) hypernatraemia irritability, skin 'doughy' circulation relatively good	Plasma Na^+ Plasma osmolality
	(b) hyponatraemia shock hypotension	Plasma Na^+ Plasma osmolality (High urine osmolality suggests inappropriate ADH secretin)
3. Acid-base	Hyperpnoea Tachypnoea	Blood gases, PH, HCO_3 or BIC
4. Loss of intracellular cation (K^+)	Weakness Hypotonia	Plasma K^+ ECG changes reflect plasma level
5. Hypocalcaemia	Neuromuscular irritability	Total plasma calcium not a good guide, Ionized calcium ideal. ECG changes helpful
6. Hypoglycaemia	Lethargy Coma Convulsion	Blood sugar

Antibiotics are not indicated unless there is evidence of systemic infection or cramping pain in campylobacter infection. Antidiarrhoeal preparations are contra-indicated in children; apart from potential toxicity, they slow gut transit time and encourage the persistence of an abnormal bowel flora increasing morbidity and mortality.

Oral rehydration therapy (ORT) works using the coupled transport system which actively absorbs glucose and sodium across even a damaged bowel wall and water follows by osmosis. ORT has been dramatically successful in reducing mortality from life-threatening diarrhoea in the developing world, and avoiding morbidity and hospital admission from less severe disease in developed countries. The regimen advocated for developing countries takes account of greater electrolyte losses, and promotes the use of WHO-UNICEF solution containing 90 mmol/l sodium. In the developed countries ORT solutions containing 30–50 mmol/l sodium are appropriate given at a rate of 150 ml/kg/day with small amounts given often. In the management of mild dehydration this solution is given in a 1:1 ratio with either water or breast milk.

Mild dehydration (under 5%). Mild dehydration can be corrected by oral rehydration solution. The infant should be allowed additional water or continuation of breast milk to satisfy thirst; the total volume should be given as frequent small volume feeds. ORT does not provide adequate energy intake and should not be prolonged beyond 24 hours without milk or light diet. Regrading the introduction of milk is unnecessary.

Moderate to severe (over 5%). Complications arise as dehydration approaches 10% of body weight and these children must be admitted. If the infant has poor perfusion (capillary refill time over 3 seconds) and/or deep breathing indicating a metabolic acidosis, obtain intravenous access, take blood for plasma electrolytes, urea and bicarbonate estimation and give 20 ml/kg 150 mmol sodium chloride over 20 minutes. The rate and type of continuing replacement fluid therapy is determined by the plasma sodium result. In hypernatraemic dehydration aim for the sodium to decease by about 1 mmol per hour. If severe, acidosis (plasma bicarbonate less than 12 mmol/l: pH < 7.0) is treated by providing about half the calculated deficit of bicarbonate:

half deficit (mmol) = weight (kg) $\times$ 0.5 $\times$ 0.3 $\times$ (24 – observed plasma bicarbonate mmol/l)

Early complications

Oliguria. The urine flow should be established within a few hours of commencing adequate intravenous rehydration. Oliguria (less than 200 ml/m² surface area per day) must first be confirmed by checking the size of the bladder, and that urine is being distinguished from watery stools. It may be necessary to introduce a bladder catheter. Once established it is essential to distinguish pre-renal from renal causes. The following investigations indicate a pre-renal cause, a urine osmolality above 500 mOsmol/kg, a urine : plasma osmolar ratio above 1.3, a urinary sodium under 10 mmol/l and a urinary urea above 250 mmol/l. The presence of haematuria and a palpable renal mass suggests renal vein thrombosis. Haematuria with fragmented red cells on blood film and a low platelet count suggests haemolytic uraemic syndrome. Urgent intravascular volume expansion is essential to correct pre-renal oliguria. Refractory oliguria may respond to repeated courses of frusemide (1–2 mg/kg) but once established, in spite of adequate plasma expansion, fluid intake must be reduced to that which corrects for rehydration but provides only 50 ml/kg/day for maintenance requirement. Potassium is omitted. The inability to correct the fluid and electrolyte status and the development of acidosis or hyperkalaemia are indications for peritoneal or haemodialysis. The majority of children recovery spontaneously with a polyuric phase.

Convulsions may be febrile, associated with electrolyte disturbance, in particular hypernatraemic dehydration and its correction, or a consequence of cerebral haemorrhages and subdural effusions. Investigations should include plasma sodium, calcium, magnesium and glucose levels and cranial ultrasound. Treatment consists of correcting the electrolyte or glucose disturbance. For prolonged convulsions give intravenous diazepam (0.2–0.3 mg/kg body weight).

Pulmonary oedema may occur without other clinical signs of fluid overload.

Late complications

The majority of recovering infants can restart their normal milk formula or mixed diet once the dehydration is corrected.

Protracted diarrhoea. A minority develop transient secondary lactose intolerance with poor weight gain and persisting diarrhoea positive for reducing substances greater than 1% and require a lactose free formula for at least a month. Other causes include transient monosaccharide intolerance, transient cows' milk protein intolerance and possibly unmasked gluten intolerance. Reinfection and persistent bacterial overgrowth of the small intestine may also be a factor. Differential diagnosis of protracted diarrhoea is discussed in the next section.

Morbidity and mortality

The mortality rate from gastroenteritis for children aged under 5 years was six per 100 000 in 1987 (England and Wales). The majority of deaths occur in young infants and hypernatraemic dehydration is the most dangerous category. Under 10% of infants surviving hypernatraemic dehydration have neurological deficits.

Problem

- Four or more loose stools per day for longer than 2 weeks.
- Failure to thrive.

Diagnosis — Protracted diarrhoea of infancy

Affected infants are usually severely malnourished and need prompt investigation and nutritional support. As it commonly occurs after gastroenteritis consider infection or re-infection. Test the stool for reducing substances present in secondary lactose intolerance. Look for features to suggest susceptibility to infection, for example refractory candidiasis. Features suggesting immune deficiency are absence of palpable lymph nodes, thymic shadow on chest X-ray and low lymphocyte count. Review the diet for possible triggers such as urticaria, stridor or vomiting after a test feed with cows' milk protein. Persistence of diarrhoea in spite of cessation of oral feeding suggests a secretory disorder, for example chloridorrhoea. Coeliac disease should be considered if on gluten diet and anti-gliadin and anti-endomysial antibodies tested. Small intestinal biopsy is indicated by endoscopy or Crosby capsule to look for: villous atrophy — patchy in cows' milk protein and soya protein intolerances and complete in gluten intolerance; microscopic examination of duodenal fluid for giardia or cryptosporidium; culture of duodenal fluid for bacterial overgrowth. The investigative procedure parallels that in the next section. Obstructive signs or abnormal anal tone suggests a structural disorder, for example Hirschsprung disease with enterocolitis.

Management

It is important to correct fluid and electrolyte status if significantly dehydrated and continue previous diet if tolerated while investigations are being performed. Adjust the diet according to clinical and investigative results, for example gluten-free diet, disaccharide-free diet, cows' milk protein-free diet. For those infants in whom the diagnosis is not obvious or where the condition does not permit extensive investigation or dietary manipulations, a cows' milk protein hydrolysate or chicken-based hypo-allergenic regimens are usually effective in providing adequate nutrition. Chicken protein is hypoallergenic and supplementing with carbohydrate, fat and a vitamin mineral preparation makes up a modular feed. If oral nutrition is not tolerated a period of intravenous feeding is necessary but every attempt should be made to continue at least some oral intake. A period on a chicken based diet should allow the child to thrive and permit investigations to be completed. A stepwise introduction of lactose, cows' milk protein and gluten should be planned over a period of several months.

CHRONIC DIARRHOEA

An initial assessment including history, examination, documentation of growth parameters and visual inspection of the stool will permit classification of the problem into one of three main categories.

Causes of chronic diarrhoea

Normal growth and general health
Toddler diarrhoea
(peas and carrots syndrome)
Irritable bowel syndrome
Anxiety
Overflow on constipation

Abnormal growth — malabsorption
(a) Mucosal abnormality
  Gluten enteropathy
  Lactase deficiency
  Cows' milk protein enteropathy
  Soya protein enteropathy
  Severe *Giardia lamblia* or
  Cryptosporidium infection

(b) Pancreatic abnormality
  Cystic fibrosis
  Exocrine failure with neutropenia
(c) Structural abnormality
  Blind loop
  Hirschsprung disease
  Lymphangiectasia
  Short gut
(d) Selective inborn errors in metabolism
  Acodermatitis enteropathica
  Congenital chloridorrhoea
  Glucose-galactose malabsorption
  Sucrose-isomaltase deficiency
  Abetalipoproteinaemia

(e) Miscellaneous conditions
  Extra-intestinal infection
  Immune deficiencies
  Tumours
  Histiocytosis X

Abnormal growth — abdominal pain and/or bloody diarrhoea
Inflammatory bowel disease
  Crohn disease
  Ulcerative colitis

Pancreatic exocrine failure has to be considered in the investigation of malabsorption. More than 95% of children with exocrine pancreatic insufficiency have **cystic fibrosis** with typically elevated sweat sodium concentration.

Problem (common)

- Normal growth.
- 3–6 loose mucous stools per day often containing identifiable vegetable material, 'peas and carrots syndrome'.
- No abnormality on examination.

Diagnosis — Benign infantile or toddler's diarrhoea
A number of mechanisms have been proposed to explain this disorder. Most evidence favours decreased whole gut transit time such that small intestinal contents reach the colon inappropriately early.

Management. This is largely reassurance of parents that growth is normal and there is 90% resolution by third year. Parents may also be reassured there is no clear association with functional bowel problems in later life. The mother should limit the intake of snacks and cold drinks which can provoke the gastrocolic reflex. Exclusion of provoking dietary factors, for example fruit juices, cows' milk, egg or cheese, may help a few but advise parents against trying inappropriate and nutritionally deficient diets. Many infants respond to a temporary reduction in dietary roughage and an increase in dietary fat including prescription of Callogen which delays gastric emptying and transit. An occasional child has such distressing symptoms particularly at toilet training that cautious use of loperamide is justified.

Problem

- Poor weight gain or short stature.
- Vomiting, diarrhoea, anorexia.
- Irritability.
- Anaemia, hypotonia.
- Abdominal distension, wasted buttocks and rickets.

Diagnosis — Suspected coeliac disease

Classically children present with malabsorption problems in the first 2 years of life. However the mean age of diagnosis has increased, probably because of the later introduction and the lower amount of gluten in our diet. Older children may present with similar features or because of growth failure with delayed bone age and puberty. The diagnosis of coeliac disease is established by typical small bowel partial villous atrophy on a gluten diet and response to a gluten free diet in children over 2 years of age. In those under 2 years of age other causes and transient gluten enteropathy should be considered. If there is any doubt, biopsy after 2 years on gluten free diet to show normal mucosa and then biopsy after a gluten challenge to show partial villous atrophy. It is also important to bear in mind the possibility of emotional deprivation and systemic disorders such as chronic renal failure.

Investigation

Anti-gliadin and anti-endomysial antibodies are useful in screening but not diagnostic for untreated coeliac disease with the former more sensitive and the latter more specific.

Small intestinal biopsy is indicated if the above antibodies are positive and if there is clinical and laboratory evidence favouring malabsorption. The diet should be gluten containing for at least 6 weeks before a biopsy to diagnose coeliac disease. While the Crosby and Watson capsules provide good quality specimens, operator experience is limited and the failure rate can be high. Upper gastrointestinal endoscopy has the advantages of a quicker procedure, provides multiple biopsies and diagnoses problems in the stomach and oesophagus. Coagulation should be tested and if abnormal corrected with intramuscular vitamin K. The following are characteristic but not diagnostic of coeliac disease:

— Flattened villi with irregular surface epithelial cells.
— An excess of chronic inflammatory cells in the lamina propria.
— Crypts showing evidence of excess proliferation.

Such changes are found in other enteropathies. The differential diagnosis includes those of cows' milk protein, soya protein, auto-immune or invasive agents of gastroenteritis.

Management

A life long gluten-free diet is recommended. This avoids wheat, rye, oats and barley. Maize, corn and rice are permitted. Supplemental iron, folate and vitamin D may be required during the recovery period. There is usually a prompt clinical response to the introduction of a gluten-free diet. Failures in treatment with a gluten-free diet usually mean non-compliance with the diet but consider also the possibility of associated cows' milk protein intolerance or lactose deficiency.

Problem

• Frequent frothy liquid acid stools causing perianal soreness.
• Vomiting, abdominal distension and pain.
• Poor weight gain.

Diagnosis — Lactose intolerance

The diagnosis is confirmed by sending fresh liquid stool for thin layer chromatography to identify lactose. A persistent reading of 1% or greater of lactose is significant. In the majority of affected children the lactase deficiency is secondary to small intestine mucosal damage; post-gastroenteritis, giardiasis, cows' milk protein intolerance, soya protein intolerance or gluten enteropathy. Inherited lactase deficiency is rare in caucasians and presents in early infancy as watery diarrhoea, while non-caucasians commonly inherit a predisposition to early loss of lactase, manifesting after age 2–3 years. An infant presenting with lactose intolerance after gastroenteritis will benefit from feeding with a lactose-free formula, e.g. the casein based preparation Galactomin 17. If the infant continues to have diarrhoea and fails to gain weight the cause could be a coexistent cows' milk protein enteropathy or giardia. A small intestinal biopsy is indicated and if a patchy partial villous atrophy is found a semi-elemental formula is prescribed as part of a cows' milk protein free diet. Older children can usually tolerate a milk-free diet based on conventional foodstuffs but will require calcium supplements. Cows' milk protein enteropathy is transient and after about 6 months the child can be reintroduced to small portions of cows' milk.

Problem

• Rarely infants present with intolerance to all carbohydrates as part of protracted diarrhoea, as a sequel of gastroenteritis or after massive gut resection.

Diagnosis — Monosaccharide intolerance

Their management is difficult and usually requires a period of total parenteral nutrition. Attempts at enteral feeding are complicated by hypoglycaemia and ketosis. Successful therapy is based on enteral feeding with carbohydrate-free preparations combined with intravenous glucose. Recovery allows the cautious reintroduction of glucose and glucose polymers.

Problem

- Profuse diarrhoea from birth.
- Glucose intolerance.

Diagnosis — Glucose/galactose intolerance

This is a rare disorder in which there is either complete deletion of or a reduction in number of the glucose-galactose transport sites. Dietary management is difficult and very restrictive. Fructose-based Galactomine-19 is the appropriate formula.

Problem

- Infants with persistent vomiting, diarrhoea and failure to thrive.
- Atopic tendency manifest by eczema.
- Facial wheals or other immediate reactions to contact with cows' milk.
- Family history of reactions to foodstuffs.

Diagnosis — Cows' milk protein intolerance

Unfortunately the picture is seldom as clear cut, and cows' milk protein intolerance (CMPI) has to be considered in the differential diagnosis of any infant with otherwise unexplained gastrointestinal symptoms. It may be a transient problem after gastroenteritis. Cows' milk intolerance may be the results of lactase deficiency, protein intolerance or a combination of both. To add to the practical problems of selecting appropriate special milk formulae, there is an increasing and misguided tendency for soya-based milks to be used in the management of non-specific feeding problems.

The only test for the confirmation of cows' milk protein enteropathy (CMPE) is the small intestinal biopsy. A patchy partial villous atrophy is typical and this, with a good response to a hydrolysate formula, equates to a diagnosis of CMPE. An empirical approach is to consider and exclude other likely causes short of the biopsy and conduct a trial of cows' milk elimination, converting the infant to a hydrolysate formula. Ten to 15% of truly intolerant infants are also allergic to soya protein and require a casein or whey hydrolysate preparation, e.g. Pepti Junior or Nutramigen. Most intolerant infants accept reintroduction of cows' milk after 6–8 months.

Problem

A small minority have:

- Steatorrhoea — parents describe stool like melted butter.
- Increased susceptibility to skin and upper airway infection.
- Intermittent or cyclical neutropenia, abnormal neutrophil mobility.
- Growth retardation and metaphyseal chondrodysplasia.
- A negative sweat test.

Diagnosis — Shwachman–Diamond syndrome

A rare condition 1 in 10 000 births which has autosomal recessive inheritance. The diagnosis is usually revealed by the combination of steatorrhoea and normal jejunal biopsy, normal sweat test, neutropenia and characteristic limb X-ray changes. The diagnosis is clinched by detailed quantitative assessment of exocrine pancreatic function by secretin-CCK stimulation which requires gastric and duodenal intubation as well as full laboratory back up.

Management. This is directed at pancreatic replacement as for cystic fibrosis and at combating the infections. Infection and malignancy are responsible for the majority of the morbidity and mortality. Chronic pancreatitis is also a complication.

Investigation of suspected malabsorption. It is not necessary to perform all of these tests. A positive sweat test would, for example, rule out the need to continue detailed investigation

Procedure	Diagnosis	Procedure	Diagnosis
Trial of normal diet	Social or emotional deprivation	**Urine** Microscopy and culture pH	Urinary tract infection Renal tubular acidosis
Blood test Hb, full blood count	Anaemia, acanthocytes, neutropenia	Reducing substances	Disaccharidase deficiency
Iron and iron binding capacity	Iron deficiency	Amino-acid chromatography	Amino-acid transport defect
Serum folate Plasma electrolytes	Folate deficiency Adrenal insufficiency Chloridorrhoea	Catecholamines, VMA	Neuroblastoma
		Sweat sodium, chloride	Cystic fibrosis
Plasma bicarbonate	Metabolic disorder Renal tubular disorder	**Radiology** Chest X-ray	Cystic fibrosis Staphylococcal pneumonia
Creatinine	Renal failure		
Calcium, phosphate, alkaline phosphatase	Vitamin D deficiency	Erect and supine plain abdominal films	Malrotation Partial obstruction Blind loop
Serum proteins Cholesterol	Hypoproteinaemia Abetalipoproteinaemia		
		Barium meal and follow -through (indicated if pain or symptoms of intestinal obstruction)	Partial obstruction Malrotation Blind loop
Low lymphocyte count and immunological studies	Immune deficiency		
Prothrombin time, partial thromboplastin time	Safe for intestinal biopsy		
Stools Culture	Pathogenic *Esch. coli*	**Endoscopy and mucosal biopsy**	Villous atrophy *Giardia lamblia*
Microscopy	*Giardia lamblia*	**Duodenal intubation studies**	Pancreatic failure
Reducing substances	Disaccharidase deficiency		
pH	Disaccharide deficiency	**Faecal alpha-1 antitrypsin**	Protein losing enteropathy
Electrolytes	Chloridorrhoea	**Gut hormone measurement**	Vipoma, Neuroblastoma

Congenital isolated defects of pancreatic exocrine enzymes are very rare. *Trypsinogen and enterokinase deficiencies* have been reported in infants presenting with severe failure to thrive, hypoproteinaemia and oedema. Specific diagnosis requires duodenal intubation and in vitro analysis of pancreatin juice activity. Less invasive tests of pancreatic exocrine function are available such as the PABA test. The compound, N-benzoyl-L-tyrosyl-P-aminobenzoate (Bz-Ty-PABA), is specifically cleaved by chymotrypsin, liberating PABA. After an oral load, the released PABA is absorbed and excreted in the urine, providing the basis for a quantitative test. However it is not consistently reliable.

There are rare but readily identifiable disorders which manifest as protracted diarrhoea. For children whose diagnosis remains unknown after preliminary investigation and trials of food elimination, it is essential to formulate a strategy of increasingly detailed investigation.

Problem

- Limb swelling, often asymmetrical.
- Periorbital oedema.
- Bulky offensive stools and poor growth.
- Subnormal plasma albumin and immunoglobulin G.
- Lymphopenia.
- Hypocalcaemia.

Diagnosis — Protein losing enteropathy due to intestinal lymphangiectasia

Areas of subcutaneous lymphangiectasia may provide an obvious clue. Gut protein loss is suggested by the hypoproteinaemia without other explanation. Measurement of faecal alpha 1-antitrypsin is a convenient confirmatory test. This protein is not digested by trypsin and marks protein leak into the gut. Endoscopic visualisation of the duodenum shows glistening white dilated lacteals which can be patchy and appropriate areas can be biopsied to show villi bulging with dilated lacteals. Therapy is directed at reducing the gut lymphatic dilatation by restricting fat intake and substituting medium chain triglycerides. Particular attention has to be paid to the adequate replacement of fat soluble vitamins.

Problem

- Early onset malabsorption with malodorous fatty stools.
- Irregular red cells with spiny projections (acanthocytes).
- Subnormal serum cholesterol.
- Subnormal vitamin A and E levels.
- Later (5 years) blindness and ataxia from vitamin A and E deficiencies.

Diagnosis — A-beta-lipoproteinaemia

Defective synthesis of beta-lipoprotein impairs particularly long chain triglyceride absorption and chylomicron formulation. Small intestinal biopsy shows villi packed with fat globules. The later manifestations of this autosomal recessive disorder, retinopathy and ataxic neuropathy, may be secondary to vitamin A and E deficiencies. A medium chain triglyceride diet with limited to essential amounts of long chain triglycerides helps the diarrhoea and, with high dose vitamin A and E supplementation, may prevent the neurological and ocular problems.

Problem

- A refractory and progressive dermatitis starting around the mouth and anus and spreading to the limbs after weaning in the breast fed.
- Loss of hair and nails.
- Malabsorption.

Diagnosis — Acrodermatitis enteropathica

This is an autosomal recessive defect of zinc absorption and deficiency. There is a dramatic response to oral zinc sulphate therapy.

ACUTE ABDOMINAL PAIN

The priority in management of acute abdominal pain is to recognise those who require prompt surgical intervention. Medical disorders cause about 10%. Urine analysis, microscopy and culture are essential. Active observation is useful in assessment but there is no place for prolonged observation in a young child where appendicitis may rapidly perforate with peritonitis or abscess formation.

Causes of acute abdominal pain

Surgical	Medical (relatively common)	Medical (rare but important)
Acute appendicitis	Mesenteric adenitis	Lead poisoning
Intussusception	Constipation	Diabetes
Intestinal obstruction	Gastroenteritis	Sickle cell crisis
Haematocolpos	Lower lobe pneumonia	Acute porphyria
Meckel diverticulum	Acute pyelonephritis	Pancreatitis
Torsion of ovary or testis	Henoch-Schönlein purpura	Primary peritonitis
Hydronephrosis	Hepatitis	Referred pain discitis
Renal calculus	Peptic ulcer	Cholecystitis
	Crohn disease	Renal stone

Problem

- Severe abdominal pain initially central then right iliac fossa.
- A low grade fever seldom exceeding 38°C.
- Vomiting and anorexia.
- Crying and irritability.

Diagnosis — Acute appendicitis

Assessment includes a search for medical disorders which imitate the features of acute appendicitis. The most common differential diagnosis is non-specific abdominal pain which includes mesenteric adenitis. Non-specific pain is usually associated with signs of an upper respiratory tract infection, a higher fever, headache and less consistent abdominal pain and tenderness. A full blood count with differential white cell count is usually carried out but is relatively unhelpful in reaching a clinical decision. Urine microscopy is essential although pyuria alone does not convincingly exclude appendicitis as it may reflect reaction to an adjacent pelvic abscess. A plain abdominal X-ray is not a routine investigation but may help in doubtful cases in the pre-school group. A faecalith in the appendix area suggests an obstructed appendix and is regarded as an indication for appendicectomy. Other radiological signs include localised ileus and the soft tissue shadow of an inflammatory mass. Consider a chest X-ray in younger children to exclude pneumonia. However the mainstay of diagnosis is active observation and clear decision making by an experienced doctor searching for rebound tenderness and reviewing the overall clinical features.

Perforated appendicitis should be considered if presentation is late, if the rebound pain is not localised and in the younger age group who can perforate rapidly. The child may have poor perfusion with a capillary return greater than 3 seconds and low blood pressure. An abdominal X-ray may show multiple fluid levels and free gas.

Appendix mass or abscess occurs usually in the pre-school child presenting after several days of pain with fever and tenderness in the right iliac fossa with or without a palpable mass. Abdominal ultrasound may be useful in cases where a palpable mass is not felt.

Perforation

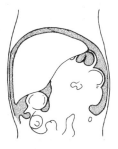

free fluid

free air

faecal peritonitis

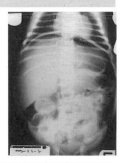

Management. Prompt appendicectomy is indicated in the acute presentation. In suspected perforation adequate resuscitation with intravenous fluids, nasogastric suction and broad spectrum antibiotics including metronidazole are crucial before surgery. Where an appendix mass or abscess is diagnosed then rest the gut, give broad spectrum antibiotics and arrange an interval appendicectomy.

Problem

- Usually an infant (66% less than 1 year old) unwell for 24 hours with irritability and disinterest in feeding.
- Spasmodic pain associated with pallor and irritability.
- Vomiting an early or delayed feature and eventually bile stained.
- The passage or rectal finding of blood stained mucous stools.
- Abdomen appears distended with palpable sausage shaped mass in the right hypochondrium or epigastrium.

Diagnosis — Intussusception

The presentation and age may be atypical and delay diagnosis, causing morbidity and mortality. Infants can present with diarrhoea and colicky pain or restlessness alternating with listlessness without showing pain. It may be possible to palpate the typical sausage shaped mass in the right upper abdomen, but this is often difficult in an irritable child. In children with stable vital signs erect and supine plain abdominal X-rays may show the characteristic signs of absence of gas in the caecum and ascending colon, a crescentic gas shadow at the apex of the intussusception and dilated loops of obstructed small intestine with fluid levels. Abdominal ultrasound is also useful in experienced hands in showing the mass.

Intussusception

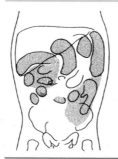

Distended small bowel absent in Lt. iliac fossa

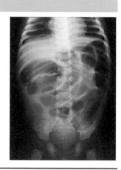

Management. Resuscitation with intravenous fluids (normal saline 20 ml/kg over 20 min if shock), control of vomiting by nasogastric tube and blood cross-matching should be done while arranging the abdominal X-ray or ultrasound. If there is no evidence of peritonitis arrange a trial of reduction by hydrostatic pressure under radiological control or ultrasound control. A barium enema will define the apex of the intussusception as a filling defect. Suitable views may demonstrate the barium lying between the inner and outer layers of the intussusception, the so-called 'coiled spring' sign. Complete reduction is demonstrated by the free passage of barium into the ileum. In appropriate patients the success rate may be as high as 80%, but there is a risk of recurrence. Surgery is indicated where hydrostatic reduction is contraindicated — clinical signs of peritonitis, fever and persistent abdominal tenderness — and if it fails. In the majority it is possible to reduce the intussusception without bowel resection. Laparotomy also permits recognition of an underlying problem which is more common in older children, for example Meckel's diverticulum, polyp, reduplication or a lymphoma. The mortality is about 1% and this is higher when the intussusception is irreducible at operation. Recurrence occurs in 1–3%.

Problem (rare)	• Nausea and vomiting. • Mild to severe epigastric pain referred posteriorly to the mid-line over D12 to L2. • Epigastric tenderness with guarding, rigidity and absent or obstructed bowel sounds. • Occasionally examination reveals ecchymoses, peri-umbilical (Cullen's sign) or in the flank (Grey Turner sign).

Diagnosis — Acute pancreatitis

The commonest causes are biliary tract problems, blunt trauma and congenital abnormalities. In some 10–20% of cases there is underlying biliary tract disease or gall stones. Blunt trauma including that due to non-accidental injury may provoke pancreatitis. It may be caused by viral infection (mumps, Coxsackie, ECHO, varicella measles), mycoplasma infection and drugs (corticosteroids, valproate, azathioprine, asparaginase). Other causes include Reye syndrome, diabetic ketoacidosis and parenteral nutrition.

Problem	• As above but recurrent.

Diagnosis — Chronic pancreatic disease

There may be a family history suggesting autosomal dominant inheritance. Predisposing disorders include anatomical abnormalities of pancreatic drainage, hyperparathyroidism, Wilson disease, alpha-1 antitrypsin deficiency, cystinuria and hyperlipidaemia.

Investigation. Plasma amylase determination is the best accepted guide to acute pancreatitis — the level rising rapidly to values over 500 iu/l. The test must however be performed early as the level falls rapidly over 72 hours even if abdominal pain persists. Salivary amylase is a closely related enzyme and can cause confusion if there is parotitis. Other investigations include a full blood count to demonstrate leucocytosis, plasma calcium seeking hypocalcaemia, glucose for hyperglycaemia and liver function tests to exclude biliary tract disease and hepatitis. The laboratory may report a milky serum. Occasionally it is justified to perform an abdominal paracentesis and the ascitic fluid may be haemorrhagic and contain a high amylase activity. Plain abdominal X-rays may be normal or show signs of intestinal obstruction and ascites. Ultrasound examination is useful for visualising the pancreatic area and for assessing adjacent organs including liver biliary tract and gall bladder. In recurrent pancreatitis appropriate investigations include abdominal CT and endoscopic retrograde cholangiopancreatography (ERCP).

Management. The emphasis of management is on the medical measures including correction of shock, analgesia (avoiding morphine and associated agents), nasogastric suction and intravenous fluid replacement. Careful monitoring is essential as patients may progress into a state of shock and disseminated intravascular coagulation. Decreasing gastric acid secretion with H-2 antagonists or proton pump inhibitors may be useful but neither blocking the proteolytic enzymes or analogues of somatostatin are of value. The problems of hypocalcaemia or hyperglycaemia need to be monitored and corrected. Surgery is seldom justified in acute pancreatitis unless there is evidence of bowel perforation or cholecystitis.

A longer term complication is the formation of a pancreatic pseudo-cyst. In these patients recovery is delayed by persisting pain, anorexia, weight loss and the development of an epigastric mass. Ultrasound is valuable in defining this pseudo-cyst. It may resolve spontaneously or require surgical drainage.

RECURRENT ABDOMINAL PAIN

Recurrent abdominal pain is amongst the most common complaints presented by school children. Although the list of possible causes is formidable, organic disorders involve only a small proportion of children and can be distinguished by a careful history, examination and appropriate tests.

The approach is to take a history directed to seeking an organic cause while asking the parent for their thoughts or worries on the cause and constructing a picture of the child, his/her family and school life. Document the periodicity, site and nature of the abdominal pain. Look for aggravating factors. Enquire regarding associated disturbances such as headache, vomiting, bowel or urinary disturbance. Careful examination must include urine microscopy and culture. Rectal examination is unnecessary unless there is a specific indication.

Causes of recurrent abdominal pain in childhood

Functional abdominal pain	Liver and pancreas	Peritoneum
Intestinal causes	Chronic hepatitis	Juvenile rheumatoid disease
Peptic ulcer	Cholelithiasis, cholecystitis	Systemic lupus erythematosis
Bezoar	Chronic pancreatitis	
Gluten enteropathy	Cystic fibrosis	**Referred pain**
Meckel diverticulum		Spine disorders
Crohn disease	**Renal**	Gonad disorders
Intestinal tuberculosis	Pyelonephritis	
Intermittent obstruction	Hydronephrosis	**Metabolic**
Food allergy	Renal calculi	Diabetes mellitus
	Bladder calculi	Porphyria
	Bladder foreign body	Lead poisoning
	Urethritis	

Only if there is still uncertainty arrange to repeat the examination during an attack of abdominal pain.

Problem (>90%)

- Age 6–9 years with a preponderance of girls.
- Normal growth although possibly slightly underweight.
- Tense, sometimes obsessive personality, succeeding well at school but socially isolated.
- Family background of ill-defined headaches, peptic or bowel disorders.
- The abdominal pain localised to the periumbilical area and no evidence of abdominal pathology.

Diagnosis — Functional abdominal pain

Apley (see Further Reading) emphasised the importance of making a positive diagnosis based on the absence of signs or symptoms of organic disease and the presence of a vulnerable personality. There is no satisfactory explanation for the disorders grouped under the heading 'periodic syndrome'. It seems reasonable to consider them as psychosomatic problems but in counselling the child and family it is worth emphasising that they are not figments of the imagination.

Dietary causes. A small subgroup of patients, usually with an atopic background, may be manifesting food intolerance. It is reasonable to enquire about foods which trigger attacks, and there may be a case for trials on and off suspect substances. Food triggers will be readily recognised by child and parents, and formal elimination diets do not work and can compromise the child receiving balanced nutrition.

Investigation

In the majority, investigations are limited to urine microscopy and culture and possibly a full blood count, ESR and CRP. An ultrasound examination of the renal tract should be considered if there are associated urinary symptoms.

Management

Explanation for parent, child and teacher. The pain is very real for the child and parents; it cannot be dismissed and needs explanation, for example increased awareness of normal bowel movements. Another explanation is increased contractions leading to spasms and pain similar to tension headaches and associated paleness of skin is caused by the same nerves shutting off the skin capillaries. Parents and school teachers can read a lot into the colour change, linking it with cancer and leukaemia. Their anxiety is then transferred to the child so increasing the perception of pain. The reverse occurs when the parents and teacher are reassured, their confidence relaxes the child and perception of pain is lessened. Consider writing to the teacher with parental permission asking how the child relates to teachers and peers, the possibility of bullying, the attendance record and academic progress. Give your view on the cause of the pain.

Reassurance. Listen then give clear advice ('Accentuate the positive, eliminate the negative and don't go for Mister in between.') Confident reassurance with satisfactory explanation are essential. Central to this is asking both parents and child what do they think or worry the cause of the pain might be. Many parents have an underlying but unexpressed fear of cancer. Uncovering this allows you to reassure them. Demonstrate your personal involvement and interest in solving the problem. Direct the family towards emphasising good rather than bad health. Stress how well the child has coped despite the pain. Medications should be avoided as it gives parent and child the mixed message of a possible disease state. Advise that the child should go to school with pain if there is no fever, if necessary using the thermometer as the decider.

Be aware of a small number of children who also have disturbance of general health, associated signs or symptoms, and in particular pain localised away from the periumbilical area.

Problem

- Intermittent bouts of epigastric pain unrelated to meals and often distressing at night.
- Relief with antacids or acid suppression.
- Associated nausea, vomiting and oesophageal reflux.
- Occasional iron deficiency anaemia or episodes of overt gastrointestinal bleeding.
- Family history of peptic ulceration in 50%.

Diagnosis — Duodenal ulcer

Helicobacter pylori is the major cause of peptic ulceration and much has to be learnt about its pathogenicity and natural history. This organism colonises the stomach of children multiplying on the mucosa under a film of protective mucus. Those children infected can develop a chronic gastritis. So far no link has been shown between *H. pylori* gastritis and recurrent abdominal pain in predicting gastritis by type or severity of symptoms and in the resolution of symptoms after proven eradication of *H. pylori*. The majority of children colonised have no symptoms.

Later many of those colonised will develop peptic ulceration usually in adult life. There is also a possibility of a causative link to some adults who later develop gastric carcinoma. The information available does not show a clear link but my pragmatic advice is that any child found to be colonised with *H. pylori* should be given an eradication regimen.

Investigations. These include haemoglobin and ferritin if there is a hypochromic anaemia. However the key investigation is endoscopy to demonstrate peptic ulceration and the presence of *H. pylori* on gastric histology or indirectly by a positive CLO test. In the CLO test an antral biopsy is put into an agar well which detects the presence of urease of *H. pylori* by a colour change of the agar.

Management. The eradication of *H. pylori* leads to ulcer healing and a very low relapse rate. The regimens to achieve this continue to be refined by clinical trials. Check local *H. pylori* resistance but a 1-week course of the triple therapy omeprazole, clarithromycin and metronidazole has about 95% eradication success in adults and should be effective.

Zollinger–Ellison Syndrome is a very rare cause of peptic ulceration, the hyperacidity is caused by a tumour of gastrin secreting cells. The extent of the disruption of the child's life due to the pain should be assessed and complications such as iron deficiency anaemia must be sought.

Problem

- Ill-defined central or lower abdominal pain.
- Diarrhoea sometimes containing blood or mucus.
- Anorexia, weight loss, growth failure.
- Fever, anaemia and a high ESR.

Diagnosis — Chronic inflammatory disease of the gut; Crohn disease and ulcerative colitis

Crohn disease is more likely to present with a non-specific illness and is frequently confused with functional abdominal pain. Later in its course, diarrhoea, abdominal pains and even palpable abdominal masses become obvious.

Ulcerative colitis typically presents with more conspicuous bowel disturbance, notably blood or mucus in the stool, but its onset may also be relatively non-specific. In both disorders there is evidence of familial susceptibility and the likelihood of an infectious trigger, but the latter has not been defined.

Crohn disease is typically a granulomatous disorder of the terminal ileum but approximately half of affected patients have large bowel involvement. Ulcerative colitis is a diffuse ulcerative process principally involving the mucosa and submucosa of the large bowel but it may also involve the small intestine. In practice it is generally possible to separate the two conditions, but there is an overlap and the two diseases may co-exist within families. First determine the extent of the systemic disturbance as manifest by growth failure, anaemia and other nutritional deficiencies. Then search for recognised associations.

Investigations

The following blood tests are indicated: full blood count and ESR; serum iron and iron binding capacity; folate and B_{12} levels; serum protein levels; and liver function tests. Stools should be sent for microscopy and culture as *Yersinia enterocolitica* is now recognised as causing a terminal ileitis. Bacillary dysentery and amoebic colitis must also be distinguished from ulcerative colitis.

Crohn disease. Barium meal with follow through and barium enema are essential for the recognition of Crohn disease and allow definition of the extent of gut involvement. In early Crohn disease, as found in childhood, involved bowel segments may not be irreversibly narrowed so that the string sign is less apparent. Affected segments of bowel are recognised by their irritability and spasticity. The contour of the terminal ileum is important and mucosal ulceration may be detectable.

Ulcerative colitis affects from the rectum upwards. It may be apparent only in the rectum and sigmoid colon and flexible sigmoidoscopy will give a tissue diagnosis. In early disease the barium enema shows multiple ulceration and pseudopolyps. In advanced disease the colon loses its typical haustral markings and becomes non-distensible. A fibreoptic colonoscopy may obviate the need for a barium enema if severity and extent are both defined.

Ulcerative colitis

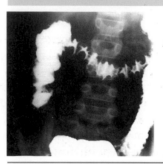 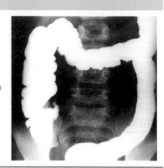

Associated findings:
aphthous ulcers
erythema nodosum
pyoderma gangrenosa
finger clubbing
arthritis
liver disease

Management

Crohn disease

Elemental diet has been shown to be as effective as corticosteroids in inducing remission in Crohn disease. It is more effective in ileal disease but worth a trial in a patient with colonic disease. A complete liquid feed of protein hydrolysate feed with carbohydrate, fat, vitamins and minerals (Peptamin) can be used. Further work suggests that a multimeric liquid diet is also effective. An 8-week period of the feed either drinking or by nasogastric tube or by gastrostomy is followed by gradual re-introduction of food under supervision by a dietitian.

Parenteral nutrition is indicated where other medical management has failed or in preparation for surgery.

Medicines. It is not known if any drug or therapy alters the eventual natural history of Crohn disease. Corticosteroids are used during relapse with widespread gut involvement. Prednisolone is commenced at a high dosage 2 mg/kg/day. There should be response by 2–3 weeks, after which the dose is gradually reduced aiming for the minimum alternate day dose able to sustain remission. The prednisolone should be tailed off completely if possible. For those patients who remain dependent on a high steroid dose, there may be a case for considering oral beclomethasone which has a high first pass metabolism by the liver greatly reducing the systemic side effects or the steroid-sparing effect of azathioprine. However azathioprine therapy introduces potentially severe complications including bone marrow suppression. If azathioprine is used the child and parents must be counselled to look out for side effects and regular blood testing for neutropenia. Mesalazine can be useful in Crohn disease to reduce the frequency of relapse. Metronidazole for 2 weeks is beneficial in settling perianal involvement.

Surgery is indicated for the management of acute complications such as perforation, fistulae, abscess formation, obstruction and severe haemorrhage. It is also justified when medical management, including a period of parenteral nutrition, fails to bring the disease under control such that the child's life is unacceptably disrupted and growth is impaired. Bowel resection should be as limited as possible. Disease limited to the small intestine has a better prognosis than ileocolitis.

Management

Ulcerative colitis

Medicines. Mesalazine has an established place in the control of ulcerative colitis. Corticosteroid enemas and foam preparations help in the relief of distal bowel disease. Loperamide can reduce the frequency and urgency of bowel actions but is contraindicated if there is a risk of fulminating colitis. Diet has a lesser role in reducing relapses but attention to general nutrition is still important. High dosage prednisolone, 1–2 mg/kg/day, should produce a response within 1–2 weeks, after which the steroid is gradually withdrawn. Azathioprine should be considered if steroid responsive but relapsing on reduction. Consider fulminating colitis and toxic megacolon in relapses marked by increased frequency of bloody diarrhoea, pain and fever and admit for careful review. Signs of deterioration include increasing abdominal distension, tenderness, diminished bowel sounds, fever, anaemia, leucocytosis and hypoalbuminaemia. These features together with abdominal X-rays showing distended colonic loops dictate that the child should be cared for in a unit with combined medical and surgical expertise in the management of ulcerative colitis. Intravenous cyclosporin may help resolution of toxic megacolon. Other major complications include massive haemorrhage and perforation.

Surgery. The issue of elective surgery is dominated by the increased risk of carcinoma of the colon. The risk is great and may not be anticipated as pre-malignant change at regular colonoscopy. Colectomy has to be considered in children with pancolitis disease with duration exceeding 10 years. Chronic ill-health in spite of medical measures may also precipitate the decision. Proctocolectomy is curative and a planned preparation programme will help adjustment to the stoma. There are also a number of ingenious surgical techniques that allow retention of anal continence.

CONSTIPATION AND SOILING

Constipation may be defined as difficulty or delay in defecation. The infrequent passage of normal stools without difficulty does not fall within this definition. Short-lived constipation is a common accompaniment of febrile illnesses and is usually amenable to abundant fluids and a stool softener. Unrecognised it can cause painful anal fissures and trigger the vicious circles of chronic constipation.

Causes of chronic constipation

Behavioural	Neuromuscular	Metabolic
Nutrition	Mental handicap	Diabetes insipidus
Low residue diet	Cerebral palsy	Diabetes mellitus (early stages)
Excess cows' milk	Spinal cord lesion	Hypercalcaemia
	Congenital absence of abdominal	Renal tubular acidosis
Anatomical	wall muscles	
Anorectal stenosis	Generalised hypotonia	
Aganglionosis	Hypothyroidism	
(Hirschsprung disease)		

The most usual presentation is that of a pre-school or young school-child whose parents have become concerned about constipation. They describe the problem as having evolved over several months with increasing intervals between satisfactory defecations. The toilet has become the focus of the family's attention and the source of an increasing amount of emotional trauma. The child is also soiling and this has interfered with attendance at school. Additional complaints may include colicky abdominal pain, anorexia, vomiting and poor weight gain. Examination reveals a healthy but withdrawn child with a mildly distended abdomen. The faecal mass is readily palpable and can be usefully demonstrated to the parents.

Vicious circles of constipation

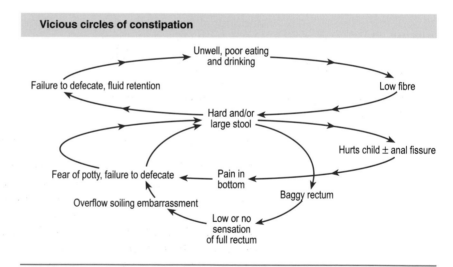

Problem

- The anal region is soiled and the sphincter is relatively lax with the faecal mass visible just above the sphincter. An active or healed anal fissure may be visualised at the anal margin. The diagnosis should be clear from the history and other examination findings and thus the rectal examination and abdominal radiograph are not necessary.

Diagnosis (1) — Constipation with acquired megacolon

Details of the neonatal history must be sought, in particular whether there was a delay in the passage of meconium and information obtained on bowel habit in earlier childhood and events surrounding the onset of constipation. Details of dietary history, child and family attitudes towards bowel habits, and secondary difficulties arising at nursery or school are also essential. The anal examination will rule out painful fissures and a rectal examination is required if there was delay in passage of meconium to assess the sphincter tone. A tight sphincter with an empty rectum but prominent abdominal distension suggests Hirschsprung disease. An abnormally lax sphincter raises the possibility of a neurogenic weakness. The sacral area may reveal a dimple or hair tuft suggestive of spina bifida occulta. Abnormally flat buttocks may be secondary to sacral agenesis. Urinary tract symptoms and infection are more common in children with chronic constipation. Investigations are unnecessary in the majority of children with chronic constipation. They should be reserved for those whose problem persists in spite of adequate medical treatment or whose history and findings point to an obstructive or neurogenic cause.

Constipation. Palpation for 'rocks' in the descending colon and rectum

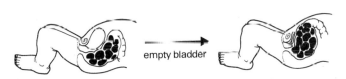

empty bladder

Children with full bladders resist abdominal palpation

Now rectal 'rocks' easily felt

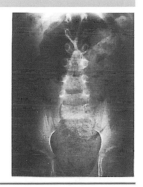

Management. The priority is to restore the child's self esteem and confidence in his or her ability to return to a normal painless bowel habit. The parents should be advised to exhibit a more relaxed attitude towards defaecation performance with an emphasis on rewarding positive results rather than dwelling on failure. Dietary measures emphasising a high fluid intake and adequate dietary residue will help achieve regular bowel actions. It is usually necessary to dislodge faecal masses with oral preparations aimed at softening the stool, for example, sodium picosulphate 0.25 ml/kg/twice daily until cleared or dioctyl sodium sulphosuccinate 5–10 mg/kg/day, lactulose 10–30 ml/day. For the minority of children in whom these measures fail, day-case admission for a phosphate enema (3 ml/kg) is usually effective. The parents must be warned that faecal soiling may be an increasing problem during this initial period of disimpaction. Measures aimed at restoring the normal bowel rhythm and amplifying the gastrocolic reflex are also important. Five to ten minutes should be set

Megacolon. There is no indication to do a barium enema, but if you do, this is what you might find! Treatment must continue until the rectum regains its tone

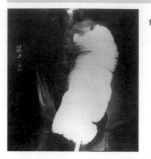

full

empty

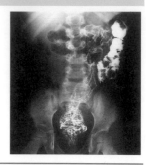

aside after breakfast and after the evening meal for a relaxed session in the toilet. Appropriate foot support may make the difference in young children. The gastrocolic reflex may be amplified with a bulk agent, for example, methylcellulose 5–10 ml with water after meals or lactulose, a stimulant agent such as Senokot 10–20 ml at bedtime or sodium picosulphate 0.25 ml/kg at bedtime. A painful anal fissure may be eased by gentle dilatation with a well lubricated finger two to three times daily and the topical application of 1% amethocaine. With sufficient care these measures are usually successful. The social and domestic disruption resulting from constipation must not be underestimated. Fortunately many of the behavioural problems resolve as the constipation and soiling improve. Soiling and inappropriate defaecation which persists in spite of normal stool consistency points to more complex psychopathology and may require the expertise of a child psychiatrist.

Problem

- Medical treatment of constipation fails.

Diagnosis (2) — Consider short segment Hirschsprung disease (aganglionosis of the colon)

If medical management fails anal dilatation under general anaesthesia in one trial has benefited some 40% of children with chronic constipation. A mucosal biopsy can be done at the same time to diagnose or exclude Hirschsprung disease. The absence of parasympathetic ganglionic cells in the submucosa and myenteric plexuses is due to defective oro-anal migration. In the affected segment, sympathetic overactivity results in hypertonus and absence of appropriate relaxation in response to proximal distension. The majority of children with Hirschsprung disease present in early infancy (over 80% in the first month and over 95% in the first year). It is among the most common causes of intestinal obstruction in the newborn period. In the newborn period the typical presentation is that of delayed passage of meconium, increasing abdominal distension, poor feeding and eventually bilious vomiting. Older children are more likely to present with chronic constipation which has been a feature since early childhood. Features which raise suspicion include poor growth and prominent abdominal distension with both gas and faecal retention. Soiling does not exclude Hirschsprung disease. The abnormally increased anal tone may or may not be clinically detectable and the relatively empty rectum may also be an inconstant feature.

Investigations. Full blood count may detect iron deficiency anaemia. Serum proteins occasionally reveal hypoproteinaemia secondary to intestinal loss. Anteroposterior and lateral plain abdominal X-ray usually confirm stool and gas retention. The absence of gas in the rectal ampulla favours Hirschsprung disease. Some authorities feel that plain abdominal X-rays provide sufficient information and that barium enemas are too unreliable to be of value. Barium enemas on unprepared colon may define the transition area between the normally innervated dilated colon and the aganglionic narrow segment. Neither investigation will be helpful in identifying the majority of short segment cases. Anal-rectal manometry demonstrates the pathophysiology by measuring pressure at the internal and external anal sphincters in response to transient rectal distension. In normal children rectal distension results in reflex relaxation of the internal sphincter and contraction of the external sphincter. In affected children the internal sphincter remains in contraction. If clinical features suggest Hirschsprung disease histological examination of the rectal mucosal biopsy is essential to confirm or exclude the diagnosis.

Management. There are a variety of surgical procedures available for the treatment of classic Hirschsprung disease. The principle aim is to bring the ganglionic bowel down to the anus. In children with short segment involvement, anal dilatation with upper partial sphincterotomy is often successful.

Hirschsprung disease

normal bowel ganglia

transitional zone

aganglionic segment

GASTROINTESTINAL BLEEDING

In the newborn period it is essential to distinguish between gastrointestinal haemorrhage and innocent regurgitation of ingested maternal

---

Causes of gastrointestinal bleeding

Check for false positive stool test

No cause identified
Straining on stool (± constipation, rarely haemorrhoids)
Fissure in ano
Infections (especially invasive bacteria, e.g. compylobacter, *E. coli* 0157)
Anatomical (polyps, telangiectasia, angioma)
Inflammatory bowel disease
Meckel diverticulum
Intussusception

Blood swallowed from the nose and throat, and bleeding from the oesophagus and stomach will also lead to 'blood in the stool'

---

blood swallowed at delivery or later from a cracked nipple. The following test distinguishes adult and fetal haemoglobin. The bloody vomitus or stool is mixed with water and the resulting solution is centrifuged. Five millilitres of the supernatant fluid is mixed with 1 ml of 1% sodium hydroxide solution. A solution which remains pink indicates infant blood and one which becomes brown indicates maternal blood (Apt test). A later section will deal with necrotising enterocolitis and the investigation of coagulation disorders in the newborn.

Problem

- Previously healthy child with haematemesis.
- Preceding upper respiratory tract infection.

Diagnosis — Haematemesis ?Cause

The priorities are the assessment of vital signs and amount of blood loss, resuscitation if required, clinical assessment for possible cause and organising appropriate investigations.

Assessment of circulation and resuscitation should follow the ABC rules.

Clinical assessment should involve a careful history to establish whether there have been previous bleeding episodes or ingestion of a non-steroidal anti-inflammatory drug, etc. General examination must include specific search for a bleeding point in the nose and throat, pigmentation over the lips and buccal mucosa suggesting Peutz–Jegher syndrome; telangiectasia over the nasal septum, face and lips suggesting hereditary haemorrhagic telangiectasia; cutaneous manifestations of chronic liver disease such as spider naevi, finger-clubbing and liver palms; splenic enlargement (this may temporarily disappear following a severe acute haemorrhage) and superficial haemangioma which may be indicative of underlying vascular anomalies.

Investigation. In the majority of children with an isolated mild haematemesis the initial assessment is compatible with bleeding from the nose or postnasal space. Investigations can be limited to full blood count and clotting screen. When more substantial haemorrhage favours intestinal pathology, endoscopy is an invaluable tool. It is particularly valuable in diagnosing upper gut problems and in emergency management of bleeding oesophageal varices. If done shortly after presentation a bleeding point and cause is more likely to be identified. Its main shortcoming is in the small intestine as unfortunately it cannot confirm bleeding from *Meckel diverticulum* other than by exclusion.

Problem

- Occasionally infants present with recurrent blood staining of vomit or faeces, and the cause remains unexplained in spite of hospitalisation and detailed investigation. The answer may be that it is a bizarre but regularly reported manifestation of child abuse.

Diagnosis — Munchausen by proxy

Problem

- Severe upper gastrointestinal bleeding may be the first sign of portal hypertension with or without underlying liver disease. Splenomegaly is a useful clue, as are cutaneous spider naevi and finger-clubbing.

Diagnosis — Oesophageal varices

Endoscopy is an important tool for both diagnosis and sclerotherapy. The latter, combined with transfusion and somatostatin infusion, controls the majority of bleeds and it is very seldom that insertion of a Sengstaken is justified. The investigations and management of portal hypertension is dealt with in the next chapter.

Problem

- A further important surgical problem is provided by young children, usually under 3 years of age, who present with copious black melaena or bright blood per rectum.

Diagnosis — Bleeding from a Meckel diverticulum

Over 50% of Meckel diverticula contain ectopic tissue, either pancreatic or gastric. A diverticulum may remain asymptomatic or present with haemorrhage, obstruction, acute inflammation, or because of a persistent communication with the umbilicus. In the absence of an obvious alternative explanation, a Meckel diverticulum is the most common cause of massive painless haemorrhage in young children. A technetium scan can identify approximately 70% of diverticula containing ectopic gastric tissue. Barium studies have a much lower yield.

Management. In the absence of another explanation, painless profuse rectal bleeding in a young child is assumed to originate from a Meckel diverticulum. The immediate priority is restoration of circulating volume and provision of a haemoglobin level safe for surgery. Imaging techniques may be justified or the surgeon may elect for an exploratory laparotomy.

FURTHER READING

Tripp JH, Candy DCA 1992 Manual of paediatric gastroenterology and nutrition, 2nd edn. Butterworth Heinemann, Oxford
Walker WA, Durie PR, Hamilton JR, Walker-Smith JA, Watkins JB 1996 Paediatric gastrointestinal disease, 2nd edn. Mosby, St Louis

12

Liver

Primary liver disease accounts for a small proportion of the general paediatrician's workload. The more frequently encountered disorders, such as biliary atresia and chronic autoimmune hepatitis, should be managed in liaison with referral centres. The wide spectrum of liver disorders have a limited repertoire of symptoms and signs. Persistent jaundice in infancy falls into one of two main categories, unconjugated or conjugated hyperbilirubinaemia.

The former are dealt with elsewhere. The latter can be recognised clinically by the presence of pale stools, and by urine which is always coloured although it is not always conspicuously dark. It is abnormal to have a positive urinary test strip response to bilirubin, or for direct or conjugated bilirubin to account for more than 10–15% of the total serum bilirubin. Unfortunately the recognition of neonatal liver disease is often delayed, not least because affected infants may appear superficially well. There are advocates for a more structured screening procedure designed to detect and investigate infants with jaundice still detectable at age 14 days.

JAUNDICE IN INFANCY

Problem

- A full-term normal birth weight infant whose early 'physiological' jaundice does not disappear and persists until age 4 weeks.
- Pale stools which remain free of green or yellow pigment over 2 or 3 days' observation.
- Yellow/brown urine which gives a positive reaction for bilirubin.
- Hepatomegaly (usual) and splenomegaly (>50%).
- Elevated conjugated bilirubin and abnormal LFTs with elevated transaminases.
- A minority present with late onset haemorrhagic disease.

Diagnosis — Conjugated jaundice ?Cause
A detailed history of pregnancy, birth, family health and exposure to drugs or infectious illnesses precedes a careful examination to detect signs of an underlying cause such as congenital infection, metabolic

Causes (Paediatric Liver Service, Kings College Hospital, London)	
Disorder	%
Biliary atresia	33
Idiopathic hepatitis	32
Alpha-I antitrypsin def.	18
Alagille syndrome	4
Others	13

disorders, and syndromatic or chromosomal disorders. The presence of a murmur compatible with pulmonary valve or pulmonary artery stenosis may point towards *Alagille syndrome* linking cardiovascular abnormalities, intrahepatic biliary hypoplasia, growth retardation, ophthalmic and minor vertebral anomalies.

A majority of infants will have either biliary atresia or idiopathic neonatal hepatitis. It is the apparently well but jaundiced infant who initially thrives and may have only modest hepatosplenomegaly who may well have biliary atresia. The risk is that false reassurance results in delayed diagnosis. The success rate of surgical intervention falls rapidly beyond age 60 days.

The priorities are to confirm conjugated hyperbilirubinaemia and hepatocellular dysfunction, detect and correct potentially dangerous complications such as deranged coagulation or hypoglycaemia, organise prompt investigation to establish the underlying disorder (infants

Investigation of conjugated hyperbilirubinaemia

	Interpretation
Biochemistry	
Total and conjugated bilirubin	
LFTs	
Transaminases AST, ALT	Hepatocellular damage
Albumin	Impaired hepatic function
Blood glucose	Hypoglycaemia due due to hepatic failure or endocrine disorder
E & U, creatinine	
Thyroxine, TSH, cortisol	Hypopituitarism
Alpha-1-antitrypsin concentration and phenotype	ZZ or Z null phenotype
Galactose-1-phosphate uridyl transferase	Galactosaemia
Immunoreactive trypsin, Δ508	Cystic fibrosis
Urine metabolic screen including succinylacetone	Tyrosinaemia (fumarylacetoacetase deficiency)
Haematology	
FBC	
Prothrombin time	Vitamin K deficiency or impaired hepatic function
Blood group	
Microbiology	
Urinalysis, culture	
Blood culture	
Congenital infection tests	
Hepatitis B, C	
Imaging	
Liver area USS	Visible, contractile gall bladder excludes biliary atresia
DISIDA scan	Rapid excretion into gut excludes biliary atresia
Echocardiography	
Skeletal X-rays	Congenital infection
Syndromatic features	
Histology	
Liver biopsy	Differentiation of biliary tract and hepatocellular disorders
Specialist	
Eye examination	Features of congenital infection or syndromatic disorders
Bone marrow aspiration	Storage disease

Causes of conjugated hyperbilirubinaemia

Structural	Infective	Endocrine
Biliary atresia	Toxoplasmosis, malaria	Hypopituitarism
Isolated	Treponema, listeria	
Syndromatic, e.g. polysplenia	CMV, rubella, herpes, coxsackie,	**Drug and TPN Induced**
syndrome	adenovirus, ECHO virus	
Intrahepatic biliary hypoplasia	Hepatitis B, C	**Hypoxic and circulatory**
Isolated	Associated infection, e.g. UTI, NEC	
Syndromatic, e.g. Alagille syndrome		**Chromosomal, e.g. trisomies**
Choledochal malformation	**Metabolic**	**13, 18, 21**
Intrahepatic biliary dilatation	Alpha-1-antitrypsin deficiency	
(Caroli syndrome)	Galactosaemia	**Idiopathic**
Progressive familial intrahepatic	Fructosaemia	
cholestasis	Tyrosinaemia	
Spontaneous perforation of	Niemann–Pick and other storage diseases	
bile duct	Peroxisomal disorders	
Haemangioma	Cystic fibrosis	

with ? biliary atresia must be referred to a centre with expertise in performing portoenterostomy, Kasai procedure, before age 60 days) and identify and provide specific correction for metabolic and endocrine disorders.

Diagnosis (1) — Biliary atresia

This is a disorder of fetal and early postnatal life in which an inflammatory sclerosing process produces progressive obliteration of the biliary tree. The cause is unknown and is seldom familial. The incidence is around one in 14 000 live births and therefore few centres gather sufficient cases to ensure surgical expertise. The pre-surgical diagnosis relies largely on excluding other recognisable causes of cholestatic jaundice, notably alpha-1-antitrypsin deficiency, and on imaging procedures which are unable to show either a contractile gall-bladder or isotopic excretion into the biliary system and gut. Percutaneous liver biopsy can be useful if an adequate sample and expert interpretation demonstrates widened portal tracts containing proliferating and distorted bile ducts as well as inflammatory infiltrate and fibrosis.

At laparotomy the majority of cases have an atretic gall bladder and an almost totally obliterated extrahepatic biliary tract. The usual procedure is a hepatic portoenterostomy in which a 30–40-cm Roux-en-Y loop of jejunum is anastomosed to a critical plane at the porta hepatis, the aim being to re-establish drainage for still patent bile channels. Success is determined by the return of bile drainage and a near normal plasma bilirubin. Elevated transaminases persist but hepatocellular synthetic function, as indicated by prothrombin time and albumin levels, should remain normal. Early success as judged by these criteria has been achieved in 80–90% of infants operated on before age 60 days but successful drainage declines rapidly as operative delay increases. Cholangitis is an early hazard.

Biliary atresia

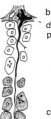

bile plugs
duct
proliferation

centrazonal
cholestasis

Early, successful surgery is associated with 70% survival without transplantation at age 10 years. For less fortunate infants the emphasis is on nutritional support and correction of events, such as variceal bleeding, likely to precipitate liver failure. Liver transplantation is now a realistic option for both infants and children, and as graft survival has improved, the threshold for transplantation to benefit quality of life has fallen. Patients with biliary atresia provide the commonest indication for transplantation. Children likely to be candidates for transplantation should be referred early before complications and malnutrition supervene.

Diagnosis (2) — Alpha-1-antitrypsin deficiency

This deficiency is the most common inherited cause of liver disease, and in European populations it is, after biliary atresia, the second most frequently identified cause for conjugated hyperbilirubinaemia. The gene on chromosome 14 determines around 80 codominant alleles, the most frequent being PiMM; deficiency and liver disease is associated with PiZZ in which there is disordered release of the peptide from hepatocyte endoplasmic reticulum. PiZZ occurs in between one in 1660 and 7000 infants of European descent but liver disease occurs in 10–15%; the additional factors which determine liver involvement are unknown.

The main presentation is with persistent cholestatic jaundice which may mimic biliary atresia. A minority have less conspicuous jaundice but present with late onset haemorrhagic disease, notably intracranial bleeding. In these dramatic presentations it is essential to collect blood for phenotype and/or genotype analysis before transfusion, or if this has been overlooked to take samples from parents. Confirmation of PiZZ requires genetic counselling with the potential for future antenatal diagnosis. The natural history of infants presenting with cholestasis is varied with 25–30% developing cirrhosis before age 20 years, which is a further major indication for liver transplantation. Older children may present with cirrhosis and its complications.

Diagnosis (3) — Idiopathic neonatal hepatitis

Published series report that, in 30–50% of infants with conjugated hyperbilirubinaemia, a specific disorder cannot be identified. The natural history is variable dependent on the severity of early cholestasis and the evolution of fibrosis or cirrhosis. A familial pattern of poor prognosis is likely to repeat itself. Consanguineous kindreds demonstrate various patterns of progressive intrahepatic cholestasis. *Byler disease*, described in a large Amish pedigree, has been linked to chromosome 18q21–q22 and benign recurrent intrahepatic cholestasis has also been mapped to this region, suggesting that it contains a gene involved in bile acid transport.

Alpha-1-antitrypsin deficiency

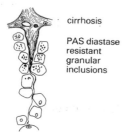

cirrhosis

PAS diastase resistant granular inclusions

Neonatal hepatitis

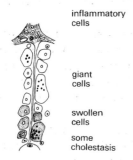

inflammatory cells

giant cells

swollen cells

some cholestasis

JAUNDICE WITH FEVER

Infectious causes of hepatitis

Hepatitis viruses (RNA and DNA groups)	A, B, C delta, GB (flavivirus-like) and others
Enterovirus	Coxsackie, Echo
Paramyxovirus	Mumps
Herpes	CMV, Epstein–Barr, herpes simplex, varicella zoster
Adenovirus	
Yellow fever	
Rickettsia	*Coxiella burnettii*
Bacteria	*Brucella, Leptospira, Treponema*
Protozoa	Toxoplasmosis, *Plasmodium*

Problem

- Anorexia, fever, headache.
- Diarrhoea, vomiting.
- A dull right hypochondrial ache and tender hepatomegaly.
- Splenomegaly and lymphadenopathy.
- Short duration jaundice which coincides with decline of other symptoms.

Diagnosis — Acute viral hepatitis type A

Hepatitis A, a picorna or enterovirus, spread by the faeco oral route produces an illness with an incubation of 15–40 days. The majority of cases are anicteric with symptoms indistinguishable from viral gastroenteritis. An icteric phase is more frequent in older children and adults. Elevated hepatic transaminases precede jaundice by 3 or 4 days, and usually return to normal within 2–3 months. A subnormal albumin or prolonged prothrombin is atypical and suggests either underlying liver disease or the rare complication of acute liver failure (less than 0.5% of hospitalised cases). Specific IgM antibody measurement confirms the diagnosis.

The majority of infected children are managed at home with either no or minimal investigation. Persistent vomiting may be a problem but antiemetics should be used with caution because of increased susceptibility to dystonic reactions. A case occurring independently of a local outbreak, or showing an atypical course with progressive or relapsing jaundice, needs laboratory confirmation. Chronic active hepatitis and Wilson disease should be considered if virology is negative. Passive immunisation with human normal immunoglobulin may be offered to household contacts of an infected child. Hepatitis A vaccine provides effective long term protection and may be warranted for children travelling to areas with high hepatitis A endemicity.

Problem

- Hepatitis B (HBsAg) positive mother or other household contact.
- Routine screening of at-risk populations.
- Investigation of chronic hepatitis or cirrhosis.
- Papular acrodermatitis.
- Associated immune complex disorders, e.g. arthritis, nephritis, polyarteritis.
- Positive HB antigen and/or antibody tests

Acute hepatitis

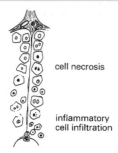

cell necrosis

inflammatory
cell infiltration

Diagnosis — Hepatitis B (HB) infection

This DNA virus has enormous epidemiological importance because it results in chronic infection with the potential for progressive liver damage, cirrhosis and hepatocellular cancer. Host immuno-competence together with viral variants are factors determining natural history. A minority of patients react to infection after an incubation of 30–180 days with an acute hepatitis and are more likely to have early spontaneous clearance of detectable HBsAg. The majority acquire infection vertically at or around birth and remain asymptomatic, or are infected later in life but again without overt illness. Persistence of HBsAg beyond 6 months implies chronic carrier status, and children infected before age 3 years are at greater risk of becoming carriers. There is a continuing spontaneous clearance rate which is greater in patients with high transaminases and histologically active disease. Treatment strategies using interferon alpha aim to enhance this clearance, and nucleoside analogues targeted at reducing viral replication are under trial.

Combined active and passive immunisation is successful in preventing vertical transmission of HB, but some authorities support a global programme rather than one based on ethnic origin or antenatal detection of maternal HB status.

Hepatitis C virus, a RNA virus, has emerged as a major cause of chronic liver disease in Europe and North America. It is thought to have been introduced relatively recently because it exhibits relatively little subtype diversity, but it has spread rapidly through at-risk populations, for example children who received multiple courses of blood products before donor screening became established. The natural history is unpredictable and ranges from mild asymptomatic infection through to cirrhosis and liver cancer. Trials of interferon alpha are being conducted but it is uncertain whether a reduction in viral load alters the prognosis.

No agent can be identified in more than 50% of patients presenting in the UK with apparent viral induced acute hepatic failure.

JAUNDICED AND VERY ILL

Main causes of acute liver failure

Infective
Hepatitis A, B, C
Epstein–Barr, Herpes simplex,
    CMV, adenovirus

Toxins and drugs
Amanita phalloides, 'ecstasy-
    agents', herbal remedies
Paracetamol, halothane, valproate

Hypoxic/circulatory
Shock related
Budd–Chiari syndrome

Autoimmune
Infiltrative/neoplastic
Leukaemia
Haemophagocytic
    lymphohistiocytosis

Metabolic
Galactosaemia
Fructosaemia
Tyrosinaemia
Alpha-1-antitrypsin deficiency
Wilson disease
Familial erythrophagocytic reticulosis
Neonatal haemachromatosis
Niemann–Pick type IIc

Investigations of cause of hepatic failure

Microbiology
Viral
    Hepatitis A, B, C antigen/antibody detection
    Viral culture and serology
Bacterial and protozoal
    Blood, urine and surface cultures
    Leptospirosis, listeriosis and toxoplasmosis serology
Biochemistry
Toxins and drugs
    Paracetamol level and drug screen
Metabolic
    Plasma ammonia
    Blood and urine metabolic screen
    Alpha-1-antitrypsin level and phenotype
    Galactose-1-phosphate uridyl transferase (infants)
    Caeruloplasmin and copper studies (age over 3 years)
    Urinary succinylacetone

Immunology
    Autoantibody screen
    Complement C3,4
Imaging
    Chest X-ray
    Abdominal ultrasound
    Echocardiography
Histology
Liver biopsy (frequently contraindicated by coagulation disorder)
Bone marrow

Problem

- Jaundice, anorexia, abdominal pain and vomiting evolving over days or weeks.
- Impaired consciousness (hepatic encephalopathy).
- Spontaneous bleeding with prolonged prothrombin time despite intravenous vitamin K.
- Hypoglycaemia.
- Ascites and reduction in liver size.

Diagnosis — Acute liver failure ?Cause

This is a rare but life-threatening disorder of childhood in which hepatic necrosis leads to multi-system decompensation. By definition there should not be recognised pre-existent chronic liver disease, but the differential diagnosis has to entertain an acute hepatitic presentation of for example pre-existent metabolic disease or autoimmune chronic active hepatitis. Encephalopathy within 8 weeks of the first sign of liver disease is a criterion for the traditional definition of *fulminant liver failure*, but in paediatric practice disease progression is often more abrupt.

Management priorities are: to establish the cause with the emphasis on metabolic disorders in infants, and on infection or toxin exposure in older children; to recognise and correct complications (especially those such as hypoglycaemia and hypotension likely to aggravate encephalopathy — this requires the resources of a fully equipped children's intensive care unit); to maximise the potential for recovery with the probability of complete return to normal liver function; and to recognise brain and life threatening deterioration so that the child is transported in time to a liver transplantation centre.

Grading of encephalopathy

1. Confused, altered mood or behaviour
2. Drowsy, inappropriate behaviour
3. Marked drowsiness , agitated, responsive to simple commands
4. Coma, unresponsive to painful stimuli

Investigation reflects two main themes: the pursuit of the primary cause and the repeated evaluation of liver and multisystem function.

Investigations of liver and multisystem function

Haematology
FBC
Coagulation studies
Blood group
(HLA typing for transplant)

Biochemistry
Blood glucose
Electrolytes, urea, creatinine, osmolality
Blood gases
LFT, ammonia, amylase
Urinary electrolytes

Microbiology
Serial blood, tracheal aspirate and surface cultures

Imaging
Cranial CT, MRI

Other monitoring
ECG
EEG
CVP
Intracerebral pressure

Management. A child with earlier stages of liver failure requires scrupulous observation with the minimum of stressful intervention, a difficult compromise given the extensive assessment necessary. Oral glucose polymer and/or intravenous dextrose is titrated to maintain a high normal blood glucose. Intravenous dextrose, 10–20% with added KCl, is limited to 60% of calculated maintenance until the potential progression of cerebral oedema has been established. Intravenous vitamin K 1 mg/day and other blood factor replacement will be guided by the extent of bleeding or coagulation disturbance. Always check that pre-transfusion diagnostic samples have been collected and preserved. H2-receptor antagonists or proton pump inhibitors may prevent gastric erosions, and lactulose reduces the evolution of encephalopathy.

The natural history of acute liver failure is variable and often unpredictable. It is essential therefore that a child with stage II or more encephalopathy is transferred to a paediatric intensive care unit equipped to manage cerebral oedema with controlled ventilation and intracerebral pressure monitoring. Renal support may also be required.

Published series have identified reliable criteria for predicting poor outcome and identifying patients in need of urgent orthotopic liver transplantation. Prior to this option, a prothrombin ratio of over 4 after vitamin K matched a mortality of 90%, and grade 3 or 4 encephalopathy developing within 7 days of onset equated with a mortality of 65–70%. Liver transplantation now offers survival rates of 60–80%.

Problem	Deliberate or accidental paracetamol ingestion

Diagnosis — Paracetamol poisoning
This is the commonest potential cause of acute hepatic failure. Well-established management protocols incorporate comparison of timed plasma levels with intervention threshold graphs and the administration of intravenous N-acetyl cysteine or oral methionine preferably within 15 hours. Persistence of nausea and vomiting, and the onset of right subcostal pain and tenderness, suggest hepatic necrosis. In cases with significant paracetamol levels 12-hourly prothrombin INR provide the best guide to the degree of liver damage. A normal 48-hour prothrombin INR predicts recovery. Poor prognostic criteria include prothrombin INR above 4, pH under 7.3 and creatinine above 300 μmol/l. In specialist units paracetamol induced acute liver failure mortality exceeds 40%.

CHRONIC JAUNDICE

Chronic hepatitis is defined as continuing liver inflammation not directly due to acute self-limiting infection. The inflammation and associated fibrosis may disrupt the liver architecture and progress to cirrhosis. Management priorities are to define the cause in order to select an appropriate treatment strategy which may include genetic counselling, establish the functional and histological status of the liver, recognise associated problems, notably malnutrition, portal hypertension, hypersplenism and ascites, and anticipate liver decompensation so as to plan liver transplantation.

Causes of chronic hepatitis

Causes	Investigation
Infective	
Viral—hepatitis B, C, D	Specific antigen and antibody detection
Parasitic—schistosomiasis	Stool microscopy, rectal biopsy
Drug induced	
Methotrexate	History
Genetic and metabolic	
Alpha-1-antitrypsin deficiency	Phenotype analysis
Wilson's disease	Caeruloplasmin and copper studies
Cystic fibrosis	Sweat test
Autoimmune	Autoantibody measurement
Associated chronic inflammatory bowel disease	Endoscopy
Biliary obstruction	Ultrasound, endoscopic cholangiography
Constrictive pericarditis	Echocardiography

Problem

- A girl, usually over age 6 years, presenting with anorexia, nausea, vomiting and cholestatic jaundice.
- Less specific features of lethargy, growth failure, vague abdominal pain.
- Hepatosplenomegaly, spider angiomata, palmar erythema.
- Associated autoimmune features, e.g. vitiligo, arthritis.
- Elevated hepatic transaminases ($\times$ 2–30 fold).
- Reduced plasma albumin and prolonged prothrombin time.
- Hypergammaglobulinaemia.
- Positive non-organ specific IgG autoantibodies, e.g. smooth muscle or antinuclear, liver/kidney microsomal (LKM associated with younger presentation and acute liver failure).

Diagnosis — Chronic active hepatitis (CAH)

The onset of CAH may be acute or insidious, and it may come to light as the result of secondary complications such as variceal bleeding. It is important not to overlook the diagnosis in a child with apparent 'infectious hepatitis' but with a past history of jaundice episodes, a persisting illness, signs of chronic liver disease, or a family history of autoimmune disorders. The confirmation of *autoimmune chronic active hepatitis* requires exclusion of other identifiable causes of CAH, and a liver biopsy showing consistent histology, namely a dense mononuclear infiltrate, piecemeal necrosis of hepatocytes, and loss of definition of the limiting plates between hepatic parenchyma and portal tracts. Reticulin stains will illustrate fibrous septa and, depending on the size of the biopsy, will give some indication of the emergence of cirrhosis. Liver specific autoantibodies may provide additional support.

Chronic hepatitis

chronic inflammatory cells

expanded portal tracts

fibrous septum

swollen, damaged cells

Management. Long-term immunosuppressive therapy reduces morbidity and prolongs cirrhosis-free survival. An initial 4-week phase of high dosage prednisolone, 2 mg/kg/day to a maximum of 60 mg/day, is given until clinical and biochemical remission is achieved, after which the dose is gradually reduced to the minimum consistent with normal transaminase levels. In cases where the required dose of prednisolone results in unacceptable side effects, azathioprine is added in a dose range 0.5–2 mg/kg/day guided by regular blood counts.

The monitoring of treatment includes attention to symptoms such as energy and appetite, growth, hepatic size and function as assessed by regular liver function tests. The target is normalisation of transaminases, albumin, immunoglobulin and prothrombin levels. The longer term strategy has to be determined by repeated liver biopsy to evaluate the persistence of aggressive hepatitis and the progression of fibrosis. The majority of patients are at risk of relapse after treatment withdrawal. Children with liver/kidney microsomal autoantibodies are reported to have a more fulminant course with poor response to treatment, and are therefore potential early candidates for transplantation.

Wilson disease is an autosomal recessive disorder (chromosome 13q) in which biliary copper excretion is defective. Accumulation of toxic products may manifest clinically as early as age 5 years, and half of children present without accompanying neurological symptoms. Wilson disease has to be considered across the spectrum of liver related presentations from the chance finding of disturbed liver function to cirrhosis. Additional clues may be provided by a history of deteriorating school performance, or by finding acute haemolysis or evidence of renal tubular dysfunction. Slit-lamp examination may reveal Kayser–Fleischer rings, a sign which is almost pathognomonic. A low plasma caeruloplasmin level strengthens the diagnosis but can also be a non-specific result of fulminant liver failure; and up to 20% of patients with Wilson disease have a normal level. Further confirmation is provided by carefully conducted urinary copper estimation before and after penicillamine, and from liver copper levels. Specific management includes reduced dietary copper, copper chelation with D-penicillamine and supplementary zinc. Patients presenting with liver failure are likely to require early liver transplantation. Genetic counselling and screening of siblings is mandatory, and emerging gene probe techniques may reduce the need for extensive biochemical testing.

POOR HEALTH ± JAUNDICE

Children with end-stage liver disease may already have been identified because of their primary disorder, e.g. alpha-1-antitrypsin deficiency, chronic active hepatitis and cystic fibrosis, or may present for the first time because of hepatocellular failure or portal hypertension.

The causes of cirrhosis fall into three main categories

1.	Billary cirrhosis—structural disorder of intra- or extrahepatic biliary tree	Billary atresis, intrahepatic biliary hyplasia, sclerosing cholangitis, Biliary and pancreatic tumours
2.	Post-necrotic cirrhosis	Postneonatal hepatitis, viral hepatitis B, C, antoimmune Irradiation or drug induced, vascular
3.	Genetic — disorders open to dietary, specific drug intervention, or genetic counselling	Alpha-1-antitrypsin deficiency, Wilson disease, cystic fibrosis, fructosaemia

Problem

- Non-specific fatigue, poor appetite and growth failure.
- A small hard liver.
- Splenomegaly.
- Cutaneous signs of liver disease, e.g. spider angiomata.

Diagnosis — Compensated cirrhosis

Assessment is directed at confirming cirrhosis together with its complications, and to identifying the underlying cause. Standard liver function tests may be normal, indicators of hepatocellular failure being a low plasma albumin and a prolonged prothrombin time. Associated hypersplenism results in a normochromic normocytic anaemia, neutropenia and thrombocytopenia. A haemolytic anaemia would raise the possibility of Wilson disease.

Ultrasound imaging with Doppler flow analysis assists in defining liver anatomy and reversed portal blood flow. It is important to exclude structural malformations of the biliary tree. Renal imaging will identify patients with polycystic changes and a probability of congenital hepatic fibrosis. Endoscopy will confirm varices and may be repeated for preventative sclerotherapy, although it is unproven that proactive measures to avoid variceal bleeding are justified.

Final confirmation of cirrhosis is provided by a liver biopsy as long as this is not contra-indicated by clotting disorders, and the sample is sufficient to interpret the distorted architecture.

Management. This is aimed at minimising further damage if the cause can be defined, and avoiding complications. Young people with cirrhosis may have little overt health impairment for months or years but may decompensate unpredictably and rapidly, often precipitated by infection or variceal bleeding. Patients require careful monitoring, preferably in liaison with a centre equipped to provide liver transplantation.

Optimal nutrition is important and must take account of the problems of anorexia, fat and fat-soluble vitamin malabsorption. High caloric supplements such as Maxijul are useful. Protein intake should only be restricted during periods of actual or threatened liver decompensation, such as when there is hepatic encephalopathy or following gastrointestinal bleeds. Children with biliary cirrhosis are especially in need of additional vitamins A, D, E and K. It is now recognised that vitamin E deficiency results in neuropathy, and that prevention may require high dosage therapy using a water-soluble formulation.

Portal hypertension is discussed later. There is debate as to whether endoscopy and sclerotherapy of oesophageal varices should be performed electively before spontaneous haemorrhage occurs.

Ascites has a complex aetiology reflecting hypo-albuminaemia, obstruction of hepatic sinusoids and the portal venous system, as well as sodium retention. It may develop gradually or acutely as the result of variceal bleeds or a coincidental illness. Ascites together with hypoalbuminaemia confirms decompensating cirrhosis but the latter may still be partially reversible. Treatment is based on sodium restriction as long as caloric intake is not penalised, and spironolactone. Spironolactone is given in an escalating dosage checking for diuresis induced hyponatraemia. Spontaneous bacterial peritonitis due to *Strep. pneumoniae* and gram-negative species is a potentially lethal complication of ascites.

Hepatic encephalopathy has gradual or acute patterns of progression. The chronic form results in increasing disturbance of behaviour and school performance. Acute encephalopathy produces drowsiness and coma. Therapy aims at controlling the precipitating factor, e.g. variceal haemorrhage or infection, reducing the protein load and maintaining body homeostasis.

Liver transplantation. Combined with modern immuno-suppressant therapy transplantation provides a viable option for children who have reached decompensating end-stage liver disease. The overall 5-year survival rate is about 80%; approximately one-third require a second liver transplant. The challenge is to recognise the stage at which the risks of continuing conservative treatment outweigh the hazards of major surgery and dependence on immunosuppression. Accepted indications include:

— Growth failure especially with muscle wasting.
— Refractory ascites.
— Gastrointestinal haemorrhage not amenable to sclerotherapy.
— Hepatic encephalopathy.
— Prothrombin INR >1.4.
— An episode of spontaneous bacterial peritonitis.

PORTAL HYPERTENSION

Problem	• Massive haematemesis preceded by acute abdominal pain.
	• Splenomegaly.
	• Normal sized or small liver.
	• Prominent periumbilical veins (seldom present in extrahepatic portal vein obstruction).

Diagnosis — Portal hypertension ?Cause

Portal hypertension is among the most common causes of massive haematemesis or melaena presenting in children. It seldom occurs before the age 2 years. There is usually little warning before the bleed, although it may be preceded by an upper respiratory tract infection. In a child without previously recognised liver disease, the vital clue is splenomegaly. An apparently normal sized liver and no features of chronic liver disease favour portal vein obstruction, but cirrhosis has to be excluded. Splenomegaly detected by chance may be the presenting feature.

Management must first focus on resuscitation and blood transfusion but an attempt must be made to store plasma for diagnostic investigations. Clinical assessment is also directed at finding evidence of established liver disease, or a history of neonatal problems which could have placed the child at risk of portal vein thrombosis. Abdominal ultrasound is a valuable tool for assessing portal venous patency and the direction of blood flow. It may detect expanded collateral drainage. An upper gastrointestinal contrast study will better define varices but is now often replaced by prompt access to endoscopy. Endoscopy has the advantage of better detection of gastric erosions as an alternative explanation for acute haemorrhage and it also enables immediate sclerotherapy.

Causes of portal hypertension

Extrahepatic	Intrahepatic	Posthepatic

Portal vein obstruction
  Congenital anomaly
  Acquired after sepsis, thrombosis, etc.
Arteriovenous fistula
	Acute and chronic hepatitis
	Cirrhosis
	Congenital hepatic fibrosis
	Schistosomiasis
	Infiltration and malignancy
		Hepatic vein obstruction
		Constrictive pericarditis
		Congestive cardiac failure

Findings

- Preliminary findings which show normal liver function, only marginal prolongation of prothrombin time and portal vein occlusion largely confirm.

Diagnosis — Extrahepatic portal hypertension

This is considered to be a developmental anomaly in the majority of cases and may be associated with cardiac, other major vessel and renal tract malformations.

Findings

- A similar clinical presentation but with firm hepatomegaly and imaging evidence of polycystic or dysplastic kidneys and a patent portal vein suggests.

Diagnosis — Congenital hepatic fibrosis

This is a histopathological diagnosis based on the liver biopsy appearance of bands of dense fibrosis joining portal tracts and separated from areas of normal hepatocellular parenchyma. There is a spectrum of associated renal findings including polycystic kidneys (both autosomal dominant and autosomal recessive), medullary sponge and medullary cystic.

Cirrhosis is discussed above and will usually be suggested by history, cutaneous signs and a small hard liver. Liver function tests may not be abnormal but a persistently low albumin and prolonged prothrombin INR favour the diagnosis.

Problem

- Haematemesis.
- Acute abdominal pain and diarrhoea.
- Rapidly evolving hepatomegaly, splenomegaly and ascites.
- Mild jaundice.
- Possible association with leg oedema.

Diagnosis — Posthepatic portal hypertension (Budd–Chiari syndrome)
This rare presentation points to occlusion of the hepatic veins, a process which may also involve the inferior vena cava. The pace of the occlusion and whether it is primarily thrombotic, inflammatory or neoplastic will modify the clinical presentation and the degree of liver and coagulation dysfunction. The exact aetiology often defies definition. Again ultrasound imaging and Doppler studies are valuable in diagnosis. The differential diagnoses include constrictive pericarditis, and veno-occlusive disease, a recognised complication after bone marrow transplantation.

Management of haematemesis. Children with active bleeding need to be managed in units equipped to provide intensive care and endoscopy. The pattern of haemorrhage is unpredictable, and patients with underlying liver disease are at risk of rapid evolution of jaundice, ascites, coagulation problems and encephalopathy. Following preliminary assessment and replacement of blood loss, endoscopy is performed to identify the source of bleeding and, if appropriate, to start sclerotherapy or banding of oesophageal varices. Continued haemorrhage will require a strategy of blood and blood factor transfusion, review endoscopy and potential use of either vasopressin or somatostatin infusion to lower portal venous pressure. Sucralfate, H2-receptor antagonists and proton pump inhibitors are used to reduce gastric and oesophageal ulceration. Balloon tamponade with a paediatric Sengstaken–Blakemore tube requires expert supervision and should only be used as part of an overall plan to gain time for repeated sclerotherapy or as preparation for liver transplantation. Patients with extrahepatic portal hypertension and intact liver function are better able to tolerate gastrointestinal haemorrhage and are unlikely to develop encephalopathy. Their management should be as conservative as possible in the knowledge that their overall natural history is of diminishing bleeding episodes with age. Beta-adrenergic blockers may result in a fall in portal venous pressure, and motility stimulants such as metoclopramide may protect from oesophageal variceal bleeding. Portosystemic shunt procedures have only a limited place, for example in patients who do not have ready access to safe blood transfusion facilities. Variceal bleeding in a child with cirrhosis adds to the case for earlier liver transplantation.

HEPATOMEGALY

The majority of children presenting with an enlarged liver do so in the context of associated systemic symptoms and signs which point to the diagnosis, for example pharyngitis, lymphadenopathy and rash favouring infectious mononucleosis; or dyspnoea, tachycardia and a murmur indicating cardiac failure. Neurodevelopmental problems, hypoglycaemia, metabolic acidosis or hyperammonaemia change the focus to a metabolic disorder.

It is important to monitor liver size in children with a wide range of chronic disorders, not only because hepatomegaly may be a marker of inadequate management such as in diabetes, but also because of superimposed complications, for example hepatitis B or C infection or haemochromatosis in children receiving blood factor replacement; or the emergence of hepatocellular carcinoma in a range of metabolic and chronic hepatitis disorders.

Occasionally hepatomegaly will be the predominant presenting sign. Examination should include careful measurement with attention to the upper as well as the lower margin. Percussion and auscultation using the scratch procedure are useful especially in defining the lower margin of soft livers. A bruit may reveal an arteriovenous malformation. Consistency, and smoothness or irregularity of the liver need to be documented. The finding of cutaneous signs of chronic liver disease or associated splenomegaly or other masses will obviously channel subsequent investigations.

Problem

- Pre-school child with soft hepatomegaly 10–12 cm below the costal margin, no splenomegaly.
- Early morning drowsiness but no overt seizures.
- Mild hypotonia and borderline delay of major motor milestones.
- Fasting blood glucose 3.2 mmol/l.
- Abdominal ultrasound confirms massive hepatomegaly with apparently normal architecture.

Diagnosis — Glycogen storage disease (not Type I)
Soft massive hepatomegaly can be missed if the examiner dismisses the protuberant abdomen as innocent and fails to define the lower

margin of the liver. This presentation without severe fasting hypogly-caemia is consistent with Types III, VI, VIII and IX; precise definition requires enzymatic analysis of a white blood sample. There is a spectrum of skeletal and cardiac muscle involvement, and additional biochemical findings include lactic acidosis and hyperlipidaemia.

Problem

- Hepatosplenomegaly with emphasis on splenomegaly.
- Hypersplenism.
- Pathological fracture(s).
- Abnormal skin pigmentation.
- Pingueculae.

Diagnosis — Gaucher disease Type 1 (glucocerebrosidase deficiency)

The majority of lipidoses present with neurological involvement, and although hepatosplenomegaly may be prominent it is seldom of major clinical significance. The hepatosplenomegaly of this chronic non-neuropathic variety may be a presenting sign, and the diagnosis may come to light when liver biopsy reveals Gaucher cells. Liver dysfunction is variable and usually modest, but can produce a picture of chronic hepatitis, portal hypertension and ascites.

It is calculated that 4–5% of Ashkenazi Jewish people carry one of the multiple alleles responsible for the enzyme deficiency. Specific replacement therapy using human placental derived enzyme is potentially available.

FURTHER READING

Caraceni P, Van Thiel DH 1996 Acute liver failure. Lancet 345: 163–169
Dusheiko GM, Khakoo S, Soni P, Grellier L 0000 A rational approach to the management of hepatitis C infection. British Medical Journal 312: 357–364
Gracey M, Burke V 1993 Pediatric gastroenterology and hepatology, 3rd edn. Blackwell Scientific Publications, Oxford
McNair ANB, Tibbs CJ, Williams R 1995 Recent advances: hepatology, British Medical Journal 311: 1351–1355
Mieli-Vergani G, Vergani D 1996 Autoimmune hepatitis. Archives of Disease in Childhood 74: 2–5
Mowat AP 1994 Liver disorders in childhood, 3rd edn. Butterworth-Heinemann, Oxford
Sherlock S, Dooley J 1993 Diseases of the liver and biliary system, 9th edn. Blackwell Scientific Publications, Oxford

Kidneys and urinary tract

Disorders of the urinary tract may be suspected when there is an obvious physical abnormality such as spina bifida but are more commonly found when investigations are initiated for urinary tract infection, haematuria or seemingly unrelated non-specific symptoms. The more routine use of urinalysis sticks and microscopy will also increase the detection rate.

Antenatal detection. Detailed ultrasound scanning of the fetus at 16–20 weeks is now routine in many centres. Abnormalities of the urinary tract occur in approximately one in 400 pregnancies. Rarely is intrauterine intervention required for obstructive conditions such as posterior urethral valves by placement of a vesicoamniotic shunt. Conversely transient mild hydronephrosis noted in some fetuses is not evident postnatally. The majority of babies are asymptomatic and those with persistent abnormality on the ultrasound (delayed until at least 48 hours) will undergo micturating cystourethrography under 48 hours, trimethoprim cover and a radionuclide investigation such as a mercaptoacetyltriglycine (MAG3) or dimercaptosuccinic acid scan (DMSA). Only if there is a mass giving rise to symptoms or significant deterioration in renal function on renal imaging will surgery be contemplated in pelviureteric junction or vesicoureteric junction obstruction. Multicystic dysplastic kidney disease (MCDK) is usually unilateral and appears to atrophy on serial ultrasound scans.

Abnormalities detected in the fetus (Nottingham data, *n* = 201)	
Abnormality	%
Pelviureteric junction obstruction	27
Multicystic dysplastic kidney	18
Vesicoureteric junction obstruction	8
Vesicoureteric reflux	7
Duplex systems	6
Posterior urethral valves	5
Others, e.g. agenesis, single kidney	15
'Transient'	14

URINARY TRACT INFECTION

Presentation

Systemic
Septicaemic
Acute cystitis
Acute pyelonephritis
Asymptomatic bacteriuria

Detection of urinary tract infections (UTI) is important because they may cause significant initial morbidity; many children have recurrent infections; they may be the clue to an underlying congenital abnormality of the urinary tract; and they may be associated with severe vesicoureteric reflux and scarring. This can lead to hypertension and chronic renal failure in a small number of patients. Although 5% of girls and 1% of boys may have a urinary tract infection before the age of 10 years, the majority will have only lower urinary tract symptoms such as frequency and dysuria. The diagnosis of UTI is based on the culture of a pure growth of organisms $>10^5$ organisms/ml (10^8 org/l). Urine collection methods are therefore crucial. This is most difficult in the younger infant where, if reflux is present, damage resulting in long term scarring is most likely to occur.

A newborn infant with a urine infection may present with prolonged jaundice, weight loss or septicaemia. There is evidence that breast feeding may be protective and infections occur more commonly in uncircumcised males. The symptoms may also be vague in the young infant and include poor weight gain, irritability, fever, vomiting and diarrhoea. A urine culture should be included in the evaluation of any child with unexplained fever. Some infants with obstruction in the urinary tract may present with signs of severe sepsis and have gross electrolytic abnormalities and acute renal failure. The clinical presentation is different in the older child.

Problem

- Frequency.
- Urgency.
- Dysuria.
- Incontinence.
- (Haematuria).

Diagnosis — Urinary tract infection

Relatively few children have the classical symptoms of loin pain and pyrexia suggestive of pyelonephritis. The diagnosis and management depends on the careful collection of urine samples. The choice of urine collection method will depend upon the age of the child and the urgency of investigation.

— *Mid stream urine collection*: appropriate in the continent child.
— *Clean catch*: requires patience and the parents should be encouraged to participate and be provided with a sterile container.
— *Urine collecting bag*: a number of types are now available and a positive result may require confirmation.
— *Suprapubic aspiration (SPA)*: this method should be employed in children less than 1 year in whom the distended bladder is an abdominal organ. It is the method of choice in the sick, septic infant to obtain urine before commencing intravenous antibiotics.

— *Catheter specimen of urine*: only as last resort because of risk in introducing infections or traumatising the urethra.

All urines for culture should be submitted to the laboratory with a minimum of delay and an SPA in a sick child should be treated with as much respect as a specimen of CSF. If there is any delay, storage at 4°C will permit an accurate diagnosis for 24 hours and possibly longer.

Dipsticks incorporating a nitrite and leucocyte detection strip can support the suspicion of a UTI. However not all urinary pathogens reduce nitrate to nitrite and sufficient bladder incubation time is necessary to produce the reaction. These sticks may be particularly useful in the out-patients setting where, if the child is asymptomatic and the dipstick is negative, then urine is not routinely cultured.

Microscopy of fresh urine can also be useful in the child with unexplained fever but pyuria and bacteria should be present. Pyuria can occur with any febrile illness and its absence does not exclude urinary tract infection. There is little place for *routine* microscopy of urine for white cells.

Dipslides incorporate plastic paddles with agar on both sides which could be immersed in urine and sent through the post to the laboratory. Because of the problems of cost and contamination the method is used much less frequently. The important practice point is that parents and medical staff should be educated about the need to obtain *proper* urine cultures in symptomatic infants.

Organisms derived from patients' own bowel flora are the main infecting agents and *E. coli* is by far the commonest. It is helpful to know the coliform organism resistance pattern in the community at the time. There are higher proportions of antibiotic resistant organisms in hospital. The recent prescription of broad spectrum antibiotics to a child may dramatically alter the bowel flora and select resistant organisms such as klebsiella.

Treatment

Early and adequate treatment is essential. Monitor clinical recovery and urine cultures to ensure effective treatment. Parenteral therapy combined with antipyretics and high fluid intake may be required in the

Antibiotics used in the treatment and prophylaxis of UTI

Antibiotic	Treatment		Prophylaxis (mg/kg single daily dose)
	Dose (mg/kg daily)	Dosing frequency	
Amoxycillin	20	3 times daily	—
Co-amoxiclav	20	3 times daily	—
Trimethoprim	8	twice daily	2
Nalidixic acid	50	4 times daily	12.5
Nitrofurantoin	3–5	4 times daily	1
Cephradine	50	2–4 times daily	—

acutely ill child but oral therapy can usually soon be introduced. The course of treatment should be at least 7 days followed by prophylactic therapy until investigations are completed in the child in whom the initial ultrasound is abnormal or who required hospitalisation. Single doses or 48 hours of antibiotics are *not* advised in any child presenting with a first infection of an uninvestigated urinary tract. Some children develop recurrent urine infections without an underlying problem and this may be associated with abnormal gram-negative colonisation of the introitus and peri-urethral areas.

It is important to stress general prevention measures to the parents of any child who develops a urine infection, the vast majority of whom will be seen in primary care and referred to the clinic. An information sheet is suggested.

Parent information sheet

Prevention of urinary tract infections

When your child has a urinary tract infection, the doctor will prescribe antibiotics. As well as the antibiotics, there are also some things you can do to help the infection to get better and also prevent another infection.

1. AVOID CONSTIPATION. You can do this by giving your child a high fibre diet to include wholemeal bread, wholewheat cereals and fresh fruit and vegetables. Ensure that your child drinks a lot and has regular exercise. The doctor may also give your child a medicine to soften the stools.

If your child has any problem with WORMS let the doctor know.

2. In young girls the tube to the bladder is very close to the back passage. WIPING should be done in a front to back direction.

3. It is better to take a shower rather than a bath. Always avoid irritating soaps and bubble baths. CLEANLINESS is very important to help prevent infection.

4. EMPTYING THE BLADDER PROPERLY IS VERY IMPORTANT. Encourage your child to sit on the toilet regularly and empty the bladder. Sometimes we ask that your child will double empty the bladder. The child will pass water then wait a few minutes before trying to pass water again.

5. Always encourage your child to DRINK as much as possible during the day, and to EMPTY THE BLADDER PROPERLY last thing at night.

6. CORRECT UNDERWEAR. Avoid tight underpants or pantyhose. They prevent air from circulating freely and encourage the warm, moist environment which favours infection. Soft cotton briefs, changed daily, are a far better choice. Consider changing the washing powder you use for the panties if irritation persists.

7. When taking antibiotics the full course must be taken at the time required. Any PROBLEMS such as burning when passing water, going to the toilet often or blood in the water SHOULD BE REPORTED to the doctor.

We hope that these ideas will help you to help your child. Please do not hesitate to ask questions or contact us if you are worried.

Investigations

All children with a proven urinary tract infection require investigation. The investigations depend on the age of the child, clues from the history and examination and the availability of local imaging facilities and expertise. There is a need to detect obstruction or other predisposing abnormalities of the urinary tract as well as defining those kidneys which are scarred or at risk from scarring due to vesicoureteric reflux. Current evidence suggests that it is the preschool child's kidney that is most susceptible to scarring and it is in this group that investigations need to be the most comprehensive. The following regimen is suggested for the initial investigation of children with proven UTI.

Ultrasound

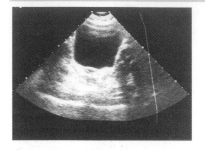 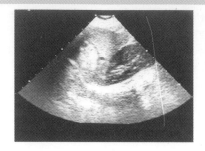 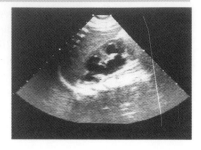

 Bladder

 Normal left kidney

 Abnormal right kidney dilated calyces

An ultrasound (US) in all ages. Ultrasound will reveal anatomical information even in the kidney without function. It will give basic information on the structure of the urinary tract and kidney sizes should be recorded with reference to centile charts based on the child's height. The ultrasound may also reveal problems of obstruction and bladder abnormality as well as stones. If these are suspected from the history or if there is a spinal abnormality, then a plain abdominal X-ray is also performed. In skilled hands the US may suggest renal scarring but is generally regarded as less sensitive than the DMSA scan in this respect. An intravenous urogram (IVU) may be requested if there is an ill defined abnormality on the ultrasound examination or if detailed upper tract imaging is required prior to surgery.

Intravenous urogram

hydronephrosis

normal kidney

dilated lower end of ureter leading into a ureterocoele

A micturating cystourethrogram (MCUG) is still routine in children under the age of 2 years with a proven UTI, as this is probably the major risk period for scarring from vesicoureteric reflux. This potentially traumatic examination is only required in those over 2 years who have recurrent infection or abnormalities on the US or IVU or a strong family history of vesicoureteric reflux (VUR) and/or renal scarring. An MCUG is requested more readily in boys, particularly if there are any reported difficulties with the urinary stream.

Micturating cystourethrogram

Grade I reflex
into ureter only

Grade II reflux
into ureter and pelvis
without distension

Grade III reflux
dilation of ureter
and pelvis +/−
intrarenal reflux

Grade III reflux

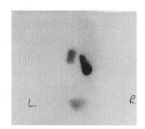

A DMSA scan is requested in those children with VUR to assess the degree of scarring in the upper tracts. It may also be employed as an early investigation in those who have suspected acute pyelonephritis where there may be focal inflammatory changes indicating the need for a MCUG and/or follow up.

DMSA scan in an 8-year-old child who presented with seizures associated with hypertension due to reflux neuropathy. Small left kidney with scarring and scarring of right upper pole. Differential function: 70% right kidney, 30% left

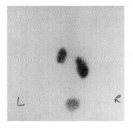
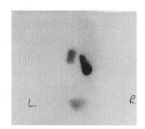
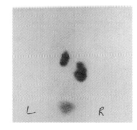

If the initial investigations (US only in the majority of older children) are negative and the follow up urine culture is sterile then the child can be monitored by the general practitioner and referred for further investigations (possibly MCUG or DMSA scan) if there are recurrent infections. Children with obvious obstructive uropathy or stones require a paediatric surgical consultation. A dilated urinary system on US or IVU may require further evaluation using a mercaptoacetyltriglycine (MAG 3) or ^{99m}Tc-Diethylenetriamine pentacetic acid (DTPA) scan. This radionuclide is often combined with an injection of frusemide to give functional information about each kidney and may help to differentiate obstruction from dilatation.

DTPA finding — vesicoureteric reflux (VUR)

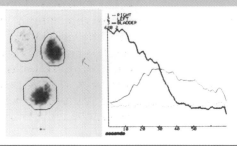

Management

The diagnosis of vesicoureteric reflux (VUR) is made by investigation! The management is still controversial. The controlled trial by the Birmingham Reflux Study Group showed no difference between operative or conservatively managed patients in terms of breakthrough infections, new scarring or progression of scarring. However, the question remains open in the very young child, especially those with gross reflux, and further studies are underway. In the meantime, in the absence of some complicating urological problem such as a bladder diverticulum, most children are managed conservatively with continuous prophylaxis using night-time doses of trimethoprim or nitrofurantoin. Surgery is considered if there are symptomatic breakthrough infections on prophylaxis or recurrent abdominal symptoms.

Antibiotic prophylaxis for VUR is generally prescribed for 2 years until the development of new renal scars or the progression of existing ones can be checked by DMSA scanning, US or IVU. If the child is old enough to co-operate with voluntary micturition (usually 4–5 years), the presence of persistent reflux can be checked using an indirect micturating cystogram following the injection of MAG3 or DTPA. Children with bilateral renal scarring (reflux nephropathy) will need long term supervision but those with normal upper renal tracts or unilateral scarring may be discharged to their general practitioner with the proviso that blood pressure is monitored annually in the scarred group where there may be up to a 10% risk of developing later hypertension.

Problem

- Frequency.
- Urgency.
- Dysuria.
- Incontinence.

Diagnosis — Frequency and dysuria syndromes

This is a diagnosis made by exclusion! It is analagous to recurrent cystitis in adults. Only 25% of children with frequency and dysuria have 'significant' bacteriuria based on the $>10^5$ bacteria/ml ($>10^8$/l) standard for voided specimens of urine. While viral infections may play a role, acute vulvitis or balanitis may be associated with poor hygeine, perineal candidiasis or contact sensitivity to nylon pants. Attention should be paid to the possibility of pin worm infestation or constipation. There are a small group of children who present with frequency only. It is possible that emotional factors are at work and generally the condition is self-limiting. Occasionally anticholinergic drugs such as oxybutinin may be required to improve bladder stability. Recurrent urinary tract symptoms associated with vulval and/or perineal signs may be pointers to sexual abuse.

WETTING

This is a common symptom. It may be the result of *enuresis* — the involuntary voiding of urine in a child over 5 years of age without structural or neurological disease of the bladder or urinary tract — or the result of *incontinence* — the leakage of urine in a child with either structural or neurological disease of the bladder or urinary tract. Enuresis is far more common than incontinence and the two can usually be distinguished easily from the history and physical examination.

Differential diagnosis of enuresis

Diagnosis	Clinical indicators
Urinary tract infection	Other urinary tract symptoms, secondary onset wetting
Neurogenic bladder	Constant severe daytime wetting, soiling, lumbosacral dimple or naevus, abnormal gait, abnormal perianal or lower limb neurology, palpable bladder
Posterior urethral valves	Poor urinary stream, daytime wetting, palpable bladder
Ectopic ureter	A constant dribble of urine between voidings
Detrusor instability	Daytime symptoms of urinary frequency, urgency and urge incontinence usually with a minor degree of wetness and worse in the afternoons
Chronic renal disease	Chronic ill health, hypertension, palpable kidneys or bladder, anaemia, polydipsia
Diabetes mellitus	Recent illness with weight loss, thirst and polydipsia

Problem

- A school aged boy with lifelong bedwetting.
- A family history of bedwetting.
- No daytime urinary symptoms.

Diagnosis — Idiopathic (primary) nocturnal enuresis
This affects 10% of 7 year old children. There is usually a family history in close relatives. The condition is the result of an inherited tendency

with environmental factors such as stress, emotional disturbances, low social class also contributing in some cases. Assessment should identify any enviromental factors that may be contributing and exclude physical disorders that may lead to wetting. Spontaneous resolution occurs at the rate of 15% per annum.

Treatment should be considered where the child is distressed by the wetting or it is leading to distress within the family. Between 5 and 7 years of age explanation, reassurance and a strategy of praise, star charts and small rewards for dry nights is usually all that is necessary. For older children conditioning therapy with an enuresis alarm is the most effective treatment, as long as the family are supervised and supported. For short term relief from wetting drugs may be useful. Desmopressin, a synthetic analogue of antidiuretic hormone, is usually of some benefit. Imipramine is also effective but has a higher incidence of side effects and is therefore not used as a first line treatment.

Problem	<ul><li>A school-aged girl with daytime wetting.</li><li>Wetting usually limited to damp underwear.</li><li>Symptoms of urgency and urge incontinence.</li><li>Some dry days.</li></ul>

Diagnosis — Diurnal enuresis due to bladder instability

This problem is usually classified as enuresis because there is no structural or neurological disorder. It is however the result of a functional disturbance of the detrussor muscle which intermittently contracts during the filling/storage phase of the bladder, a time the detrussor muscle is normally relaxed. The child has difficulty suppressing these contractions (normally an involuntary reflex) which therefore result in leakage of urine and urgency/urge incontinence before the child contracts the pelvic floor to stop micturition. It may be associated with urinary tract infections and constipation. Emotional stresses may precipitate the problem in some children.

Treatment is aimed at establishing a routine of complete and regular emptying of the bladder to restore their confidence. Star charts and rewards may be helpful. Constipation must be treated and urine infections eradicated. An anticholinergic drug such as oxybutinin is usually effective but should not be used until the aforementioned strategy has been tried.

POLYURIA

The normal daily urine volume is highly variable and is determined by fluid intake, the amount of solute generated requiring excretion via the kidneys and the renal concentrating capacity. Average urine output increases from approximately 500 ml/day at 1 year to 1.5 litres by 15 years of age. Polyuria is usually associated with urine volumes exceeding 1 litre in preschool children and 2–3 litres in school age children. Polyuria is almost invariably accompanied by polydipsia, nocturia and nocturnal drinking. A careful clinical history and simple urinalysis with baseline biochemistry will be strong pointers as to whether further investigations are needed.

Causes of polyuria in children

Increased fluid intake
Behavioural/psychogenic
Hypothalamic polydipsia

Failure of ADH production — central diabetes insipidus, e.g.
Idiopathic — congenital or familial type
Post-traumatic
Neoplasia — leukaemia, craniopharyngioma, histiocytosis X
Infections — encephalitis, meningitis

Increased osmotic load
insipidus, e.g.
(i) Glucose — diabetes mellitus
(ii) Urea — relieved obstructive uropathy
— hypercatabolic states (burns)
— chronic renal failure
— following renal transplantation
(iii) Mannitol infusion

Tubular unresponsiveness to ADH — nephrogenic diabetes
insipidus, e.g.
Sex-linked inherited
Acquired — obstructive uropathy
chronic renal failure
potassium depletion
hypercalcaemia
sickle cell disease

Drugs
e.g. Theophylline, amphotericin

Diabetes. *Diabetes mellitus* is easily detected on urinalysis and confirmed by the blood glucose levels. *Diabetes insipidus* is more difficult to diagnose. The distinction between central and nephrogenic diabetes insipidus requires a carefully supervised water deprivation test to determine whether the kidneys produce appropriately hyperosmolar urine in response to an elevated plasma osmolality. If the urine does not become hyperosmolar then the vasopressin analogue desamino-8-D-arginine vasopressin (DDAVP) is administered to see if the kidneys are capable of responding to vasopressin. In infants a water deprivation test may be hazardous and so if diabetes insipidus is strongly suspected measure urine and blood osmolality prior to a feed (i.e. after a 3–4 hour fast). If the plasma osmolality is *high* and urine osmolality is *low* then proceed straight to a DDAVP test.

Finding

- Urine osmolarity does not increase with fluid deprivation and elevated plasma osmolality but does so in response to DDAVP.

Diagnosis — Central diabetes insipidus
Urine volumes in cranial diabetes insipidus may be 4–10 litres with osmolalities between 50 and 200 mosmol/l. Renal function is otherwise normal. Further investigations such as CT or MRI scanning and testing of other pituitary hormonal functions may be required to establish the underlying cause.

Management. Intranasal DDAVP once or twice daily will normalise the urine output. Strict attention to fluid balance is essential in the acute stages of management.

Finding

- Urine osmolarity does not increase with fluid deprivation and elevated plasma osmolality or in response to DDAVP.

Diagnosis — Nephrogenic diabetes insipidus (NDI)

Isolated NDI is due to a primary unresponsiveness of the distal tubal and collecting ducts to vasopressin and follows an X-linked recessive inheritance, hence affecting boys. It usually presents in infancy with poor growth and feeding due to the excessive thirst, and affected infants may suffer repeated episodes of hypernatraemic dehydration before the diagnosis is made.

Management. Free access to water day and night is the mainstay of management. The urine output can be decreased by dietary restriction of sodium and protein in order to reduce the renal solute load. Further reduction of urine output may be achieved by thiazide diuretics and a prostaglandin synthetase inhibitor such as indomethacin. Control can be relaxed in the older child who has easier access to fluids, is less susceptible to dehydration and may cope with the polyuria and polydipsia without drug therapy.

Findings

- Thriving.
- Low plasma and urine osmolalities before fluid deprivation.
- Urine osmolality partially responsive to fluid deprivation.

Diagnosis — Excessive water intake (psychogenic polydipsia or compulsive water drinking)

This is relatively common, particularly in the toddler age group. In severe cases there can be confusion with diabetes insipidus because prolonged excessive water intake can reduce the renal medullary solute concentration with impaired urine concentrating capacity in response to both fluid deprivation and DDAVP. If there is doubt about the diagnosis it may be necessary to admit the child to hospital for a couple of days in order to observe the pattern of fluid intake and moderately restrict fluids before the formal testing. It may also give an opportunity to observe family interactions and the child's behaviour.

Findings

- Poor appetite.
- Elevated blood urea and creatinine levels.

Diagnosis — Chronic renal failure (CRF)

Polyuria due to reduced concentrating ability occurs early in the course of CRF when tubular damage is present, e.g. reflux nephropathy or obstructive uropathy. Infants may fail to thrive whilst older children may have persistent bed wetting as well as other signs of CRF.

Findings

- Glycosuria and generalised aminoaciduria.
- Rickets and poor growth.
- Metabolic acidosis, hypokalaemia, hypophosphataemia.

Diagnosis — Tubular defect

This is a very rare problem, cystinosis is the commonest cause of a generalised proximal tubular defect (Fanconi syndrome) in childhood, the antifungal agent amphotericin and cancer chemotherapeutic agents such as ifosfamide may also cause a Fanconi-like syndrome. Cystinosis arises from a lysosomal transport defect resulting in the accumulation of cysteine within cells. The diagnosis is supported by finding cystine crystals in the cornea by slit lamp examination of the eyes and is confirmed by the presence of increased levels of cysteine in white blood cells or in skin fibroblasts. Therapy consists of fluid and electrolyte replacement, correction of acidosis, nutritional support. The

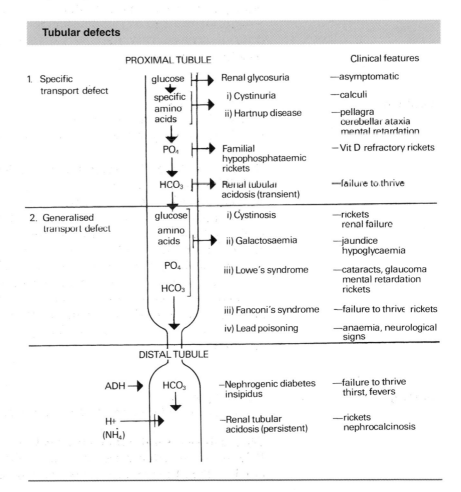

Tubular defects

	PROXIMAL TUBULE		Clinical features
1. Specific transport defect	glucose	Renal glycosuria	—asymptomatic
	specific amino acids	i) Cystinuria	—calculi
		ii) Hartnup disease	—pellagra cerebellar ataxia mental retardation
	PO₄	Familial hypophosphataemic rickets	—Vit D refractory rickets
	HCO₃	Renal tubular acidosis (transient)	—failure to thrive
2. Generalised transport defect	glucose amino acids PO₄ HCO₃	i) Cystinosis	—rickets renal failure
		ii) Galactosaemia	—jaundice hypoglycaemia
		iii) Lowe's syndrome	—cataracts, glaucoma mental retardation rickets
		iii) Fanconi's syndrome	—failure to thrive rickets
		iv) Lead poisoning	—anaemia, neurological signs
	DISTAL TUBULE		
ADH →	HCO₃	—Nephrogenic diabetes insipidus	—failure to thrive thirst, fevers
H⁺ (NH₄) →		—Renal tubular acidosis (persistent)	—rickets nephrocalcinosis

administration of cysteine depleting agents such as cysteamine or phosphocysteamine may improve the long term outcome and slow the progression of renal disease which if left untreated results in end stage renal failure by around 10 years of age.

Bartter syndrome is a rare childhood disorder presenting with failure to thrive, polyuria and polydipsia. A hypokalaemic metabolic alkalosis is noted on blood biochemistry. Blood pressure is normal despite high plasma renin and normal plasma aldosterone levels, which usually rise when the plasma potassium is normalised. Treatment of this chronic disease is with potassium supplements and indomethacin.

HAEMATURIA

Macroscopic haematuria is a dramatic symptom and is usually quickly brought to medical attention. The description may be of tea or 'coke' coloured urine, but it may be bright red, suggesting more of an extra renal or lower urinary tract source. Haematuria confined to the start or end of the urinary stream also suggests lower urinary tract pathology. Dark urine can also be due to haemoglobinuria, myoglobinuria, beeturia or confectionary dyes. Urate crystals appear red or reddish brown and may be present on the napkin of a neonate.

The history may give important clues as to the cause of the haematuria such as a preceding upper respiratory infection (nephritis), urinary symptoms (urinary tract infection), abdominal pain (stones or obstruction). A detailed family history should also be elicited, particularly with respect to familial nephritis. Microscopy of freshly voided urine should be carried out in all cases of haematuria to confirm the presence of red blood cells. Cellular casts and dysmorphic red blood cells indicate a glomerular source for the bleeding. Increased white blood cells or motile bacteria suggest urinary tract infection, which needs to be confirmed by urine culture.

Investigation of unexplained haematuria

Urinalysis for blood and protein	Urea electrolytes and creatinine
Urine calcium : creatinine ratio	Full blood count
Urine microscopy and culture	ASO titre
Renal tract ultrasound +/− abdominal X-ray	C3 and C4

Microscopic haematuria. This is increasingly detected on routine urinalysis and may be present in 4% of children. It is usually a transient finding in healthy children that is more likely in the context of heavy exercise or any febrile illness. Urine may also be contaminated with blood from the external genital area, urethral meatus or menstrual blood. Microscopic haematuria should be confirmed on several samples as persistent haematuria, which is present in 0.3% of children, is more likely to be significant.

Fictitious haematuria has been recognised as part of the Münchausen syndrome by proxy where symptoms and signs are manufactured by the care givers, usually the mother. The diagnosis should be considered if other clinical pointers are present.

Persistent asymptomatic microscopic haematuria and recurrent macroscopic haematuria usually originate from the glomeruli therefore invasive urological investigation is rarely needed. The most likely diagnoses are IgA nephropathy, thin basement membrane nephropathy or Alport syndrome. The presence of proteinuria, hypertension or elevated serum creatinine are indicators of serious renal disease and a renal biopsy may be necessary. If asymptomatic microscopic haematuria is the only sign of disease then the prognosis is far better, with very few children progressing to more serious problems. A renal biopsy may be considered after 1–2 years in order to make a diagnosis and determine the need for long term follow-up.

Problem

- Sudden onset of haematuria with a history of upper respiratory tract infection in the previous 2–3 weeks.
- Oedema with puffiness often first noticed in the periorbital region.
- Hypertension which may lead to headaches and even convulsions.
- Raised urea and creatinine.

Diagnosis — Acute glomerulonephritis

This is a clinical syndrome with a number of causes. Urine microscopy will reveal numerous red blood cells with granular and red cell casts. Classical *post-streptococcal glomerulonephritis* still occurs in western countries following infection with nephritogenic strains of group A beta haemolytic streptococcus in the throat or skin. An elevated antistreptolysin O titre with a low C3 and normal C4 level confirms the diagnosis. A number of other bacteria and viruses can also give rise to a post-infectious glomerulonephritis.

Investigations. These should include full blood count, urea, electrolytes, creatinine, liver function tests, throat swab, complement levels, antinuclear factor, antistreptolysin O and viral titres and hepatitis B associated antigen.

Management. The child with significant renal impairment will require sodium and fluid restriction with strict attention to fluid balance, a protein and potassium restricted diet with high calorie intake. Antihypertensive therapy may be required. A 10-day course of penicillin should be commenced while awaiting the result of the throat swab. Very rarely dialysis may be required for fluid overload, uraemia or severe electrolyte disturbance (see 'Management of acute renal failure below'), in these circumstances a diagnosis other than post infectious nephritis is likely.

Prognosis

Most children with post-streptococcal or post-infectious glomerulonephritis make an excellent recovery, with over 90% resolving without significant renal impairment. Renal biopsy in a child with nephritis is only justified if the clinical presentation is very atypical, the serum complement is normal in the presence of renal insufficiency (which makes post-streptoccocal nephritis unlikely) or there is persistent hypo-complementaemia. Glomerulonephritis can occur in other diseases including Henoch–Schönlein pupura and systemic lupus erythematosus.

Henoch–Schönlein purpura. Seventy per cent of children with this condition have haematuria (mainly microscopic) and/or proteinuria early in the course of their illness which in most cases resolves. Some children do develop chronic progressive nephritis; therefore those children with a nephrotic syndrome picture or persistent renal impairment require a biopsy. The finding of a rapidly progressive nephritis with crescents may justify immunosuppressive therapy. Children with persistent urinary abnormalities following Henoch–Schönlein purpura should continue to be followed in the outpatient clinic to detect the late development of hypertension and renal impairment.

Systemic lupus erythematosus. Lupus nephritis if inadequately treated may lead to end stage renal failure. A biopsy may be required to document the degree of renal involvement, as this will be the major factor in the choice of immunosuppressive treatment employed.

Problem

- Recurrent attacks of painless haematuria.
- No evidence of urinary tract infection.
- Normal complement levels.
- Normal ultrasound of the renal tract.

Diagnosis — IgA nephropathy (Berger disease)

This may present with asymptomatic microscopic haematuria or more characteristically with episodes of macroscopic haematuria coincident with intercurrent respiratory infections. Many children labelled as having benign recurrent haematuria fall into the category of IgA nephropathy and although the prognosis is generally very good the children do need to be followed up because long term studies demonstrate a minority can progress to chronic renal damage. The diagnosis can only be made on renal biopsy where mesangial deposition of IgA is seen. There is no proven treatment for this condition, although immunosupressive therapy may help in the child with a severe proliferative nephritis.

Other diagnoses

Some children with recurrent haematuria have also been found to have hypercalciuria which can be screened for on a spot urine calcium to creatinine ratio (should be <0.7 mmol/μmol). Benign familial haematuria due to thin basement membrane nephropathy is suggested by the finding of microscopic haematuria in other family members. The outlook is excellent in this condition but any suggestion of renal impairment or sensorineural deafness in the family would lead to consideration of renal biopsy to define a condition such as Alport syndrome which is usually of X-linked recessive inheritance, hence affecting males more than females. Males with this condition usually develop chronic renal failure as young adults.

Problem (common)

- Urinary frequency and dysuria.
- Pyuria and bacteriuria.

Diagnosis — Urinary tract infection

This is the commonest cause of haematuria in childhood. Acute cystitis, either viral or bacterial, can result in gross haematuria. It is important to prove a bacterial cause by appropriate urine cultures before treating with antibiotics.

Rarely the haematuria is associated with an **abdominal mass**. An abdominal ultrasound will establish whether the mass is a hydronephrosis from a lesion such as pelviureteric junction obstruction or is solid due to nephroblastoma (Wilms tumour) which in 30% of cases gives rise to haematuria that is usually microscopic.

OEDEMA

Oedema is a clinical finding which indicates overexpansion of the interstitial fluid compartment. It is most noticeable in the ankles, genitalia overlying the sacrum or in the periorbital region. Ascites will develop in more advanced cases. After the history and examination, the most important investigation is the urinalysis. Heavy proteinuria immediately points towards nephrotic syndrome, whereas moderate proteinuria and heavy haematuria suggest acute glomerulonephritis. The absence of or minimal proteinuria suggests a non-renal cause.

Causes of oedema include

Increased capillary pressure as occurs in acute renal failure, acute glomerulonephritis or in cardiac failure

Decreased colloidal oncotic pressure as in protein losing states, e.g. nephrotic syndrome, protein losing enteropathy, burns or in severe protein-calorie malnutrition (kwashiorkor)

Increased permeability of the capillaries, e.g. septic shock, allergic reactions, burns, trauma

Blockage of lymphatics, e.g. malignancy, post surgical

Problem

- Oedema.
- Heavy proteinuria.
- Hypoalbuminaemia.

Diagnosis — Nephrotic syndrome

This is an uncommon condition with an incidence of two 2 per 100 000 Caucasian children. The incidence in the Asian population in the UK is higher with 9–16/100 000 being affected. The typical child is preschool (1–5 years) with males more commonly affected (2 : 1). They will present with increasing oedema over a few days or weeks and there may be lethargy, poor appetite and sometimes abdominal pain and mild diarrhoea. Since it is an uncommon condition, many children are treated for allergic conditions before the true cause of the periorbital oedema is recognised.

Investigations

Classification	
Membranous	1.5%
Mesangio-proliferative	2.5%
Membrano-proliferative	8%
Focal segmental	10%
Minimal change	78%

Nephrotic syndrome should be confirmed by documenting the proteinuria in a random urine protein to creatinine ratio (>200 mg/mmol) and the hypoalbuminaemia (plasma albumin <25 g/l). Renal function and a full blood count should be checked along with the hepatitis B surface antigen and the Varicella immunity status. Urine should be taken for microscopy to look for signs of glomerulonephritis such as cellular casts and haematuria and for culture to exclude infection (a cause of steroid resistance). Further tests such as ASO titre, serum complement and antinuclear factor are only needed if the clinical features are not typical. *Renal biopsy* is undertaken in two circumstances where pathology other than minimal change disease is suspected. The first is when there are unusual clinical features such as being very young (under 1 year) or relatively old (greater than 12 years) or there is persistent heavy haematuria, hypocomplementaemia, hypertension or renal failure. The second is where the nephrotic syndrome does not respond to a therapeutic trial of prednisolone 60 mg/m²/day within 28 days.

Management

Fluid balance. In the child who is oedematous, excessive sodium intake should be avoided and a moderate fluid restriction can be prescribed. Diuretics such as frusemide and spironolactone should be used with great caution, as children are likely to have a contracted plasma volume due to the low plasma oncotic pressure and symptomatic hypovolaemia may be precipitated. Careful clinical assessment of the circulatory status is required during the initial oedematous phase of the illness.

Albumin infusions should be reserved for the child with signs of hypovolaemia (abdominal pain, tachycardia, cool peripheries, oliguria, raised haematocrit) or the presence of severe symptomatic oedema or ascites refractory to other measures. Twenty per cent albumin (1 g/kg) can be infused over 1–2 hours to expand the circulating volume followed by frusemide 1–2 mg/kg. A hypercoagulable state exists in the nephrotic child and hypovolaemia may lead to major thrombotic events.

Diet. A well balanced 'healthy eating', no added salt diet is encouraged. Calorie supplements may be required during the acute illness but excessive weight gain may become a problem later on because of the corticosteroid therapy.

Infection. Oedematous children are at risk of serious infections and in particular they are susceptible to the pneumococcus. Oral penicillin should therefore be prescribed in the grossly oedematous child as prophylaxis. Corticosteroid therapy leaves children susceptible to potentially life threatening infections such as chickenpox; their immunity status should therefore be known and parents be warned of the risks of this infection in order that prophylaxis with zoster immunoglobulin can be given if they are in contact and acyclovir be given should chickenpox develop.

Medication. A trial of corticosteroids is usually undertaken after the initial investigations have been performed. The recommended regimen is: prednisolone 60 mg/m^2/day divided in 2–3 doses until the urine is free of protein for 3 consecutive days, followed by prednisolone 40 mg/m^2 as a single dose on alternate days for 4 weeks.

Prognosis

Steroid *responsive* nephrotic syndrome. Ninety per cent of children with minimal change nephrotic syndrome will respond to the recommended regimen of prednisolone, within 7–10 days. Three-quarters of children who respond initially to prednisolone will have a subsequent relapse (recurrence of proteinuria) and about one-third will suffer from frequent relapses. The parents are therefore instructed to carry out regular monitoring of the urine and record the results in a diary. Those who are relapsing frequently are prescribed an alternate day steroid regimen which is only slowly reduced over several months. Children who are becoming steroid dependent, especially if they are manifesting toxic steroid side effects, may be considered for alternative immunomodulating therapy such as levamisole, cyclophophamide or cyclosporin. As long as the child responds to steroids the prognosis for renal function is still excellent and relapses become less frequent as the child grows older. However, a few children continue to have relapses into late adolescence and adulthood. The 1–2% documented mortality from nephrotic syndrome is due to infection and thrombosis, usually occurring during the initial episode.

Steroid *resistant* nephrotic syndrome. The prognosis for FSGS and other pathological conditions causing steroid resistant nephrotic syndrome is very different with a less good favourable response to immunosuppressive therapy. Although some will remit, as many as 50% will progress to chronic renal failure over the years.

Congenital nephrotic syndrome. This is very rare and presents in the first few months of life. It may be familial with an autosomal recesive inheritance pattern such as the Finnish type where there are microcystic changes in the renal cortex. Antenatal diagnosis is possible based on alpha fetoprotein estimations in serum and amniotic fluid. Diffuse mesangial sclerosis and FSGS may also present in the first few months of life. Previously the condition was fatal before 2 years of age, but dialysis and transplantation is now available.

Secondary causes of nephrotic syndrome. Any chronic nephritis may give rise to a nephrotic state if the proteinuria is sufficiently heavy to result in hypoalbuminaemia. Examples are Henoch–Schönlein purpura, SLE, quartan malaria and schistosomiasis. Heavy metal poisoning, congenital syphilis and drugs are other potential causes.

OLIGURIA

Oliguria is the reduction in urine output to less than 300 ml/m²/day, which is inadequate to excrete the normal solute output. This figure equates to approximately <1 ml/kg/h (<0.6 ml/kg/h in the neonatal period). Oliguria requires prompt assessment to define any readily reversible cause and to decide whether emergency treatment of fluid and electrolyte or metabolic disturbance is necessary. The history and examination usually provide major clues as to the cause. Urgent investigations will include urinalysis and urine microscopy as well as blood and urine samples for electrolytes, urea, creatinine and osmolality. Renal tract ultrasound imaging is mandatory if the cause of ARF is not readily apparent.

Causes of acute renal failure

Prerenal *Circulatory insufficiency*	Intrarenal (renal parenchyma)	Postrenal
Gastroenteritis	Haemolytic uraemic syndrome	Posterior urethral valves
Septic shock	Acute glomerulonephritis	Bilateral obstruction, e.g.
Haemorrhage	Acute interstitial nephritis from drug	pelviureteric junction or
	hypersensitivity	vesicoureteric junction
Cardiac failure	Nephrotoxins, e.g. antibiotics, anticancer drugs	obstruction
Burns	Bilateral acute pyelonephritis	Stones
Hypovolaemia associated with	Vasculitis, e.g. polyarteritis	
nephrotic syndrome	Myoglobinuria, haemoglobinuria	Neurogenic bladder
Bilateral renal artery or	Acute crystalline nephropathy, e.g. uric	
vein occlusion	acid, oxalosis	

Problem

Oligura with:

- Clinical signs of hypovolaemia.
- Urine osmolality >400 mosmol/kg.
- Urinary sodium <20 mmol/l.
- Urine/plasma osmolality ratio >1:2.

- Urine/plasma urea ratio >4:1.
- Fractional excretion of filtered sodium (FeNa) <1%.

$$Fe\,Na = \frac{UNa}{UCr} \times \frac{PCr}{PNa} \times 100$$

Diagnosis — Prerenal failure

These indices suggest the kidney is attempting to excrete the solute load in highly concentrated urine whilst conserving sodium. Prerenal failure should be considered in all oliguric children as parenchymal damage will ensue if adequate renal perfusion is not restored. The urinary indices quoted above are only a guide and the results become difficult to interpret if there has already been administration of intravenous fluids or diuretics. If prerenal failure is suspected then prompt administration of 20 ml/kg normal saline or plasma or blood over 30–60 minutes may result in increased urine output. The boluses may have to be repeated until circulation is restored and may be combined with a trial of frusemide 2 mg/kg i.v. (up to a maximum of 5 mg/kg) to initiate a diuresis. If there is no response, consider established renal failure and avoid fluid overload.

Findings

Oliguria or anuria with a history and urinalysis to suggest a renal parenchymal damage:

- Urine osmolality <350 mosmol/kg.
- Urinary sodium >40 mmol/l.
- Urine/plasma osmolality ratio <1:1.
- Urine/plasma urea concentration ratio <4:1.
- Fractional excretion of filtered sodium >1%.

Diagnosis   Acute renal or obstructive renal failure

It can be difficult to distinguish renal parenchymal from obstructive causes for renal failure on the above tests. If an ultrasound examination suggests obstruction, urethral, suprapubic or nephrostomy drainage will be required. A marked diuresis may occur with relief of the obstruction and the fluid balance must be strictly monitored.

Management

Fluids. Circulating volume should be maintained with colloid. In the oliguric child with acute renal failure (ARF), fluid input should be limited to insensible losses (400 ml/m²/day) plus any ongoing losses. Sodium intake should be minimised. Hidden sources of fluid and electrolyte intake such as drugs and arterial lines should not be neglected. Hyponatraemia is usually the result of water overload and will respond to fluid restriction. Central nervous system symptoms do not usually occur until the plasma sodium is <120 unless the sodium has dropped very rapidly. If the patient is symptomatic, the sodium can be raised by about 3 mmol/l by administering 30% sodium chloride (5 mmol/ml) in a dose of 2 mmol/kg bodyweight. Daily weighing, careful monitoring of fluid balance and electrolyte monitoring are necessary to guide subsequent therapy.

Hyperkalaemia requires immediate emergency treatment if ECG changes are present (peaked T waves, prolonged PR interval and widening of the QRS complex). Treatment measures that shift potassium into cells provide only temporary respite and need to be followed by measures to remove potassium from the body. Potassium intake should be limited and adequate calories should be given to prevent tissue catabolism.

Hypocalcaemia seldom leads to symptoms but these may be precipitated by the liberal use of alkali therapy. Reduction of high phosphate levels may also improve the serum calcium.

Treatment of hyperkalaemia

Drug	Dose	Onset	Mode of action
10% calcium gluconate	0.5 ml/kg body weight i.v. over 5–10 min	Immediate	Antagonizes the effect of potassium
8.4% NaHCO3	2–3 mmol/kg weight i.v.	5 min	Shifts potassium into cells
Glucose ± insulin	Intravenous glucose (0.5 g/kg) insulin 1 unit: 4 g glucose more than 10 mmol/l	30 min	Shifts potassium into cells
Ion exchange resins	1 g/kg body weight calcium resonium orally or rectally	2 h when given orally 30 min when given rectally	Removes potassium from body
Dialysis	Haemodialysis Peritoneal dialysis	Rapid Gradua	Removes potassium from body

Metabolic acidosis is treated when the plasma pH falls below 7.25 using intravenous and then oral bicarbonate therapy. This however results in a significant sodium load and therefore metabolic acidosis in the anuric child may be an indication for dialysis.

Hypertension may be due to fluid overload, intrinsic renal disease or drugs such as prednisolone. If hypertension exists after correction of fluid overload then antihypertensive medication (see later) is required. Severe hypertension should be managed with a carefully controlled infusion of labetolol or sodium nitroprusside, aiming for slow reduction of blood pressure over 24–48 hours.

Nutrition. The aim is to provide adequate nutrition for the patient's metabolic needs and to prevent catabolism. Protein restriction is only needed if the child is not on dialysis or has a high intake. Daily energy intake should be between 50 and 100 kcal/kg body weight depending upon age. The diet is also restricted in potassium, phosphate and sodium. Since patients with renal failure are usually anorexic, a period of nasogastric or intravenous feeding may be required. The amount of fluid may be a limiting factor and dialysis may be required to allow for a fluid volume sufficient to provide adequate kilocalories.

Anaemia. This is almost inevitable and a blood transfusion is indicated if the haemoglobin concentration is less than 6 g/dl or is dropping rapidly.

Drugs. Dosages may need modifying in the presence of renal failure and nephrotoxic drugs should be avoided.

Dialysis

The need for dialysis should be anticipated to allow transfer to a unit experienced in such treatment. Absolute indications are: severe hyperkalaemia, hyponatraemia or fluid overload or symptomatic uraemia. Dialysis should be commenced earlier in the treatment of an acutely ill child when fluid restriction will compromise care by reducing nutritional intake or when blood products need to be administered and where the fluid and potassium load may precipitate problems.

Peritoneal dialysis is the preferred treatment in most situations as it provides satisfactory metabolic control and fluid removal and is well tolerated. Initial treatment is with continuous cycling peritoneal dialysis, although when the child is stable it may be restricted to overnight.

Haemodialysis is the most rapid and efficient mode for solute removal and fluid removal but is technically demanding and may not be well tolerated in the acutely ill child in whom very rapid fluid and solute removal can lead to hypotension and convulsions.

Continuous arteriovenous haemofiltration is an alternative therapy in the critically ill. It is well tolerated and very effective in fluid removal but less good in solute removal. It is only suitable for immobile children.

Prognosis

ARF is a treatable state and the prognosis is determined by the underlying condition and by comorbidity. Mortality rates are high in neonatal ARF but the outcome is generally good in the older children although chronic renal damage can occur.

Problem

- Oliguria and anuria following a prodromal illness of diarrhoea which is often bloody.
- Increasing pallor and sometimes mild jaundice.
- Thrombocytopenia and red cell fragments on blood film.

Diagnosis — Diarrhoea associated haemolytic uraemic syndrome (HUS)

This is the commonest cause of ARF in children. It predominantly effects young children but can occur at any age. It is commoner in the summer months and may occur in small epidemics. It is usually associated with a verotoxin producing *E. coli* 0157. The toxin causes damage to vascular endothelial cells in the kidneys. Encephalopathy, the most serious extra-renal manifestation, can occur but is uncommon; haemorrhagic colitis is more frequently encountered. The prognosis is

Follow-up HUS (BAPN survey)	
complete recovery	177
alive ?follow-up	48
chronic renal failure	26
acute death	15
hypertension only	5
on dialysis	4

usually good with recovery in 1–2 weeks. A minority are left with significant long term renal damage. It is important to remember this uncommon condition in a child who is slow to recover from a diarrhoeal illness (particularly bloody diarrhoea).

A non-diarrhoea associated HUS also occurs and carries a less good prognosis. Major extra-renal manifestations are more likely and may be fatal. Chronic renal damage is also more common. Fresh frozen plasma, prostacyclin infusions and plasma exchange may be employed in severe cases although there is no conclusive evidence of effectiveness.

Acute on chronic renal failure. In any child with acute renal failure for no obvious cause, the possibility of acute on chronic renal failure should be considered. Signs which would be suggestive of chronicity include growth retardation, renal bone disease (osteodystrophy) and anaemia. Radiographs of the hand, wrist and knee should be examined for evidence of metabolic bone disease. Small scarred kidneys on ultrasound are pathognomonic of a chronic renal problem.

CHRONIC RENAL FAILURE

Renal insufficiency exists when function is reduced to below the critical level at which the kidney is able to maintain normal homeostasis. Chronic renal failure (CRF) is said to be present when there are symptoms and signs such as lethargy and anorexia, growth failure, bone disease and anaemia. It is important to remember that the blood urea and creatinine levels may not be elevated until the glomerular filtration rate (GFR) is reduced by 50%. Children are defined as having end-stage renal failure (ESRF) when the GFR is <10 ml/min/1.73 m^2. They require renal replacement therapy, i.e. dialysis and transplantation.

Chronic renal failure may be anticipated shortly after birth in a neonate whose mother had oligohydramnios or in whom there are obvious clinical problems such as prune belly (a syndrome associated with mega-cystis mega-ureter and often dysplastic kidneys). Pulmonary hypoplasia is often the cause of death in children with congenital abnormalities of the urinary tract in the neonatal period. However, if the respiratory function is adequate then the child need not necessarily die of chronic renal failure as maturation of the remaining renal function may take place in the first year of life and chronic dialysis is available for all ages.

The majority of children with **hypoplastic/dysplastic kidneys** or **chronic reflux nephropathy** present only later with growth failure, anorexia or an acute or chronic crisis. This may be precipitated either by infection in the urinary tract or extra renal site with an increase in metabolic demands and an acute decline in the glomerular filtration rate. One of the commonest group causes of CRF is **chronic nephritis**, of which focal segmental glomerulosclerosis is the most prevalent.

Inherited and metabolic problems are important because genetic counselling and antenatal detection can be offered.

Investigations

— Urine microscopy, osmolality, culture; 24-hour urine collection for volume, sodium and protein excretion.
— Plasma electrolytes, bicarbonate, urea, creatinine, calcium, phosphate, alkaline phosphatase, albumin, total protein, haemoglobin, white cells, platelets, blood film.
— Radiology, ultrasound of urinary tract, X-ray of wrists, hands and knees for bone age and changes of renal osteodystrophy.
— The glomerular filtration rate (GFR) calculated from

$$\text{GFR (ml/min/1.73 m}^2) = \frac{38 \times \text{height (cm)}}{\text{Plasma creatinine (}\mu\text{mol/l)}}$$

(A more accurate GFR is better performed using a radionuclide method such as chromium ^{51}EDTA or ^{99m}Tc-DTPA. Twenty four hour urine collections for creatinine clearance are too unreliable.)
— Other investigations, e.g. MCUG, DMSA scan, renal biopsy, will depend upon clinical pointers.

Monitoring

In kidneys that have a reduced renal mass, deterioration of GFR with time may be due to hyperfiltration in the remaining glomeruli leading to progressive glomerulosclerosis. Factors which may hasten progression of chronic renal failure include:

— Infection: urine cultures should be checked in children with abnormalities of the urinary tract.
— Correction of electrolyte abnormalities: sodium depletion and dehydration can occur in children with salt losing renal conditions such as obstructive uropathy or dysplasia.
— Hypertension: should be strictly controlled with drugs such as propanolol, atcnolol and nifedipine, or ACE inhibitors such as enalapril (used with caution).
— Obstruction in the urinary tract: close liaison with paediatric urologist is essential.
— Drug toxicity: all drug doses should be checked in renal impairment. Many drugs can cause interstitial nephritis.
— Hypercalcaemia: the use of vitamin D analogues can cause hypercalcaemia which can hasten renal deterioration.

Management

Nutrition and growth. The causes of poor growth in children with CRF are multifactorial. Growth potential lost in the first few years cannot be regained easily, so the tendency is to aggressively feed young infants with close supervision by the renal dietitian. Energy supplemented feeds are delivered by nasogastric tube or gastrostomy button feeds in younger children, and oral energy supplements are used in older children. In the conservative pre-dialysis phase protein in the diet is generally restricted to 1–1.5 g/kg body weight/day which also helps restrict hyperphosphataemia. A low protein diet has been advocated to slow the progression of renal disease in adult patients, but is not employed in children. Children with CRF are not growth hormone deficient but they do respond to daily injections of supra-physiological doses of growth hormone. Growth hormone has recently been licensed for use in children with chronic renal insufficiency.

Renal osteodystrophy. Renal rickets or osteodystrophy is a combination of both growth zone lesions and hyperparathyroidism. The mechanism of renal osteodystrophy is believed to involve phosphate retention leading to hypocalcaemia and secondary hyperparathyroidism, combined with a lack of 1,25-dihydroxycholecalciferol from the kidneys. Treatment consists of:

— Dietary phosphate restriction under supervision of dietitian.
— Use of phosphate binders such as calcium carbonate given three times a day with meals; aluminium hydroxide treatment has now been abandoned because of the risk of aluminium toxicity.
— Vitamin D analogues such as 1-alpha hydroxycholecalciferal or 1,25-dihydroxycholecalciferol prescribed daily.

and is monitored with assessments of plasma calcium, phosphate, alkaline phosphatase and whole molecule parathyroid hormone assay. This last has reduced the need for regular X-rays. Usually a hand and wrist X-ray are performed every 6–12 months depending on clinical status. Parathroidectomy is rarely required.

Metabolic acidosis and electrolytes. Acidosis can be a major contributor to failure to thrive, bone mineralisation and hyperkalaemia. Treatment is with oral sodium bicarbonate supplements, approximately 2 mmol/kg/day and titrated to each child's needs. Some children, particularly infants, are salt wasters and require additional sodium supplements. Others who have a low urine output and are prone to hypertension may require frequent advice about restricting sodium and potassium intake.

Anaemia. This is typically nomochromic and normocytic but iron and folate supplements are generally prescribed. Recombinant human erythropoietin can be given by subcutaneous injection once or twice a week.

Psychosocial support. Children and parents may have to live with the uncertainty of progressive CRF for many years. It is essential that they are given appropriate information and education which is supported by a discussion with multi-disciplinary members in the CRF clinic.

Dialysis

The number of patients who reach end stage renal disease in childhood (<16 years) requiring dialysis and transplantation is approximately 10 per million child population. Dialysis and transplantation is now feasible at any age, but it does impose considerable burdens upon the patient, family, staff and resources. It requires a fully integrated team approach to decide the best treatment option for each individual. Sometimes it is feasible to undertake kidney transplantation without the child being on dialysis, but generally most children pass through a period of chronic dialysis. The timing of chronic dialysis depends upon a number of factors but it is best to avoid waiting before the patient becomes symptomatic. Good preparation of the patient and family is essential.

The method of choice is continuous cycling peritoneal dialysis (CCPD), where the child has continuous peritoneal dialysis overnight using an automatic cycling machine which accurately records input and output volumes. The child is disconnected from the machine in the morning and still has some fluid in the abdomen during the day. This technique avoids the need for three or four bag changes during the day which was part of the original continuous ambulatory peritoneal dialysis (CAPD) technique that was introduced in 1978. The child is therefore freer during the day to attend school and participate in all activities. Peritonitis remains the major risk of CCPD/CAPD and is recognised by cloudy bags, abdominal pain and/or fever.

Prior to chronic peritoneal dialysis haemodialysis was usually the technique of choice. This is still used as a back up for chronic peritoneal dialysis when there are complications or for those children who cannot undertake chronic peritoneal dialysis. Haemodialysis is technically more difficult and requires access to the circulation. Traditionally this was by means of an arterial-venous fistula, but we now prefer the use of an indwelling jugular venous catheter.

Transplantation

Dialysis is only a holding measure until a suitable renal transplant becomes available. A transplant offers the best option in terms of physical and psychological rehabilitation. The offer of a suitable cadaveric transplant will depend upon blood group and tissue type match. The alternative is a living related donor transplant from either parent or sibling.

The transplant is usually placed in the iliac fossa position with anastomoses to the common iliac vessels. Occasionally in the smaller child it is placed intra-abdominally but this makes access for procedures such as biopsy very difficult. The child will need intensive monitoring in the postoperative situation and immunosuppression is with a combination of cyclosporin, prednisolone and azathioprine. Patients are carefully monitored for signs of rejection (fever, reduced urine output, graft tenderness and rise in serum creatinine). Other potential post transplant problems include:

— Susceptibility to infection, particularly cytomegalovirus and varicella.
— Hypertension due to drug therapy, chronic rejection, stenosis of the transplant renal artery or persistently high renin levels from the native kidneys.
— Weight gain and hirsutism association with prednisolone and cyclosporin treatment.

Present cadaveric graft survival rates are in the region of 85% at 2 years with 93% graft survival at 5 years using living related donor transplants. Unfortunately transplants are still lost to chronic rejection for several years afterwards but it is possible to undertake transplantation two or more times if necessary.

HYPERTENSION

In children this is defined as persistent or repeated elevation of the systolic and/or diastolic blood pressure above the 95th centile for age and sex. The prevalence of hypertension in childhood is probably between 1 and 3% but the majority of children will have mild increases and can be regarded as having primary (essential) hypertension. Elevated blood pressure in childhood may persist into adult life, where it is a risk factor for cardiovascular disease and so early recognition may enable appropriate advice and monitoring to be offered. Measurement of blood pressure should therefore be included in the examination of all children. Blood pressure varies with age and sex and reference should be made to appropriate centile charts just as for growth.

To avoid spuriously high readings, the blood pressure should be recorded with a cuff that is at least two-thirds of the length of the upper arm and has a bladder that encircles the arm. Obviously, blood pressure measurements should be repeated if high in a distressed patient (pain is a common cause of elevated blood pressure in the post-surgical situation), but just because a patient is restless, it should not be assumed that the blood pressure is falsely elevated. Elevated blood pressure may be making the patient restless and may be a sign of impending hypertensive encephalopathy. A much smaller number of children will have severe sustained hypertension which carries a high risk of morbidity and mortality. Renal diseases account for 80–90% of cases, with the commonest problem being the coarse renal scarring of reflux nephropathy.

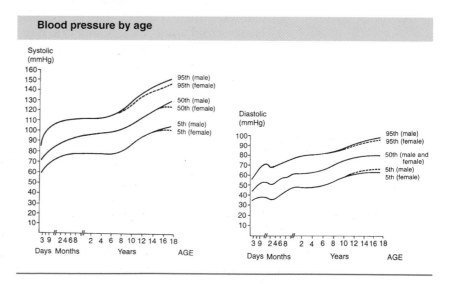

Blood pressure by age

Assessment. There may be a few clues in the history to account for the severe hypertension or there may be a story of previous urinary tract infections or unexplained fevers to suggest the possibility of vesicoureteric reflux. Examination should pay particular attention to abdominal masses; radial–femoral arterial pulse difference (suggesting coarctation) or the presence of abdominal bruits (suggesting renal vascular disease). Few children will have any evidence of clinical cardiomegaly and the fundi are usually normal but may show evidence of haemorrhages with or without papilloedema in severe cases. Investigations and treatment will often have to run concurrently.

— Urinalysis and urine culture.
— Full blood count, urea, electrolytes, including chloride and bicarbonate, creatinine, calcium, phosphate, albumin.
— A blood sample for plasma renin and aldosterone prior to any treatment would be useful if it can be arranged with the specialist laboratory in time.
— Radiological investigations will include a chest X-ray, an abdominal X-ray, and renal tract ultrasound. Further investigations will depend upon clinical suspicions and initial investigations, e.g. DMSA scan to look for renal scars of reflux nephropathy or renal arteriogram for renal artery stenosis.
— Urine for VMA and HVA creatinine ratio (also saved for toxicological analysis or steroid profile).
— ECG or preferably echocardiogram.

Management. Blood pressure needs to be adequately controlled while investigations proceed. If there is symptomatic hypertension, then the blood pressure needs to be carefully reduced using either sublingual nifedipine, or continuous intravenous nitroprusside or labetalol infusion. Oral therapy can then be introduced using vasodilators such as nifedipine or hydralazine in combination with beta blockers such as propanolol or atenolol. An angiotensin converting enzyme inhibitor such as captopril or enalapril is logical treatment when there is a high renin output state. Hypertension due to renal artery stenosis may need a direct surgical approach or balloon angioplasty.

Drug therapy in hypertensive crises

Drug	Administration	Onset of effect	Side-effects
Nifedipine	Sublingual hrly prn 0.2–0.5 mg/kg	minutes	headaches, tachycardia
Sodium Nitroprusside	0.5–10 mcg/kg/min as infusion	seconds/minutes	V rapid effect, titrate dose, cyanide accumulates after 48 hrs of use
Labetolol	1–3 mg/kg/hr	10–30 min	postural hypotension
Hydrallazine	slow i.v. or i.m., 0.2–0.8 mg/kg	10–30 min	tachycardia, flushing, headaches

STONES

The incidence of renal stones in children in the UK is about 1.5 per million population. Stones are much commoner in other parts of the world and this is probably attributable to high infection rates and dietary factors. They may be asymptomatic or result in haematuria, abdominal pain, urinary infection or even renal failure if there is obstruction of a single kidney or both kidneys. Stones in the urinary tract (urolithiasis) may or may not be associated with nephrocalcinosis which is the deposition of calcium salts within the renal parenchyma.

Investigations

— Urinalysis: a pH of <5.3 excludes distal renal tubular acidosis. A low specific gravity suggests tubular defect and chronic renal failure.
— Urine microscopy may identify red cells, white cells, bacteria. Specific crystals may be identified.
— Urine culture (to exclude associated infection; *proteus mirabilis* commonly associated with stones in boys)
— Urine amino acid screen: finding of cystine, ornithine, lysine and arginine ('cola') suggests cystinuria.
— Electrolytes, bicarbonate, urea, creatinine: may indicate renal failure or tubular acidosis.
— Fasting serum calcium, phosphate, alkaline phosphatase and urate-hyperparathyroidism and other causes of hypercalcaemia. Uric acid stones.
— PTH level only if calcium is elevated (hyperparathyroidism).
— Screen urine with calcium/creatinine and oxalate/creatinine ratios. May then need 24-hour collections.
— Plain abdominal X-ray, ultrasound, ± IVU, ± MUCG.
— Stone analysis (the commonest stone is magnesium ammonium phosphate associated with urinary infection).

Management

This is usually in conjunction with a paediatric surgeon. Stones causing obstruction or persistent infection require removal by pyelolithotomy or ureterolithotomy. Very small cystoscopes are now available for use in children and low ureteric stones can be captured in a dormia basket. Extracorporeal shock wave lithotripsy has been carried out in children but large stones are still best dealt with by a direct surgical approach. A high fluid intake is always advised in any stone former and occasionally thiazide diuretics may be contemplated in patients with hypercalciuria.

FURTHER READING

Cohen et al 1996 Pediatric urolithiasis. Urology 47: 292–303
Consensus statement on management and audit potential for steroid responsive nephrotic syndrome. 1994 Archives of Disease in Childhood 70: 151–157
Edelmann CM 1992 Pediatric kidney disease. Little Braun, Boston
Evans JHC 1992 Nocturnal enuresis. The Practitioner 236: 780–784
Fine RN et al 1995 Recombinant human growth hormone in infants and young children with chronic renal insufficiency. Pediatric Nephrology 9: 451–457

Holliday MA, Barratt TM, Avner CD 1994 Pediatric Nephrology, 3rd edn. Williams & Wilkins, Baltimore

Milford DV, Taylor CM, Guttridge B et al 1990 Haemolytic uraemic syndromes in the British Isles 1985–88: association with vero cytotoxin producing *Escherichia coli*. Part 1: clinical and epidemiological aspects. Archives of Disease in Childhood 65: 716–721

Postlethwaite RJ 1994 Clinical paediatric nephrology, 2nd edn. Butterworth-Heinmann, Oxford

Taylor CM, Chapman S 1989 Handbook of renal investigations in Children. Wright, London

Tripp BM, Homsy YL 1995 Neonatal hydronephrosis — the controversy and the management. Pediatric Nephrology 9: 503–509

Uldall R 1988 Renal nursing, 3rd edn. Blackwell Scientific Publications, Oxford

Watson AR 1993 Renal transplantation in children. Current Paediatrics 3: 141–155

Watson AR 1994 Urinary tract infection in infancy. Journal of Antimicrobial Chemotherapy 34S: 53–60

14 Blood

Haematological problems present in a limited number of ways, as anaemia with or without jaundice, petechiae or bruising, with or without anaemia and the chronic bleeding disorders. Congenital and acquired effects in white cell function result in recurrent and chronic infections.

ANAEMIA

The commonest presentation of anaemia remains that of the toddler or young child who has:

Problem

- A history of poor dietary intake of iron-containing foods sometimes with items in the diet which inhibit iron uptake.
- A hypochromic peripheral blood film with microcytosis and a normal reticulocyte count.

Haemoglobin	Film	Reticulocytes	WBC	Platelets
6 g/dl	Hypochromia	40×10^9/l	5.1×10^9/l	250×10^9/l

Diagnosis — Iron deficiency anaemia

In most cases the iron deficiency will be secondary to poor iron intake. There are other causes: a blood loss of more than 8 ml a day causes the loss of more iron than can be replaced. The serum ferritin is usually reduced and red cell protoporphyrin levels increased.

Causes of iron deficiency in children	
Diet	Poor iron intake
Increased requirements	During periods of rapid growth
Blood loss	Gastro-oesophageal reflux
	Meckel diverticulum
	Colonic polyps
	Cows' milk intolerance
Malabsorption	Coeliac disease

Changes in serum ferritin

Rise with	Rise with	Fall with
Increased body iron stores Iron-loading anaemia (e.g. thalassaemia)	**Increased ferritin synthesis** Inflammation/infection Malignancy: acute leukaemias, hepatoma, Stage IV neuroblastoma Hyperthyroidism	**Decreased body iron stores** Iron deficiency
Redistribution of body iron Anaemia not due to iron deficiency or blood loss (eg megaloblastic or hypoplastic anaemias)	**Release of tissue ferritins** Cell necrosis: hepatic necrosis, chronic liver disease, spleen or bone marrow infarction (e.g. sickle cell disease)	**Decreased ferritin synthesis (rare)** Ascorbate deficiency Hypothyroidism

Iron preparations

Elemental Fe content	
	mg/10 ml
Ferrous sulphate	24
Ferrous fumarate	90
Ferrous succinate	74
Ferrous glycerine sulphate	50
Sodium iron edetate	55
Polysaccharide iron	200
Ferrous gluconate	35
	mg/tab

Management. Take a full dietary history and exclude possible blood loss. Give dietary advice, and commence on oral iron therapy. Iron therapy should consist of up to 5 mg/kg/day elemental iron. Reticulocytes peak by day 7–10. Treatment with iron should continue for 3–6 months to replenish iron stores. If there is not a good response to iron therapy then investigations should be directed against malabsorption (after excluding a failure to take the iron medicine!) and might include examining the stool for fat globules, xylose tolerance test or jejunal biopsy. If there is a history of blood loss, then investigation of the gastrointestinal tract might include radioactive technetium to show site of bleeding; barium swallow and meal and possibly endoscopy; barium enema and sigmoidoscopy. Occasionally if the haemoglobin is very low, below 4 g/dl, a transfusion may be needed. Microcytosis persisting once iron replete suggests a thalassaemia trait.

Problem (rare)

- Anaemia developing in the latter part of the first year.
- Progressive pallor.
- Loss of energy.
- Macrocytic anaemia.
- Low serum and red cell folate.

Haemoglobin	Film	Reticulocytes	WBC	Platelets
6 g/dl	Macrocytosis	20×10^9/l	5.1×10^9/l	250×10^9/l

Diagnosis — Megaloblastic anaemia of infancy
This results when folic acid demand exceeds supply and responds rapidly to oral folic acid given in doses of 5 mg each day. This type of anaemia is also occasionally seen in children on cytotoxics, anti-convulsants and other drugs.

Problem (even rarer)

- Onset of progressive lethargy and pallor in late childhood.
- Atrophy of the papillae of the tongue and recurrent glossitis.
- Sometimes neurological signs of ataxia, paraesthesiae and absence of tendon reflexes.
- Macrocytic anaemia with megaloblastic marrow.

Diagnosis — Juvenile pernicious anaemia

A reduced serum Vitamin B_{12} level in the presence of Intrinsic Factor Antibodies and impaired B_{12} absorption (Schilling test) confirms the diagnosis. Treatment is with parenteral Vitamin B_{12} 250–1000 every 1–2 months. Surgical resection of the terminal ileum requires similar B_{12} replacement therapy.

Drugs known to cause megaloblastosis

Anticonvulsants	**Antituberculous drugs**
Phenytoin (Dilantin, Epanutin)	Para-amino salicylic acid
Primidone (Mysoline)	Pyrazinamide
Barbiturates	Cycloserine
Antimetabolites	**Antibacterial drugs**
Azathioprine	Nitrofurantoin
6-Mercaptopurine	Co-trimoxazole
Methotrexate	
Pyrimethamine (Daraprim)	**Other**
Vitamin B_{12} antagonists	Cyclophosphamide
Cytosine arabinoside	Phenylbutazone
	Arsenic

Problem (common)

- Pallor since infancy often associated with jaundice, beginning in the neonatal period.
- Often with splenomegaly.
- A family history of mild anaemia and jaundice.

Diagnosis — Congenital haemolytic anaemias

These may be due to a defect in the red cell membrane or the haemoglobin within the cell.

Finding (1)

- Presence of large numbers of spherocytes and a reticulocytosis, e.g.:

Haemoglobin	Film	Reticulotyes	WBC	Platelets
6 g/dl	Spherocytes and micro-spherocytes	230×10^9/l	5.0×10^9/l	250×10^9/l

Diagnosis — Hereditary spherocytosis

This is usually due to spectrin deficiency in the red cell membrane and the diagnosis can be made on the well known triad of spherocytosis, increased osmotic fragility and dominant inheritance. Testing for osmotic fragility involves adding washed red cells to progressive dilutions of saline showing that the red cells have abnormal fragility. Unfortunately the test is not specific for hereditary spherocytosis and other causes of spherocytosis must be excluded. Spherocytes may be seen in the peripheral blood in neonates particularly with ABO incompatibility, so the diagnosis is not always easy. Incubation for 24 hours increases the sensitivity of the test. There may be clinical jaundice in the neonatal period or at any other time — but the child is more yellow than sick. Cholelithiasis is very common.

Management. Folic acid 5 mg daily is usually given to most children with chronic haemolytic anaemias. Aplastic crises can occur, possibly associated with parvo-virus infections. If symptoms justify it then

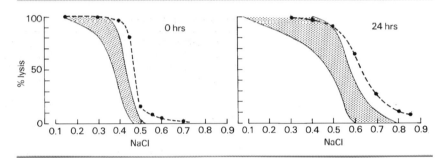

Red cell fragility showing normal range (shadow) and an abnormal response

splenectomy is recommended but whenever possible this is delayed until late childhood. Splenectomy removes the symptoms, reduces haemolysis, jaundice clears and cholelithiasis and aplastic crises do not occur. Splenectomy in young children, particularly 5 years of age and under, is associated with a significant increase in infections, septi caemia and meningitis most commonly caused by the pneumococcus. If splenectomy is planned Pneumovax and Hib vaccine are administered and penicillin 250 mg bd is given post-operatively at least until the age of 16 years if not for life. Aplastic crises usually require blood transfusion and antibiotics. Genetic advice is needed.

Finding (2)

- The red cells become sickle shaped under conditions of low oxygen tension: the sickle test is positive.

Diagnosis — Sickle cell disorder

This test does not distinguish between sickle cell trait — the heterozygous state — and sickle cell anaemia — the homozygous state — nor between HbSS and HbSC or S Thalassaemia. Haemoglobin electrophoresis is needed and often the picture will only become clear when family studies have been done. Those with sickle cell trait (HbAS) usually run haemoglobins of 10–12 g/dl and do not require any treatment other than advice to avoid situations where they are likely to come into contact with low oxygen tensions such as flying at high altitudes and some anaesthetics. Those with any of the homozygous or double

Differential diagnosis of sickle cell disease

S.S
  80–95% S
  2–20% F
  2–4% A_2
SB°Thal
  80–95% S
  0% A
  1–15% F
  3–6% A_2
SB+Thal
  55–75% S
  10–30% A
  1–13% F
  3–5% A_2
SD
  50% S
  50% D
SC
  50% S
  50% C

heterozygous diseases are more likely to have symptoms and signs. In HbSS the haemoglobin usually runs between 5 and 9 g, depending upon how much HbF is present. The liver is often enlarged, the spleen which is enlarged for the first few years of life then shrinks due to infarction by the end of the first decade. The child is functionally hyposplenic. There are often flow murmurs and venous hums and there is an inability to concentrate urine so that dehydration may occur easily. The child may subsequently present with the following variety of acute problems:

Painful crisis. This is the most common and is usually due to infarction either in bone, in the spleen or in the lungs, the 'chest' syndrome. They can be provoked by infection, cold or dehydration and treatment is with fluids, antibiotics, analgesis and oxygen.

Aplastic crisis. This is usually associated with an infection, often Parvo-virus. The haemoglobin falls and there is no reticulocyte response. Blood transfusion, fluids and antibiotics are normally required.

Megaloblastic crisis. This is due to folate deficiency.

Haemolytic crisis. The haemoglobin falls, jaundice increases but there is a good reticulocyte response. Fluids and antibiotics are usually given.

Hepatic crisis. This is rare but is usually fatal. Severe obstructive jaundice develops for no known reason. Other clinical problems include persistent ulceration around the ankles, infection with tetanus and salmonella which may cause osteomyelitis, persistent signs of pneumonia which are probably infarctive in origin, and priapism. Stroke can occur.

Management

There is no specific treatment for sickle cell crises. Management consists of adequate fluids, warmth, antibiotics, analgesia and oxygen. Blood transfusions are only needed if the haemoglobin falls. Apart from painful episodes, it should be possible for people with sickle cell anaemia to lead a fairly normal life. Splenectomy is not indicated and indeed recurrent infarcts in the spleen reduce its size so that it may be impalpable by mid childhood. The sickling episodes are often followed by a transient jaundice and occasionally lead to an aplastic crisis when blood transfusions may well be required. Folic acid supplements are given and prophylactic penicillin is recommended from 3–4 months of age. For this reason many areas are now carrying out a screening programme on all relevant neonates. The problems that can arise during an anaesthetic, whether for emergency or elective surgery, can be greatly reduced by giving a transfusion before surgery. Sickling is then less likely to occur but the anaesthetist should still be forewarned.

Findings (3)

- Onset of severe anaemia at about 6 months of age.
- Familial origins in the Mediterranean, Middle East or Asia.
- A hypochromic microcytic anaemia very similar to that seen in iron deficiency but with target cells.
- Raised fetal haemoglobin >5%.
- Absence of HbA on electrophoresis.

Diagnosis — Beta thalassaemia major

The homozygous state usually presents within the first 6 months of life, the heterozygous state may not present at all. Children with beta thalassaemia trait may have haemoglobins of 10–12 g/dl, but the film will look very like iron deficiency. No specific treatment is needed. Those with thalassaemia major require blood transfusions from the age of 6 months every 4–6 weeks for life. The aim is to keep the haemoglobin above 10 g/dl as this reduces endogenous red cell production. The side effects of severe iron overload can be reduced by giving desferrioxamine (400 mg i.v.) with each transfusion, and 35 mg/kg/day 5 nights each week. This is given by subcutaneous infusion in the anterior abdominal wall using a syringe pump and a butterfly needle. Despite chelation, affected children get progressive iron overload leading to growth failure, diabetes mellitus, cardiomyopathy, hypoparathyroidism and marked skin pigmentation can occur. Poor compliance with chelation is a common problem.

Thalassaemia major is inherited as an autosomal recessive. Recent advances in identifying the point mutations responsible for the different beta thalassaemias have made it possible to identify the homozygote in a chorionic villous biopsy during the first trimester, permitting an early termination if indicated.

Bone marrow transplantation from an HLA compatible sibling can effect a cure of homozygous beta thalassaemia but there is some morbidity and a reducing but significant mortality rate. The dilemma is that using transfusions and chelation, patients can be given a reasonable life for about 20 years. There is always the hope that more definite therapy may be developed in the meantime. Decisions to transplant must be based on a realistic awareness of all the facts.

Findings (4)

- If the congenital haemolytic anaemia does not fit into any of the clinical pictures described so far, the most likely cause is due to an enzyme defect leading to instability of the red cell membrane. A typical full blood count would be:

Haemoglobin	Film	Reticulocytes	WBC	Platelets
6 g/dl	'Bite' cells	$1401 \times 10^9/l$	$5.0 \times 10^9/l$	$250 \times 10^9/l$

Diagnosis (1) — Glucose-6-phosphate dehydrogenase deficiency (G6PD)

This condition often produces haemolytic episodes in the neonatal period associated with jaundice. Outside this period the red cells still have an abnormally short life span but this produces few problems unless the child comes in contact with a variety of drugs and organic compounds. Nothing can be done to increase the life span of the red cells other than to advise the parents on drugs and situations which should be avoided. A particularly severe haemolysis that may be fatal occurs with fava beans (favism).

Some drugs reported to produce haemolysis in patients with G-6-PD deficiency

Antimalarials
Primaquine
Pentaquine
Quinocide
Quinacrine
Quinine (C)

Antipyretics and analgesics
Acetylsalicylic acid
Acetanilide
Phenacetin
Antipyrine (C)
Amidopyrine
p-Aminosalicylic acid

Sulphonamides
Sulphanilamide
N_2 Acetylsulphanilamide
Sulphacetamide
Sulphamethoxypyridazine
Sulphasalazine
Sulphafurazole
Sulphapyridine

Others
Dimercaprol (BAL)
Methylene blue
Naphthalene
Phenylhydrazine
Acetylphenhydrazine
Probenecid
Vitamin K (large doses of water soluble analogues)
Chloramphenicol (C)
Fava beans (C)
Chloroquine
Nalidixic acid
Tolbutamid

Nitrofurans
Nitrofurantoin

Sulfones

Diagnosis (2) — Pyruvate kinase deficiency

Children with pyruvate kinase deficiency also have red cells with shortened life-spans. They occasionally have haemolytic episodes, often precipitated by infection and run low haemoglobin levels, though the anaemia is rarely very severe.

Problem

- The infant or child becomes irritable, lethargic, pale, often jaundiced.
- Fever and abdominal pain may occur.
- The liver is enlarged and the spleen is palpable (50% of cases).
- The blood picture usually shows a normocytic, normochromic pattern of variable severity with a reticulocytosis and macrocytosis. Spherocytes are seen but not in the numbers found in congenital spherocytosis. Heinz bodies and fragmented erythrocytes may be present.
- Haemoglobinuria may be present.

Diagnosis — Acquired haemolytic anaemia

The commonest acquired haemolytic anaemia in the neonate is undoubtedly rhesus iso-immunisation. This is discussed in the neonatal section. It is often not possible to find an aetiological diagnosis in haemolytic anaemia presenting during later childhood. Red cell fragmentation with thrombocytopenia suggests the haemolytic uraemic syndrome.

Some drugs which have been associated with acute haemolytic anaemia

Drugs
Antimalarials
Sulphonamides
Antibiotics — penicillin, amphotericin B, chloramphenicol, novobiocin, oxytetracycline, streptomycin, sulphones, nalidixic acid, nitrofurantoin, nitrofurazone
Antituberculous drugs — para-aminosalicyclic acid, sodium salt (PAS), Isonicotinic acid hydrazide (INAH)
Anthelminthics — betanaphthol, stibophen
Antipyretics — aspirin, phenacetin
Vitamin K and synthetic analogues

Miscellaneous drugs
Antihistamines
Barbiturates
Amphetamine sulphate
Chlorpromazine
Methion
Methylene blue
Quinidine
Resorcinol
Thiazides

Organic chemicals
Naphthalene
Aniline
Benzene
Carbon tetrachloride
Insecticides
Nitrobenzene
Para-dichlorbenzene
Phenols
Trinitrotoleune
Zinc ethylene bisthiocarbamate

Inorganic chemicals
Lead
Chlorate
Copper sulphate

Problem

- Previous history of infection which is often respiratory.
- Identification of cold agglutinins in the blood, with Anti I activity.

Diagnosis — Haemolytic anaemia due to cold agglutinins (mycoplasma infection)

The haemolysis is self-limiting and although initially it may be severe enough to require transfusions the antibodies do not persist for more than 6 months and rarely recur.

Problem

- A child with haemoglobinuria in the morning with bruising, jaundice and anaemia.

Diagnosis — Paroxysmal nocturnal haemoglobinuria

In these children intravascular haemolysis occurs as the pH drops. It is a stem cell disorder which can evolve to aplastic anaemia and it is characterised by a positive Ham test.

Problem

- A persistent anaemia lasting for weeks or months.
- A persistent reticulocytosis and normal or raised WBC and platelet counts.
- A positive direct Coomb test.
- Sera which will produce agglutination of red cells at 37°C.

Diagnosis — Immune haemolytic anaemia

This condition is autoimmune in origin. Some are drug induced but often the triggers responsible for the onset of this condition cannot be identified. Transfusions may be needed but should be reserved for situations when the haemoglobin is less than 6 g/dl and there are anaemic symptoms. Prednisolone (2 mg/kg/day) can be given and the dose reduced once response is seen. Alternate day maintenance steroid may be required but eventual spontaneous resolution usually occurs. The few children with persisting haemolysis despite steroids may require splenectomy. This results in a lasting remission in about 75% of children. An immune haemolytic anaemia characterised by a cold (Donath-Landsteiner) antibody, often with Anti P specificity, can occur in children after a non-specific viral infection. Paroxysmal cold haemoglobinuria is a benign self-limiting condition and requires only supportive therapy.

PETECHIAE AND BRUISING WITH OR WITHOUT ANAEMIA

Spontaneous onset of petechiae and bruising in a child who has otherwise been well is a relatively common symptom in childhood. It is usually fairly easy to make the right diagnosis and commence appropriate therapy. Several different patterns of disease are seen.

Problem (common)

- Onset of petechiae and spontaneous bruises particularly on the anterior aspect of the shins, extensor surfaces of the forearm and buttocks.
- Often associated abdominal pain.
- Often associated swollen painful joints, particularly the ankles, knees, wrists and elbows.

Diagnosis — Henoch–Schönlein purpura

The lesions of the skin usually commence as papules which then become frankly haemorrhagic. The condition can easily be distinguished from the other causes of purpura as the platelet count is in the normal range $(150–300 \times 10^9/l)$. It is usually benign and settles within 5–10 days. However, the children should be admitted to hospital for observation if there is: abdominal pain (occasionally they develop intussusception as a result of lesions in the gut wall and may need surgery); severe arthritis (the arthropathy is always benign and self-limiting but can cause the children a great deal of discomfort). Most will develop microscopic haematuria but if the haematuria is frank this indicates the presence of glomerulonephritis. In this particular form of nephritis approximately 15% will progress to chronic renal failure.

Management. Apart from surgery for intussusception, the only treatment needed is to provide the children with analgesics for their abdominal pain and arthritis. The majority will improve within 5–10 days although some continue to have a relapsing course for weeks or months. Steroids are occasionally given for very extensive lesions but there is little evidence that they alter the course of the disease and they are not advisable if there is renal involvement.

Causes of thrombocytopenia in the newborn

Newborn	Intrauterine infections	Rubella, cytomegalovirus, herpes simplex, toxoplasmosis, syphilis
	Platelet antibodies	Autoimmune: maternal ITP and SLE
		Alloimmune: fetomaternal incompatibility
		Drug induced
	Disseminated intravascular coagulation	Maternal pre-eclampsia
		Hypothermia, asphyxia, shock, sepsis
		Rh isoimmunisation
		Necrotizing enterocolitis
	Congenital megakaryocytic hypoplasia	TAR syndrome
		Maternal drug ingestion
	Hereditary thrombocytopenias	Wiskott–Aldrich syndrome
		May–Hegglin anomaly
	Others	Giant haemangioma
		Congenital and neonatal leukaemia
		Histiocytosis
	Metabolic disorders	Hyperglycinaemia, methyl-malonic acidaemia
Childhood	Idiopathic thrombocytopenic purpura	Acute
		Chronic
	Acute leukaemias	
	Bone marrow aplasia	Hereditary (Fanconi anaemia)
		Acquired
	Hereditary thrombocytopenias	Wiskott–Aldrich syndrome
		Bernard–Soulier syndrome
		May–Hegglin anomaly
	Others	Haemolytic uraemic syndrome
		Acute viral and rickettsial infections
		Septicaemia, purpura fulminans
		Giant haemangioma
		Splenomegaly
		Cyanotic congenital heart disease
		Osteopetrosis

Problem

- Often a previous history of infection.
- A grossly reduced platelet count often less than $10 \times 10^9/l$ associated with a normal or only slightly reduced haemoglobin and a normal white count. The blood film is normal apart from the lack of platelets.

Diagnosis — Idiopathic thrombocytopenic purpura (ITP)

It is usually possible to make a confident diagnosis of this condition on the clinical picture and the peripheral blood film but the diagnosis is essentially one of exclusion of other causes of thrombocytopenia. If there is any doubt then a bone marrow aspiration should be carried out, this shows increased numbers of megakaryocytes. There are other causes of thrombocytopenia, best divided into those occurring during the neonatal period and those occurring in childhood. It is now generally agreed that thrombocytopenic purpura is an immune disorder characterised by platelet bound antibody. The sudden appearance of platelet bound antibody is probably caused by a preceding viral infection.

Management. In 90% of childhood ITP the thrombocytopenia will resolve within 3 months, this is true of less than 20% in adult ITP which is more commonly chronic. The main anxiety is that a serious bleed may occur before the natural remission comes about. Many clinicians believe treatment is indicated if there are haemorrhagic symptoms such as mouth bleeds. Both steroids and intravenous immunoglobulin have been shown to shorten the duration of thrombocytopenia. A bone marrow should be done before giving steroids and i.v. IgG is expensive and not without risks and side effects. Other immuno-suppressives such as azathioprine are no longer used in children. Immunoglobulin may be useful in emergencies or prior to surgery, the platelets rise within 2–5 days of administration.

Chronic idiopathic thrombocytopenic purpura (ITP), persisting for more than 6 months, requires treatment if overt haemorrhagic symptoms are present. Some children are steroid responsive but dependent. Splenectomy may eventually be indicated but late spontaneous remission remains a possibility.

Problem (the worst)	• Progressive anaemia and petechiae over a period of weeks.

• Progressive anaemia and petechiae over a period of weeks.
• Onset of purpura and spontaneous bruising occurring all over the body often with ulceration of the gums.
• History of increased susceptibility to infection.
• Often associated enlargement of liver, spleen and lymph glands.
• Peripheral blood picture showing anaemia of variable severity, with thrombocytopenia and a grossly raised or reduced white count usually but not always, with the presence of very immature white cells, e.g.:

Haemoglobin	Film	Reticulocytes	WBC	Platelets
5.3 g/dl	Blast cells	31×10^9/l	28×10^9/l	8.0×10^9/l

• Bone marrow showing almost total replacement of normal cells with uniform immature cells which are either lymphoid or myeloid.

Diagnosis — Acute leukaemia
For management see Chapter 13.

Problem (rarer but as bad) • Onset of anaemia.
• History of increased susceptibility to infection.

- Peripheral film showing reduction in all components, e.g.:

Haemoglobin	Reticulocytes	WBC	Platelets
5 g/dl	zero	$1.0 \times 10^9/l$	$25 \times 10^9/l$

- Sometimes petechial rash with spontaneous bruising due to severe thrombocytopenia.
- Bone marrow showing grossly hypocellular picture.

Diagnosis — Aplastic anaemia

There are a number of drugs and conditions which undoubtedly cause aplastic anaemia. It is a rare but well recognised complication of infective hepatitis. However, in the majority of cases the aetiological agent cannot be identified. The severity may be a guide to prognosis. The criteria for severe aplastic anaemia are:

— Granulocytes $<0.5 \times 10^9/l$
— Platelets $<20 \times 10^9/l$
— Reticulocytes $<1\%$

Drugs causing aplastic anaemia

Therapeutic use	Definite association	Possible association
Antibiotics Sulphonamides	Chloramphenicol Methicillin Nitrofurantoin	Streptomycin
Anti-inflammatory agents Amidopyrine Gold salts	Phenylbutazone Oxyphenbutazone Colchicine	Indomethacin D-penicillamine
Anti-epileptic drugs Troxidone	Phenytoin sodium Methoin	
Oral hypoglycaemic agents	Tolbutamide Chlorpropamide	
Drugs used for parasite infections	Mepacrine Organic arsenicals	Amodiaquine Pyrimethamine
Antithroid drugs	Potassium perchlorate Thiouracil	Carbimazole
Antihistamines	Tripelennamine	Chlorpheniramine
Psychoactive drugs	Chlordiazepoxide Meprobamate	
Diuretics	Chlorothiazide Hydroflumethiazide	Acetazolamide
Others		Quinidine

Chemicals causing aplastic anemia

Proven
Solvents
  Benzene
  Toluene
  Stoddart solvent
Insecticides
  DDT
  Gammabenzene
    hexachloride
    (Lindane)
Possible
Model aeroplane glue
Hair dyes

Management. Treatment involves providing total support while waiting for the bone marrow to recover, and attempting to help it recover. Blood transfusions using packed cells are required and over a period of weeks it is usually possible to prevent the patient becoming severely anaemic by regular transfusions. Platelet transfusions are likely to be needed. Red cell and platelet transfusions should be filtered to remove white blood cells. Febrile episodes require prompt treatment with broad spectrum intravenous antibiotics. Take blood from the child, siblings and parents for blood groups and HLA tissue types as compatible bone marrow transplant may offer the only long term possibility of cure.

The prognosis has improved significantly in recent years with the combined use of antilymphocyte globulin, cyclosporin A and steroids giving response rates in excess of 60%. Relapses can occur and bone marrow transplant may still be required.

Fanconi anaemia is a familial form, associated with other congenital abnormalities, abnormal skin pigmentation, short stature, skeletal and renal malformations and raised HbF. This does not respond to the above combined therapy and although the anaemia may show initial response to androgens, bone marrow transplant offers the only cure. There is a predisposition to leukaemia and other malignant tumours. The characteristic laboratory finding is of increased chromosomal fragility particularly in response to stress by agents such as Mitomycin C.

Abnormalities associated with Fanconi anaemia	
Short stature	80%
Hyperpigmentation of the skin	75%
Malformation of the skeleton (e.g. aplasia or hypoplasia of the thumb)	66%
Microsomy	60%
Microcephaly	40%
Malformation of kidneys	28%
Cryptorchidism	20%
Mental retardation	17%
Deafness	7%
Growth hormone deficiency*	

*This has been reported.

CHRONIC BLEEDING DISORDERS

There are many children who appear to bruise more easily than their peers. The large majority are entirely normal. Those who bruise spontaneously or have prolonged excessive bleeding following cuts or dental extraction require further investigation. Take a careful history including details of all close relatives. Clotting studies will usually include: (1) platelet count, if normal this excludes ITP; (2) prothrombin time tests extrinsic clotting factors, this is usually normal in haemophilia A and B, and abnormal in liver disease; (3) partial thromboplastin time (PTT) which tests intrinsic clotting factors and is abnormal in haemophilia, A and B, and some von Willebrand; (4) thrombin time which detects disorders of fibrinogen quantity and quality. If the PTT is prolonged Factor VIII and Factor IX levels should be measured. A level <50% indicates haemophilia. The Factor VIII level may be normal

Laboratory diagnosis of inherited bleeding disorders

Disorder	Screening tests* (UNITS/DL)				Specific assays †
	PT	PTTK	TCT	BT	
Haemophilia A	N	↑	N	N	Factor VIII less than 50% VWF:AgN Ricof.N
von Willebrand	N	↑ or N	N	↑ or N	Factor VIII N or ↓ VWF:Ag less than 50% Ricof.less than 50%
Haemophilia B	N	↑	N	N	Factor IX less than 50%
Factor XI deficiency	N	↑	N	N	Factor XI less than 35%
Factor X deficiency	↑	↑	N	N	Factor X less than 50%
Factor V deficiency	↑	↑	N	N	Factor V less than 50%
Factor VII	↑	N	N	N	Factor VII less than 50%
Factor II	↑	↑	N	N	Factor II less than 50%
Afibrinogenaemia	↑	↑	↑	↑	Fibrinogen undetectable
Dysfibrinogenaemia	↑	↑	↑	N	Fibrinogen N or ↓
Factor XIII deficiency	N	N	N	N	Fibrin solubility ↑

Factor XIII less than 1
*PT=prothrombin time; PTTK=activated partial thromboplastin time; TCT=thrombin clotting time; BT=bleeding time.
† Factor VIII (formerly VIII:c). VWF: Ag=von Willebrand factor antigen (formerly VIIIR: Ag); Ricof.=ristocetin cofactor.
↑=increased; ↓=decreased; N=normal.

in von Willebrand disease but the Factor VIII VWF Antigen and Ristocetin Cofactor levels are reduced. Platelet function tests may be required to demonstrate abnormal platelet function despite a normal platelet count, i.e. thrombasthenia.

Findings

- Normal platelet count.
- Normal prothrombin time.
- Raised partial thromboplastin time.
- Level of factor VIII below 20%.

Diagnosis (1) — Haemophilia A

Before the age of 1, haemophilia may present as excessive subcutaneous bruising, or bleeding following circumcision or herniotomy. Later, when mobile, haemarthroses are common. Tonsillectomy provides a severe haemostatic challenge. The level of Factor VIII correlates with the severity of the illness. Inheritance is sex linked.

Management. Haemophiliacs have to visit hospitals so frequently that it becomes a major part of their life. Each visit should be as rapid and as pleasant as possible. Replacement therapy with high purity specific Factor VIII concentrates is the norm. Most boys with severe haemophilia A are on regular home prophylactic treatment three times/week. This reduces the frequency of spontaneous joint bleeds and the resulting potentially crippling arthritis. Concern over potential viral transmission from human plasma derived products persists and

Haemophilia A: clinical severity. This table is also applicable to factor IX, X, VII and II deficiencies but not to factor XI, V, XIII or von Willebrand factor deficiencies

Factor VIII (units/dl)	Bleeding tendency	Relative incidence (% of cases)
less than 2	Severe; frequent spontaneous bleeding* into joints, muscles and internal organs	50
2–5	Moderately severe; some 'spontaneous bleeds', bleeding after minor trauma	30
more than 5–30	Mild; bleeding only after significant trauma, surgery	20

*Spontaneous bleeding refers to those episodes where no obvious precipitating event preceded the bleed. No doubt minor tissue damage consequent on every day activities actually initiates bleeding.

recombinant human Factor VIII is now available and the Factor IX product is on the horizon.

Specific bleeds

Head injuries. Always admit and give Factor VIII concentrate aiming for a Factor VIII level of 100%. Consider CT scan.

Major trauma/surgery. Aim for 100% and top up doses 12 hourly for several days.

Dental extractions, well established joint bleeds and major soft tissue bleeds. Aim for 50%. A repeat dose the following day may be needed.

Simple joint bleeds, subcutaneous haematoma. Aim for 30%. A single treatment may be adequate. In the acute phase of a joint bleed rest is recommended, however gentle exercise after recovery is important to maintain muscle strength and joint support. Avoid aspirin and non-steroidal anti-inflammatory analgesics.

All major surgery, including dental extractions, should be done under controlled conditions at a recognised haemophilia centre with liaison between surgeon, anaesthetist, haematologist and paediatrician.

Units of Factor VIII required = 1/2 (wt (kg) × desired rise in units/dl

Tranexamic acid is useful in the additional control of mouth and dental bleeds in particular. It is contra-indicated in the presence of haematuria. Boys with mild haemophilia A often reach the desired Factor VIII level after DDAVP infusion (0.3 μg/kg i.v.) and thus avoid exposure to Factor VIII concentrates. The nature of the disease and Factor VIII requirements must be explained in detail to the child and his parents and arrangements for visits streamlined as far as possible. Social workers may need to be involved and genetic counselling is required. Education and career advice is vitally important. Psychological support is often required.

Diagnosis (2) — Haemophilia B (Christmas disease)

Factor IX deficiency is clinically indistinguishable from haemophilia A. Replacement is with Factor IX concentrate which has a longer half-life than Factor VIII.

Units of Factor IX required = wt (kg) × desired rise in Factor IX U/dl

Boys with Factor IX deficiency do not respond to DDAVP and so need factor concentrate replacement.

Diagnosis (3) — von Willebrand disease

This is the most common inherited bleeding disorder. Inheritance is usually autosomal dominant and the bleeding pattern that of a platelet defect, i.e. easy bruising and epistaxis rather than soft tissue and joint bleeds. Several subtypes exist but the most common responds to DDAVP infusion (0.3 µg/kg i.v.). Factor VIII concentrate may however be required to cover major surgery or trauma.

Diagnosis (4) — Glanzman thrombasthenia

This is an inherited disorder in which there is abnormal bleeding though all the routine tests are normal. Platelet function tests are required. There is no specific treatment. Platelet transfusions may be needed for significant bleeds.

Incidence of inherited bleeding disorders

Factor deficiency	Name	Inheritance	Incidence
VIII	Haemophilia A	Sex-linked	1 in 30 000
IX	Haemophilia B	Sex-linked	1 in 150 000
XI	PTA	Autosomal recessive	1 in 150 000
X	Stuart Prower	Autosomal recessive	1 in 500 000
VII	Proconvertin	Autosomal recessive	1 in 1 000 000
I	Fibrinogen	Autosomal recessive	
II	Prothrombin	Autosomal recessive	
XII	Hageman	Autosomal recessive	Very rare
XIII	Fibrin stabilizing factor	Autosomal recessive	
VIII:VWF	von Willebrand Disease	Autosomal dominant	Probably at least 1:1000
Other defects			
Hereditary haemorrhagic telangiectasia		Autosomal dominant	Rare
Ehler–Danlos syndrome		Autosomal dominant	Rare

RECURRENT INFECTIONS

In many countries children are infected because of poor hygiene, undernutrition and lack of immunisation. In well nourished, immunised children in clean environments, recurrent infections are more likely to be due to defects in defence such as structural abnormalities — ureteric reflux, functional abnormalities — abnormal ciliary activity or due to specific defects of the immune system. The first two are considered in other chapters. The immunodeficiency states affecting children are most commonly congenital. Acquired immunodeficiency

Congenital immunodeficiencies

Antibody defects	Combined immuno-deficiency	Immunodeficiency associated with other defects	Complement deficiency	Defects in phagocytic function
X-linked and autosomal recessive agammaglobu-linaemia	Severe combined immunodeficiency (SCID — reduced T- and B-cell numbers)	3rd & 4th arch anomalad — Di George syndrome	Family deficiencies of C1r, C2, C3, C4, C5, C6, C7 and C8	Neonatal neutrophils
				Chronic granulomatous disease
	Reticular dysgenesis	Wiskott–Aldrich syndrome	Complement pathway dysfunction	
Common variable immune deficiency	Adenosine deaminase (ADA) deficiency	Ataxia telangiectasia	(e.g. neonates, SLE, diabetes mellitus, C5 dysfunction, chronic haemodialysis, glomerulonephritis)	Chediak–Higashi syndrome
Ig deficiency with increased IgM (Hyper IgM syndrome)	Purine nucleoside phophorylase (PNP) deficiency	Transcobalamin II deficiency		Specific granule deficiencies
		Partial albinism		Leucocyte adhesion deficiency
IgA deficiency	MHC Class I and II deficiency	Hereditary defective response to EBV		
IgG subclass deficiency				
kappa chain deficiency				

is most commonly secondary to splenectomy and the use of long term steroids or chemotherapy. Acquired HIV infection by transmission from blood products or via vertical transmission has a widely variable prevalence, linked to risk factors in the local community.

Immunodeficiency in childhood is characterised by a history suggestive of excessive frequency and abnormal types of infections coupled with abnormal laboratory tests of immune function. Modern immunology has defined components of the immune system, classification of defects requires each component to be investigated.

After birth, organisms colonise the infant and the infant's immune system matures and responds to a host of foreign antigens — natural immunisation. In the pre-school years minor infections are very common with an average around nine and a range of 6–12. The majority are respiratory and occur in clusters in winter. Recurrent infections demand further investigation if they are virtually continuous, unusually severe or cause repeated systemic illness, are associated with failure to thrive, are caused by organisms with low pathogenicity, or there is a family history of susceptibility to unusual infections. The use of infection diaries by parents is particularly valuable for assessing frequency of infections for diagnostic or monitoring purposes. Careful examination for any lymph nodes, not only enlarged ones, and the presence of tonsils should be made. An X-ray of the neck for evidence of tonsils and adenoids may be justified; the chest X-ray should be scrutinised for the presence of a thymus.

Investigation of the immune system

Innate immunity	Humoral immunity	Cell-mediated immunity	Combined immunity	Phagocytic function
Complement subtype assays	Quantitative serum immunoglobulins, including IgG subclasses	T lymphocyte numbers (CD3, CD4, CD8)	Total lymphocyte count ($< 2.8 \times 10^9$/L — abnormal)	Granulocyte count in blood and bone marrow
CH50 assay — assay of classical + terminal complement pathway	Functional antibody responses to immunisations (e.g. Tetanus, Hib) common	T-cell response to mitogens (e.g. phytohaemagglutinin)	MHC Class expression	Granulocyte morphology
AP50 assay — assay of alternate and terminal complement pathway	bacteria (e.g. Streptococcus) and red cell antigens	Skin sensitivity testing (depends upon prior exposure to antigen)	Adenine deaminase (ADA) levels	Nitrobluetetrazolium (NBT) screening test — test of bacterial killing
			Purine nucleoside phosphorylase (PNP) levels	Chemotaxis assay
Natural Killer Cell numbers	Plasma B lymphocyte numbers (CD19, CD20)			Opsonisation, phagocytosis + killing assays
				Chromosomal abnormalities secondary to defects in DNA repair

Successful management depends upon swift recognition of clinical immunodeficiency, thorough characterisation of the full range of immune function, initiation of specific treatments where indicated and meticulous attention to bacteriological and virological investigation of all infectious episodes. Where indicated, immunoglobulin replacement can be very effective but needs specialist supervision of product selection, adjustment of dosage during growth and home administration. Antibiotics may need to be used prophylactically for bacterial infections. Immunisations can be given in some conditions but seroconversions should be documented. Live vaccines should be avoided. Where there is humoral deficiency and immunoglobulin is not being used, case contacts with chickenpox should be treated either with prophylactic acyclovir (for up to 3 weeks) or Zoster Immune Globulin (within 72 hours of contact). Case contact with measles should be treated with Human Immunoglobulin within 72 hours of contact. Co-trimoxazole should be used for pneumocystis prophylaxis if there is a humoral defect. In severe combined immunodeficiencies, blood products should be irradiated to prevent graft versus host disease.

Problem

- Recurrent sinopulmonary infection.
- Recurrent otitis media.
- Bronchiectasis.
- Giardiasis infection.

Diagnosis — Panhypogammaglobulinaemia

This may be 'early onset' in the first 2 years, which is almost always the

X-linked disorder described by Bruton, or 'late onset' where the presentation is more variable and the inheritance pattern less certain. Failure to thrive, gastrointestinal disorders and autoimmune disorders may complicate the clinical course but they are not common. Gamma globulin replacement therapy often results in a dramatic improvement.

Children with defects of complement (C3) may present in an identical way. C3 conversion is the bulk reaction of the complement pathway and it is at this stage that the most important biological activities are generated — chemotaxis, immune adherence and mast cell degranulation.

Problem

- Recurrent upper and lower respiratory and gastrointestinal tract infections.

Diagnosis — Selective IgA deficiency

Low IgA levels are found in 1 : 400 to 1 : 700 children, but deficiency disorders only occur in around 1 : 15 000. The reason is that this smaller group have associated abnormalities in IgG. They too benefit from gamma globulin administration.

Problem

- Frequent and severe infections with herpes simplex, overwhelming infections with measles, varicella, cytomegalovirus, pneumocystis and fungi — nocardia, candida and aspergillus.

Diagnosis — T cell deficiencies

These deficiencies may be isolated, with normal levels of immunoglobulin, alternatively they may be part of more extensive immunodeficiency states. Di George syndrome is an example of an isolated T cell deficiency associated with congenital absence of the thymus. T cell function is defective in Wiskott–Aldrich syndrome, ataxia telangiectasia and chronic mucocutaneous candidiasis, amongst others. Bone marrow transplantation may be used to replace T cell deficiencies, although is of high risk, especially in patients with a strong previous history of recurrent infections.

Problem

- Failure to thrive in the first year of life, recurrent sinopulmonary infection, persistent candidiasis, pneumocystis infections, persistent diarrhoea, severe recurrent systemic infections, disseminated viral infections — chicken pox , measles etc.

Diagnosis — Severe combined immune deficiency (SCID)

This rare condition is genetically determined, may be inherited as autosomal recessive or X-linked. First cases in families are difficult to diagnose and almost always have established infection. A low lymphocyte count ($<2.8 \times 10^9$/l) is an important clue, worthy of further investigation. Subsequent siblings should be investigated at birth.

Deficiencies of adenine deaminase (ADA) or purine nucleoside phosphorylase (PNP) are critical findings. Assay of these enzymes may be used in antenatal testing. For children with SCID successful treatment depends upon the presence of an HLA matched bone marrow donor. Haplo-identical donors may be used, associated infections pose the greatest risk to the procedure. Enzyme replacement therapy is under trial.

Problem

- Recurrent neisserial infections.

Diagnosis — Complement (C 5,6,7 and 8) deficiencies

These deficiencies do not normally present with recurrent infections, however recurrent neisserial infections is an exception and is due to the specific need for this component of complement to clear this group of organisms.

Problem

- Recurrent staphylococcal infections with abscesses — in and around liver, lungs and bones.
- Infection with uncommon organisms — *Serratia marcescens*, aspergillus, nocardia and atypical mycobacteria.
- Chronic lymphadenopathy and hepatosplenomegaly.

Diagnosis — Phagocyte defect: chronic granulomatous disease (CGD)

CGD is a X-linked disease in which phagocytes can ingest pathogens but are unable to mount the oxidative burst of intracellular metabolism necessary to kill them. It used to be fatal, but anti-bacterial agents like trimethoprim, used continuously, together with vigorous antibiotic therapy for each new infection has improved the outlook in children diagnosed early and monitored closely.

Problem

- Infants of an HIV positive mother.

Diagnosis — Human immunodeficiency virus (HIV) infection

All babies born of HIV positive mothers will have antibodies to HIV, and whilst on average they disappear by 10 months, they may linger until 18 months. The infant is considered to have the infection if the antibodies persist after 18 months or the child develops the clinical features of AIDS. However these are of no help in deciding whether to commence a vigorous programme of prophylaxis. Some laboratories are now able, using a range of virological tests, to identify the HIV infection with reasonable confidence. Prophylaxis with co-trimoxazole, intravenous immunoglobulin and zidovudine (ZDV) should be used. There are other anti-viral agents undergoing trial so management demands a knowledge of the current literature and involvement with current clinical trials.

Problem

- An infant with opportunistic infections especially interstitial pneumonia due to pneumocystis carinii.
- Recurrent bacterial infections especially with the polysaccharide encapsulated bacteria.
- Failure to thrive with intractable diarrhoea and mouth infections.
- Encephalopathy.

Diagnosis — HIV infection

These are all presentations of vertically transmitted HIV infection. The finding of HIV antibody in the mother, virus in the infant or antibody in an infant over 18 months strongly suggests the diagnosis. The discovery of the infection for the first time in a sick infant creates a major challenge for all concerned. The whole family will need understanding and support. What is needed is a team approach by those with knowledge of the disease, its effects and management, and for that reason, in the UK, they should be cared for in centres with the necessary expertise.

Problem

- Fever for 7 days without localising signs.
- 1 week in hospital fails to identify the cause.

Diagnosis — Pyrexia of unknown origin

The symptoms and signs of a febrile response are perhaps the most common presentation of illness in childhood. Usually after careful examination the site of the infection can be identified and appropriate treatment given. The management of these disorders is considered in the appropriate sections. If despite a thorough examination and preliminary investigations the cause is not obvious, then the child

---

Causes of a prolonged fever

Bacterial diseases	**Viral diseases**	**Malignancies**
Abscesses: dental, liver, pelvic, perinephric, subdiaphragmatic	Cytomegalic inclusion disease	Hodgkin disease
Bacterial endocarditis	Hepatitis (chronic active)	
Brucellosis	Infectious mononucleosis	Lymphoma
Leptospirosis		Neuroblastoma
Mastoiditis (chronic)	**Fungal diseases**	
Meningo-encephalitis	Blastomycosis (non-pulmonary)	**Miscellaneous disorders**
Osteomyelitis	Histoplasmosis (disseminated)	Periodic fever
Pyelonephritis		Drug fever
Salmonellosis	**Parasitic diseases**	Serum sickness
Sinusitis	Malaria	Fictitious fever
Tuberculosis	Toxoplasmosis	Familial dysautonomia
	Visceral larva migrans	Colitis
		Ulcerative colitis
	Collagen diseases	Pancreatitis
	Juvenile rheumatoid arthritis	Thyrotoxicosis
	Polyarteritis nodosa	
	Systemic lupus erythematosus	

requires careful re-assessment, neither 'blunderbus' investigations nor antibiotics given 'on spec' are in the child's interests. There is no alternative to a careful attention to detail. Often the fever settles and the child recovers without the cause becoming obvious. If the child remains ill and the fever persists consider the possibilities given in the list. Some children have larger diurnal variations in body temperature than others and this can lead to unnecessary investigations. In this situation and in fictitious fever the child remains well.

FURTHER READING

Crawley J, Gibb D 1993 Clinical features and management of HIV infection in children. Current Paediatric 3: 164–167
Hoffbrand AV, Lewis SM Postgraduate haematology, (3rd edn.) Heinemann Professional Publishing, Oxford
Lee C (ed) 1996 Haemophilia. Clinical Haematology 9(2)
Lilleyman JS, Hann IM 1992 Paediatric haematology, Churchill Livingstone, Edinburgh
Nathan DG, Oski FA Haematology of infancy and childhood, 4th edn. WB Saunders, Philadelphia
Roberton D 1993 Basic investigations of children with recurrent infections. Current Paediatrics 3: 6–9
Serjeant GR, Sickle cell anaemia, 2nd edn. Oxford University Press, Oxford

15 Cancer

Childhood cancer affects one in 600 children; its incidence is comparable to that of diabetes and cerebral palsy. It can arise in many systems and is in the differential diagnosis of many clinical presentations. Wherever it arises, the care of the child demands a precise diagnosis and appropriate therapy sensitively administered. Those who provide that care, the family doctor, local paediatrician and the specialist and the teams within which they work, must share a common approach if the harm to the child and family are to be kept to a minimum.

Childhood cancers develop in the tissues undergoing the greatest rates of growth and development. The role of exposure to environmental carcinogens in the development of childhood cancers is not proven. There is some evidence that exposure of parental germ cells to radiation might lead to leukaemia. A small number are due to genetic predisposition.

Age at presentation of the commoner childhood cancers

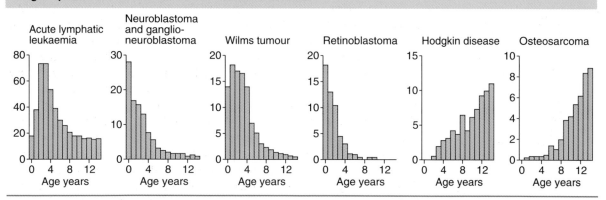

Screening. Identifying a child at risk of developing cancer poses serious difficulties for parents and doctor. Neuroblastoma is currently the only tumour where population screening is being considered. Any screening for cancer in childhood is likely to generate considerable anxiety in the child and family. Parents may have to consider their own risk of developing cancer. The balance, the benefits and the risks need to be carefully assessed before a screening programme is introduced.

Making the diagnosis. A family or hospital doctor may be the first to realise that the child has a cancer. Usually a lot more information has to be gathered before deciding optimal treatment and giving advice on the prognosis. Each tumour entity has a known pattern of spread. Experience from clinical trials has identified optimal methods for grouping patients according to patient factors (age, sex, presenting symptoms) and tumour factors (tumour size, histological grade, cellular or chemical markers and the presence of metastases). These staging systems follow international guidelines. Defining the clinical stage, therefore, frequently involves the full range of imaging scans as well as biopsies of draining lymph nodes, bone marrow and examination of spinal fluid cytology. Where the child presents with a tumour mass, the selection of optimal imaging techniques should be directed at defining the tissue of origin if possible, and to look for evidence of tumour dissemination. Tumour markers should be measured early where indicated. Biopsy using minimally invasive techniques needs to be discussed between the pathologist, radiologist and surgeon, as it is crucial that a reliable answer is obtained with the minimum of delay. It may not always be necessary to biopsy the primary tumour if there is evidence of tumour dissemination. In such cases obtaining malignant cells from bone marrow, blood or effusion fluid may be adequate for diagnosis either on its own or in conjunction with serum or urinary tumour markers.

Treatments

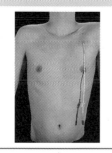

Central venous line

Surgery. Complete tumour resection remains a most powerful treatment and improves the prognosis of a wide range of tumours. But surgery may also be required for tumour biopsy, urinary diversion, the insertion of a central venous catheter, placing of intracranial ventriculo peritoneal shunt as well as formal resection of the tumour.

Chemotherapy plays a major part in childhood cancer because of the enhanced sensitivity of leukaemias and cancers to chemotherapy in childhood compared to the experience in adulthood. The specific combinations of drugs have evolved over many years as a result, initially, of empiricism. Subsequently, clinical trials and ongoing national and international collaborations have led to refinements. The drugs are used in some situations as the sole method of treatment and are directed at achieving a cure (e.g. leukaemia). In others, tumour shrinkage by chemotherapy agents permits the surgeon to achieve a complete resection with less risk of either tumour spillage or functional damage to the organ of origin or surrounding tissues. Administering intrathecal chemotherapy permits treatment of meningeal and spinal dissemination of cancer cells, a crucial process in the prevention of CNS relapse of acute lymphoblastic leukaemia. In certain situations, chemotherapy has a role in terminal care to control tumour-related symptoms.

Radiotherapy has an established role in the treatment of many childhood malignancies, in particular those involving the brain and spine. It is also used for treating residual tumour, metastatic tumour and in palliative care. Its value is limited by difficulties in the administration of treatment in young children as well as inevitable radiation damage to growing tissues.

In general, it is always best to await confirmation of diagnosis with full imaging and histology before starting any specific anti-cancer treatment. Where pain is severe or there is a deterioration in organ function (e.g. superior vena cava obstruction or renal failure), then anti-cancer treatment may be started early. Specific anti-cancer therapies should be selected from recognised guidelines or trials. Where trials are open it is considered optimal to use them as they provide a mechanism for both clinical audit and research. Over 80% of children in the UK are treated within the framework of a national or international clinical trial.

Children with cancer should be treated in specialised units aimed at delivering coordinated care in a child-orientated environment. Within such a chronic illness team there are many specialist doctors, nurses and allied professionals who have a part to play. The oncologist has the role of chemotherapist and co-ordinating paediatrician during initial treatment and subsequent follow up.

The child and family need emotional support and understanding through the initial diagnosis, the delivery of treatment and recovery after treatment. The range of reactions is wide and on occasions the reaction may be extreme and require the help of psychologists or psychiatrists. It is very important that families have easy access to accurate information about the illness and its treatment and that their general practitioners, school teachers and other local carers are kept informed of developments. Visits home during therapy hold great importance and are essential to reassure child and family alike.

± LUMPS, ± MALAISE, ± BLEEDING

Problem

- A 4-year-old child presents with bilateral cervical lymphadenopathy and generalised malaise. There are no other specific symptoms and no abnormalities on examination.

Diagnosis — Suspected malignant lymphadenopathy

This is a common problem in paediatric clinics and one which causes great anxiety to parents and professionals alike. This concern is understandable as the range of causes is legion and includes potentially life-threatening illnesses. Agreement on the definition of enlarged lymph nodes is elusive but many would take nodes greater than 1 cm as abnormal. Important historical details should include the duration, extent and course of the lymph node enlargement, preceding infectious episodes, systemic symptoms (exanthema, fever, weight loss, night sweats and arthralgia), underlying illness (i.e. eczema) and travel abroad. Examination needs to determine the size and extent of the lymphadenopathy, seek local sources of inflammation and look for evidence of systemic illness. Where a precipitating cause, other than malignancy, is suspected investigations and treatment should be directed accordingly. In the absence of obvious signs of associated disease it is reasonable to prescribe a course of oral antibiotics prior to review. If the lymphadenopathy is unchanged after 4-8 weeks then further investigations, including biopsy, should be carried out.

Problem

Immunocytochemistry

CD 2	7%	T cell marker
CD 4	5%	T cell marker
CD 7	6%	T cell marker
CD 10	92%	Common marker
CD 13	0%	myeloid marker
CD 14	0%	myeloid marker
CD 19	92%	B cell marker
CD 33	0%	myeloid marker

- A 5-year-old girl has had generalised lymphadenopathy, pallor and recurrent infections for 3 weeks. Examination shows widespread petechiae and spontaneous bruising, hepato-splenomegaly. A full blood count reveals: Hb 3 g/dl , WCC $150 \times 10^9/l$ (neutrophils $0.5 \times 10^9/l$, lymph cells $3.9 \times 10^9/l$, blast cells $146.6 \times 10^9/l$), platelets $30 \times 10^9/l$.

Diagnosis — Common acute lymphoblastic leukaemia (common all)
The problem posed by this child is one of making a complete oncological diagnosis, anticipating complications at the time of presentation so that they can be treated early and planning optimal treatment for her leukaemia associated with best chances of long term survival and, hopefully, cure.

Symptoms and signs of acute leukaemia

Symptoms	Signs
Anorexia / lethargy	Pallor
History of fever / infections	Herpes infections, mucosal candidiasis, signs of systemic bacterial infection
Spontaneous / easy bleeding	Petechiae, eccymoses, epistaxis
Bone and joint pain	Bony tenderness
Skin rash, swollen gums, enlarged glands	Infiltrative skin rashes, gum hypertrophy, lymphadenopathy
Headaches, vomiting, double vision	Papilloedema, cranial nerve palsies
Disturbed appetite	Weight loss or gain
Difficulty in breathing	Superior vena cava obstruction

Acute leukaemia is characterised by a malignant, clonal, proliferation of white cell precursors (blast cells) which occupy and inhibit the function of the bone marrow. They may circulate in the blood and form leukaemic deposits in any tissue. There are two main types, lymphoid and myeloid. In acute lymphoblastic leukaemia (ALL) which accounts for 85% of childhood acute leukaemia, blast cells morphologically resemble primitive precursors of lymphoid cells which can be classified into three categories (L1, L2 and L3). Additionally, there are characteristic cytochemical and immunocytochemical reactions which permit further classification. The acute myeloid leukaemias (AML) account for the remaining 15% of childhood acute leukaemias. The malignant cells resemble myeloid precursors morphologically and can also be further classified with cytochemical and immunocytochemical 'markers'. The wide range of normal myeloid precursors is mirrored in the seven morphological classes of myeloid leukaemias (M1–M7).

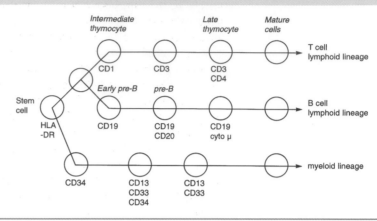

Cell surface markers showing lineage

The clinical diagnosis, in the majority of cases, is suspected from presenting symptoms and physical signs.

Making an oncological diagnosis requires the collection of the correct specimens. Typing the leukaemia requires an adequate number of blast cells. If the peripheral blood blast cell count is high, as in the example above, then a peripheral blood sample will suffice, but if not a bone marrow aspirate will be necessary. Diagnostic bone marrow samples can be difficult to obtain and so an experienced doctor should be responsible for its collection. Samples for cytogenetic studies should be processed urgently. When there are no symptoms or signs of raised intracranial pressure, a diagnostic CSF sample is collected to look for blasts cells in the CSF which if present indicate CNS involvement. If there are signs of raised intracranial pressure a CT scan of the brain should be performed to exclude an intracranial space occupying lesion.

Presenting complications. At the time of diagnosis a child with acute leukaemia is often very ill. This may be because of bone marrow failure, and anaemia, infection or bleeding. They may have a metabolic disturbance due to tumour lysis syndrome. Deposition of leukaemia cells in organs or body cavities can lead to disturbances of organ function like superior vena cava obstruction, pleural effusion, cardiac tamponade, pleural/ascitic effusions, renal, hepatic or splenic infiltration. They may have neurological disturbances secondary to either intracranial bleeding, tumour deposition or metabolic disturbances.

Management of ALL

The objectives of ALL therapy treatment are

— Remission induction.
— Intensification.
— CNS directed therapy.
— Continuing therapy.

Remission induction is the phase of therapy which results in the achievement of a resolution of clinical signs and symptoms as well as achievement of bone marrow remission, where less than 5% of nucleated cells in the bone marrow are blast cells.

Intensification therapy consists of combinations of chemotherapy agents directed at further reducing the leukaemic cell population, assuming that undetectable leukaemia cells remain in an initial 'remission' marrow sample. Such intensification treatments use different drug combinations to remission induction courses and subsequently lead to marked myelotoxicity.

CNS directed therapy is designed to eradicate leukaemia cells within the CNS which are partially protected from the actions of systemic drugs by the blood–brain barrier. Methods used include intrathecal chemotherapy, high doses of systemic drugs which penetrate the blood brain barrier (e.g. methotrexate) or cranial radiotherapy in selected cases.

Continuing therapy consists of low dose, continuous, oral chemotherapy in combination with monthly steroid courses and vincristine. Such treatment may be given for long periods. Current UK protocols for ALL take 2 years to complete.

ALL treatment indicators

Patient features	Therapeutic actions
Age < 1 year	Intensify systemic treatment Delay/omit radiotherapy
Age > 12 years	Greater risk of relapse: no change to treatment approach
Sex	Girls do better than boys: no change to treatment approach
White cell count > 50×10^9/L	Intensify systemic treatment
CSF involvement	Intensify CNS-directed therapy
Biological features	
T-cell type	Risk of recurrence linked to blast count: counts are often high
Mature B-cell leukaemia/ lymphoma	Intensify chemotherapy, modified regimens
Common ALL antigen	Standard risk
Pre B cell	Standard risk
nul cell (commonly, infant leukaemia)	Higher risk of relapse
Cytogenetics	
Hyperdiploid	Good prognosis — standard treatment
Diploid/pseudodiploid	Higher risk of relapse
t(8;14)(q24;q32) commonly mature B cell: t(4;11)(q21;q23) (congenital leukaemia) t(9;22) Philadelphia chromosome t(1:19)	Intensify treatment, consider bone marrow transplant in first remission
Slow remission induction (by day 28)	Higher risk of relapse. Modify treatment

Management of other leukaemias and lymphomas

In AML and B cell leukaemia/lymphoma different drugs are effective. They are used in higher doses, in more intensive combinations and over shorter periods (typically 6–8 months). The high dose, intensive drug combinations are associated with greater risk of life threatening toxicity. Bone marrow transplant may be considered in first remission if a related bone marrow donor is available. Selection of the optimal treatment approach is currently dictated by the availability of a range of randomised clinical trials run by the Medical Research Council. Exceptional cases may need an individualised approach. Such decisions can only be taken by those fully familiar with the most recent information.

Bone marrow transplantation (rescue) use in children is limited by the effectiveness of conventional treatment, its significant toxicities and the difficulties of finding a matched sibling donor. The use of unrelated donors remains experimental. The principle is to give myeloablative treatment with high dose chemotherapy and total body irradiation to eradicate the disease and the bone marrow, and then 'rescue' the patient with an HLA matched marrow from either a sibling (related, allograft) or an unrelated donor (matched unrelated donor — MUD). The consequences of related and unrelated donor transplants can be serious and include life-threatening infection, graft versus host disease (GvHD), prolonged immunodeficiency, graft failure, leukaemia relapse and growth and development problems due to damage by total body irradiation. Typical mortality rates from related donor transplantation would be 10%, whilst the risk is considerably greater for MUDs. Using marrow from the patient (autograft) has fallen from favour in the treatment of leukaemia. The use of peripheral blood stem cells as a source of marrow rescue is gaining popularity as a method to intensify chemotherapy doses in patients with solid tumours, e.g. neuroblastoma, disseminated rhabdomyosarcoma and brain tumours.

Prognosis

In the late 1960s only 1% of children with ALL survived for 5 years or more. Most died within 2 years and in half of these the first relapse was in the CNS. Now we can expect more than 70% of children to survive in first remission for 5 years. Eighty-five per cent of these will survive into adult life and could be considered cured. The long term sequelae are discussed later and may be a major problem.

Non-Hodgkin lymphomas are predominantly lymphoblastic in children and can therefore be classified similarly to ALL. Children with widespread lymphadenopathy and more than 25% of blast cells in the marrow are classed as having leukaemia rather than lymphoma. Treatment is with the same approaches recommended for the corresponding leukaemic cell type. T cell lymphomas present most commonly with mediastinal masses (see 'Thoracic mass' below). B cell lymphomas frequently present with massive and rapidly enlarging abdominal lymphadenopathy. Other types can present as enlarged lymph nodes with visceral, marrow or bone involvement.

CML/Myelodynplasia

Juvenile chronic myeloid leukaemia
Myelodysplasia (FAB classification)
Philadelphia chromosome negative CML
Philadelphia chromosome positive CML
Polycythaemia vera
Essential thromboocythaemia
Myelofibrosis

Chronic leukaemias and myelodysplasia can occur in childhood and their presenting signs and symptoms may mimick acute leukaemias. Diagnosis is dependent upon careful assessment of peripheral blood and bone marrow including chromosomal analysis. Treatment may be directed at controlling excessive cell production where this is causing problems. Bone marrow transplantation is commonly the only treatment offering a chance of cure.

BRAIN MASS

Brain tumours are the commonest group of solid tumours in childhood. Because the onset is slow and the symptoms vague, there is often a delay between symptom onset and the diagnosis. The diagnosis is usually made by CT/MR scan. Many of the treatment recommendations are under review, so best practice can only be achieved by those with a working knowledge of the latest literature. Once a brain or spinal tumour is diagnosed then the potential for neurological damage by the tumour should be assessed and appropriate action taken.

Severe symptoms of raised intracranial pressure may be eased temporarily by dexamethasone. Operations might relieve raised intracranial pressure by tumour resection or drainage of a hydrocephalus. Emergency spinal cord decompression may be necessary. Staging

---

Symptoms and signs intracranial tumours

Focal neurological signs:

Raised intracranial pressure	**Infratentorial tumours**	**Supratentorial tumours**
Headache (early morning)	Cerebellum / 4th ventricle	Cortical
Vomiting	Ataxia	Seizures
Mood changes	Nystagmus	Spasticity
Depressed or fluctuating	Diplopia	Focal fits
consciousness level	Brainstem	Deterioration in memory/concentration
Papilloedema	Facial weakness	Disturbed behaviour
VI nerve palsy	Dysphagia	
Reduced visual acuity	Ocular palsies	Mid-line
Head tilt	Spasticity	Disturbed growth — short stature or
	Altered consciousness level	excessive growth
		Disturbed development — precocious
		or delayed puberty
		Disturbed eating and drinking —
		altered appetite and thirst
		Disturbed behaviour — school
		performance, patterns of temper, day
		Night patterns, hyperactivity —
		unresponsive to behaviour
		modification
		Disturbed vision — visual field loss,
		dysconjugate eye movements

Distribution of tumour type by site

Cerebellum / 4th ventricle	Cortical	Spinal
Astrocytic tumour — low grade	Astrocytic tumours — high grade	Intrinsic
MB/PNET	Astrocytic tumours — low grade	Astrocytic tumours — low grade
Ependymal tumours	MB/PNET	Ependymal tumour
Astrocytic tumour — high grade	Lymphoma	Extrinsic
	Meningeal tumours	Neuroblastoma
Brainstem		Ewing's tumour
Astrocytic tumour — high grade	**Midline supratentorial**	Lymphoma
Astrocytic tumour — low grade	Astrocytic tumours — low grade	
MB/PNET	Astrocytic tumour — high grade	
Ependymal tumour	Craniopharyngioma	
	Choroid plexus tumours	
	Germinoma (non-secreting AFP/HCG)	
	Non-germinomatous germ cell tumour	
	(secreting AFP/HCG)	
	Pinealoma/pineocytoma	

involves identifying the anatomical site, the dimensions of the tumour and the presence or absence of neuro-axial metastasis. Where possible neuroaxial imaging with MR should be performed prior to resection of the tumour to reduce false positive scans due to postoperative imaging artefacts. CSF may be looked at for circulating malignant cells but should be collected at the time of operation and not by lumbar puncture.

Problem

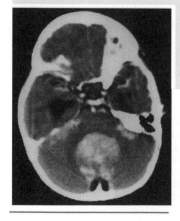

- An 8-year-old boy presents with a 3-month history of intermittent headaches, 1 month history of disturbed vision, intermittent squint and increasing unsteadiness. He started vomiting in the early morning. On examination he has cerebellar ataxia, a 6th nerve palsy, bilateral papilloedema, brisk knee reflexes, absent ankle reflexes.

Diagnosis — Cerebellar tumour with hydrocephalus and spinal secondary

Primary surgical resection is attempted after relief of hydrocephalus. Postoperative anti-cancer treatment depends on the histology of the tumour. Low grade astrocytomas need no further treatment if they are completely resected (80–90% survival), whilst MB/PNETs require cranio-spinal radiotherapy, chemotherapy is also given in the majority of centres (60–70% survival). The need for adjuvant treatment with chemotherapy or radiotherapy in ependymal tumours (ependymoma) is not so clear cut (50% survival).

Problem

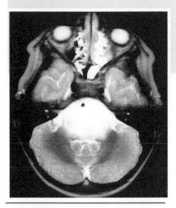

- A 6-year-old girl presents with a 3-month history of an intermittent squint and more recent development of choking, fluctuating sleepiness, episodic vomiting and weakness of the legs. On examination she has bilateral bulbar palsies, internuclear ophthalmoplegia and weakness of her lower limbs with brisk reflexes and up-going plantars.

Diagnosis — Diffuse pontine tumour (glioma)

Surgical resection is almost always incomplete and can be extremely hazardous. There are some situations where resection can be attempted with success. No drugs are known to work. Radiation therapy is used to palliate symptoms. All the children die.

Problem

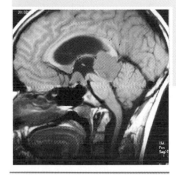

- A 14-year-old boy presents with a 4-month history of blurred vision, intermittent headaches and deteriorating school performance. On examination, he has dysconjugate eye movements with loss of upward gaze, bilateral papilloedma, he is withdrawn, his height is on the 3rd percentile, he has stage 2 penis and pubic hair and testicular volume of 8 ml. On investigation his AFP is 30 000 μ/l.

Diagnosis — Pineal germinoma

Germinomas commonly develop in puberty and early adulthood within the pineal gland and adjacent hypothalamus. Large tumours may press upon adjacent structures leading to neurological and endocrinological disorder. Germinomas do not secrete AFP or beta HCG, whilst non-germinomatous tumours do. Their location often precludes complete resection. In contrast to many other brain tumours they are highly sensitive to both chemotherapy and radiotherapy. Long term survival is best with germinomas (80–90% survival) which may be achieved with radiotherapy alone. Chemotherapy and radiotherapy is given for non-germinomatous germ cell tumours, the survival rates are poorer.

Problem

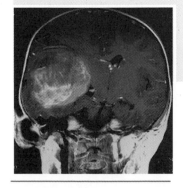

- A 5-year-old girl presents with a 2-week history of frequent focal fits affecting her left arm and face, associated intermittent headache, vomiting and a tendency to walk into furniture. She is confused after the fits, anti-convulsants have not been effective in controlling them. On examination she is weak in all movements of her left arm, she has a right temporal hemianopia and bilateral papilloedma.

Diagnosis — Parietal lobe astrocytomic tumour : high grade (glioblastoma multiforme)

Presentation varies with the lobe involved. Focal fits are a common presentation, as well as loss of motor function and deteriorating school performance. Completeness of surgical resection is limited because of the risk of damaging the surrounding brain. Adjuvant therapy is dictated by the histology of the tumour. Low grade tumours are less likely to recur and if resection is complete, close monitoring of the tumour is all that is required. High grade tumours have a greater tendency to recur locally and spread throughout the neuro-axis. Radiotherapy is used routinely. The place of chemotherapy and the whole brain radiation are under investigation.

Problem

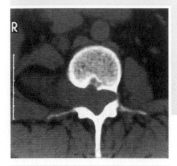

- A 6-month-old baby presents with persistent crying and loss of movement of her lower limbs. On examination she was distressed, had a flaccid paraparesis, patulous anus, absent knee and ankle relexes and equivocal plantar responses. A mass was palpable in her right upper abdomen, urinary catecholamines were elevated, an abdominal ultrasound showed a suprarenal mass growing into the intervertebral foramen, a spinal MRI showed spinal cord compression by a 'dumbell' tumour.

Diagnosis — Spinal cord compression secondary to neuroblastoma

Extrinsic spinal tumours are unusual. In infants and younger children neuroblastoma is more common, in older children, lymphoma and Ewing's tumour predominate. Intrinsic tumours of the spinal cord are most commonly astrocytic or ependymal in origin. Treatment is primarily by surgical resection, adjuvant therapy being used if they are incompletely resected or recurrent.

Problem

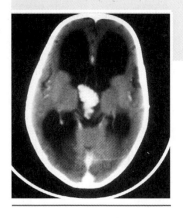

- A 2-month-old baby presented with poor feeding, a bulging fonatanelle rapid head growth and visual inattention. Cranial ultrasound demonstrated a large mass within the left lateral ventricle and associated hydrocephalus of the 3rd and right lateral ventricle.

Diagnosis — Choroid plexus papilloma/carcinoma

Clinical management is dictated by the clinical condition of the child at diagnosis, the resectability of the tumour and the extreme sensitivity of the young child's brain to damaging side effects of radiotherapy. For tumours where local recurrence or dissemination is predicted, adjuvant chemotherapy is recommended for prolonged periods. Radiation is reserved until recurrence occurs or the child has achieved their 3rd birth-day, by which time the majority of brain growth involving cell division has occurred.

ABDOMINAL MASS

Problem	• A 10-year-old boy presents with a 2 week history of poor appetite, constipation, pallor and sudden onset of abdominal distension. On examination he is lethargic, has wasted limbs but a distended abdomen. There is a central abdominal mass, hepatosplenomegaly and free fluid detectable clinically. He has widespread lymphadenopathy, a mid-systolic murmur, pulse of 110/min, BP 120/95.

Diagnosis — Abdominal B cell lymphoma / leukaemia

Investigations are needed to exclude obstruction of the renal tract or renal infiltration. Careful monitoring of renal function are important. Blood pressure may be raised and require controlling prior to surgery. Haematological investigations should be directed at identifying

Abdominal tumours

Organ of origin	Tumour diagnoses		
Renal tumours	Wilms tumour — favourable histology (triphasic tumours, epithelial-rich tumours) Wilms tumour — unfavourable histology (anaplasia, rhabdoid, clear cell sarcoma) Mesoblastic nephroma Intrarenal neuroblastoma Renal cell carcinoma Benign renal tumours		
Abdominal lymphadenopathy	Non-Hodgkin lymphoma Hodgkin disease Neuroblastoma Benign lymphadenopathy (LCH, sarcoidosis, viral infections, Castleman disease)		
Adrenal mass	Neuroblastoma Adrenal adenoma Adrenocortical carcinoma Phaeochromocytoma As part of multiple endocrine neoplasia syndrome		
Pelvic mass	Soft tissue sarcoma (STS) of urogenital tract Germ cell tumour (ovary, sacroccygeal teratoma) Neuroblastoma		
Hepatic masses	**Malignant tumours** Hepatoblastoma Hepatocellular carcinoma Fibrolamellar carcinoma	**Infiltration** Leukaemia/lymphoma Myelodysplasia / myeloproliferative disorders Metastatic neuroblastoma, nephroblastoma, rhabdomyosarcoma	**Benign tumours** Haemangioma Haemangioendothelioma Mesenchymal hamartomas
Splenic masses	Leukaemic/lymphomatous infiltration Myelodysplasia/myeloprolferative disorders Haemangioma		
Rare tumours	Gastrointestinal carcinomas Ca female genital tract Neuroepithelioma Mesothelioma Pancreatic tumours		

leukaemia, coagulopathies due to disseminated intravascular coagulation (DIC) or thrombocytopenia in preparation for any invasive procedures. Tumours in the upper abdomen may obstruct biliary or portal drainage or may grow through the diaphragm into the chest. Retroperitoneal tumours may cause upper intestinal obstruction, they may grow into the spinal canal and cause cord compression or may extend laterally on both sides and present as bilateral abdominal masses. Renal tumours can grow intravascularly up the vena cava and into the right heart where there may be associated vena caval obstruction or cardiac arrhythmias. Tumours arising in the pelvis may obstruct the viscera or compress vessels or nerves traversing the pelvis. Once the tumour's tissue of origin is established then investigations for tumour markers or metastases should be planned.

Problem

• The parents of a 3-year-old boy felt a lump in his abdomen during a bath. On examination he has a left loin mass, microscopic haematuria and a blood pressure of 110/70.

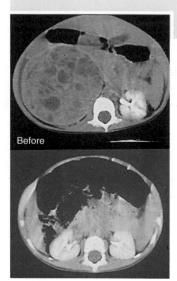

Before

After radiotherapy

Diagnosis — Wilms tumour

Tumour staging can only be completed at the time of surgery. The timing of attempted resection is controversial. Some groups favour initial surgery whilst others prefer pre-surgical chemotherapy to induce tumour shrinkage.

Subsequent treatment is based upon staging the resected specimen and sampling regional lymph nodes. The more extensive the tumour, the longer the course of chemotherapy. Stage 3 and 4 patients also receive postoperative radiotherapy to tumour bearing tissues; the renal bed and lungs. Bilateral tumours require careful assessment and therapy should aim to conserve as much renal tissue as possible.

Wilms tumour

Histological type	Sites of metastases	Biological/Tumour markers
Favourable histology	May be bilateral	Ploidy — Tumour tissue
Unfavourable histology (focal anaplasia, clear cell variant, rhabdoid)	Lung, liver	
	Bone (clear cell variant) Brain (rhabdoid variant)	del 11p13/del 11p15
Mesoblastic nephroma	Metastasises rarely	
Renal cell carcinoma	Bone	Erythropoietin

Wilms tumour staging

Stage 1: Tumour limited to kidney and completely excised
Outcome: Favourable histology >95% overall survival
Unfavourable histology 90% overall survival

Stage 2: Tumour extends beyond the kidney but is completely removed, involvement of blood vessels outside the kidney, tumours that have been biopsied
Outcome: Favourable histology 90% overall survival
Unfavourable histology 67% overall survival

Stage 3: Residual tumour confined to abdomen. This includes lymph node involvement, peritoneal involvement or spillage and incompletely resected tumours due to invasion of adjacent structure
Outcome: Favourable histology 83% overall survival
Unfavourable histology 60% overall survival

Stage 4: Haematogenous metastases, e.g. lung, liver, bone and brain
Outcome: Favourable histology 64% overall survival
Unfavourable histology 0% overall survival

Stage 5: Bilateral renal involvement at diagnosis
Outcome: Favourable histology 80% overall survival
Unfavourable histology 50% overall survival

Note: Survival figures are 6-year survival rates from UK studies.

Problem

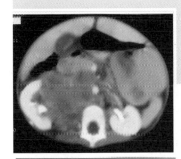

- An 18-month-old boy presented with a 3-week history of increasing misery, pallor and easy bruising. On examination there was a right sided abdominal mass, hepato-splenomegaly and boney tenderness. There was widespread bruising over extensor surfaces and periorbital swelling, associated bruising. Investigations identified pancytopenia, a consumptive coagulopathy and raised urinary catecholamines.

Diagnosis — Sympathetic nervous system tumours

Clinical presentation is linked to the site of the primary tumour and the extent of tumour metastasis. Seventy-five per cent of the tumours are metastatic at the time of presentation. The children are frequently very miserable, failing to thrive and may have extensive bruising, mimicking the appearance of a physically abused child. Hypertension is commonly a complication at presentation.

Neuroblastoma

Paraneoplastic syndromes
Chronic watery diarrhoea (VIP secretion)
Opsiclonus (dancing eyes syndrome)
Hypertension, flushes, sweating, tachycardia

Primary tumour sites
Sympathetic chain (posterior mediastinum, paraspinal, pelvic brim)
Adrenal gland
Nasal (esthesio-neuroblastoma)
Intracranial

Histological grading
Ranges from benign ganglioneuroma to highly malignant neuroblastoma
Shimada histological grading system predicts metastatic potential

Diagnosis is dependent upon the presence of a typical mass, elevation of catecholamines in the urine and the identification of tumour cells in the marrow or biopsy of a tumour mass if no cells are seen. Presentation in the first 6 months of life is remarkable for its rapid progression and potential for spontaneous resolution.

Sympathetic nervous system tumours metastases and biological markers

Histological type	Sites of metastases	Biological/tumour markers
Sympathetic nervous system tumours (neuroblastoma ganglioneuro-blastoma)	Bone marrow Liver Brain Bones and Skull Periorbital tissues Direct infiltration of other organs Cortical bone, skin and liver may be involved in infancy with stage 4s presentation	Tumour tissue Chromosome 1p del n-*myc* oncogene amplification Serum Elevated ferritin, elevated neuron, specific enolase Urine VMA and HMMA
Ganglioneuroma (benign variant)	Does not metastasise	

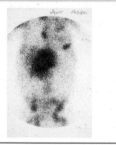

mIBG Scan

Treatment is dictated by the stage at presentation. Localised tumours are resected and adjuvant chemotherapy and radiotherapy given to eradicate residual disease. Infants with stage 4s disease are treated conservatively, with chemotherapy only being given if tumour progression is relentless or potentially life-threatening. In the over 1-year age group, disseminated disease requires high dose multiagent chemotherapy but is still associated with a poor prognosis (20–30% survival). Novel treatment approaches are being explored, including targeted radiotherapy using mono-iodo-benzyl-guanidine (mIBG), a breakdown product of nor-adrenaline, which is taken up by neuroblasts. Recent work has identified biological markers which predict resistance of the tumour to treatment. These include amplification of the n-*myc* oncogene, deletion of chromosome 1p, elevated serum NSE and elevated ferritin.

Problem

- A 10-month-old boy with Wiedmann–Beckwith syndrome presents with feeding difficulties and a progressively enlarging abdomen. On examination the baby had a tight abdominal wall, wasted limbs and was miserable. There was an upper abdominal mass. On investigation Hb 10 g/dl, WCC 6×10^9/l and platelets 1245×10^9/l. AFP 10 000 iu/l.

Diagnosis — Hepatoblastoma

Hepatoblastoma is an embryonic tumour affecting children less than 3 years of age and is associated with hemihypertrophy and family cancer syndromes. On the other hand, hepatocellular carcinoma occurs later in childhood and is associated with pre-existing cirrhosis brought about by infection (hepatitis B), longstanding biliary obstruction, alpha$_1$ anti-trypsin deficiency or some inborn errors of metabolism, e.g. hereditary tyrosinaemia. In both these tumour types a combination of primary chemotherapy and surgical resection has resulted in improved success rates. Liver transplantation should be considered in tumours unsuitable for resection.

Hepatic tumours

Histological type	Sites of metastases	Biological/Tumour markers
Liver tumours — malignant		
Hepatoblastoma	May be multicentric within the liver	Serum alpha-fetoprotein
Hepatocellular carcinoma	Lung	Serum/urine beta human chorionic gonadotrophin
Fibrolamellar carcinoma		Urinary cystathionine

Adrenal adenomas and carcinomas can present with a combination of a cancer predisposition syndrome such as hemihypertrophy, Wiedmann–Beckwith syndrome or precocious puberty. Treatment of the tumour requires control of steroid release, shrinkage with chemotherapy and subsequent surgical resection. Despite such therapy 5-year survival rates nationally remain at 25%.

Gastrointestinal carcinomas may complicate immunodeficiencies and be associated with familial adenomatous polyposis syndrome. Treatment with primary surgical resection and chemotherapy is used, although success rates are poor.

Pleural and abdominal mesotheliomas do occur in childhood, although the histology is different from that seen in adulthood. The outlook is very poor as they are difficult to resect and do not respond in a sustained fashion to chemotherapy or radiotherapy.

Pancreatic tumours often present a diagnostic challenge as symptoms may be related to the release of a variety of intestinal peptides. Treatment with chemotherapy may shrink the tumour and facilitate subsequent tumour resection.

Rare tumour types

Histological type	Sites of metastases	Biological/Tumour markers
Adrenal carcinoma	Lungs	17 ketosteroids
Carcinomas of stomach, large bowel, rectum and female genital tract	Liver, lungs and bones	
Mesothelioma	Local mesothelial spread	
Pancreatic tumours	Liver, lungs and bones	Serum insulin, glucagon, somatomedins, ACTH, gastrin, vasoactive peptide (VIP)

THORACIC MASS

Thoracic masses

Anterior mediastinum	Posterior mediastinum	Lung parenchyma	Chest wall and pleura
T-cell NHL	Neuroblastoma	Adenocarcinoma	Soft tissue sarcoma
Hodgkin disease	Ganglioneuroma	Pulmonary blastoma	Neuroepithelioma/Askin's tumour
Soft tissue sarcoma	Phaeochromocytoma		
Germ cell tumour			Mesothelioma

Problem

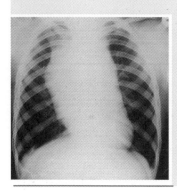

- An 11-year-old girl presented with a 4-week history of cough and progressive dyspnoea. She had been treated for a 'chest infection' with antibiotics. On examination she had a tachycardia and soft heart sounds. There were palpable, painless lymph nodes in the cervical chain, groin, axillae with a maximum size of 2 × 3 cm. Her trachea was deviated to the right, the left side of her chest had reduced expansion, was dull to percussion and there was reduced air entry in both lower zones. (on chest X-ray shown). Pleural fluid was obtained and histological review described a cell population of small round blue cells which demonstrated the following surface markers on immunochemical analysis: CD3 = 98%; CD4 = 97%; CD10 = 3%; CD19 = 2%.

Diagnosis — T-cell non-Hodgkin lymphoma

The child with a thoracic mass needs careful assessment. The anatomical position of the mass is critical to both the tumour type but also the optimal method of investigation.

Obtaining tissue may need thoracotomy, although other sources of pathological material should be sought. Lymph nodes, pleural fluid, peripheral blood or bone marrow and serum tumour markers may all contribute to the diagnosis. Tracheal and vascular compression can make anaesthesia hazardous. In typical anterior mediastinal lymphoma impirical chemotherapy may be justified without a biopsy.

Problem

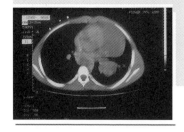

- A 12-year-old boy presented with a recent history of recurrent candidal and viral infections, weight loss, lethargy and extensive lymphadenopathy. On examination he had numerous herpetic lesions on his lips, massive cervical lymphadenopathy. A chest X-ray showed a mediastinal mass, a blood count showed a marked eosinophilia.

Diagnosis — Hodgkin disease

Clinical presentation of Hodgkin disease is generally insidious with marked lymphadenopathy, typical 'B' symptoms and sometimes a history of recurrent infection typical of cell mediated immunodeficiency. The disease typically spreads from one of a group of lymph nodes to contiguous groups. Treatment is highly effective. Localised disease in a single group of lymph nodes is treated by local radiotherapy whilst more extensive disease justifies the use of multi-agent chemotherapy. Cure rates exceed 95% at 5 years. Relapses can occur but are frequently amenable to subsequent therapy with similar treatments.

Hodgkin disease

Histological type	Sites of metastases	Biological/tumour markers
Lymphocyte predominant	Lymph nodes Bone marrow Direct infiltration of other organs	Elevated ESR Eosinophilia Associated cell-mediated immunodeficiency

Chest wall tumours. Tumours may also arise from the structures of the chest wall although these are very rare. Soft tissue sarcomas, bone tumours and a peripheral neuro-ectodermal tumour (Askin's tumour) should all be considered.

Tumours of lung parenchyma. Most parenchymal tumours are secondary deposits. Primary tumours of the lung parenchyma are rare, pulmonary blastoma and adenocarcinoma have been reported.

BONE TUMOURS

Problem

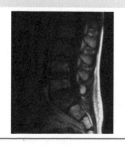

• A 9-year-old boy presented with a 5-month history of worsening low back pain. A diagnosis of structural backache had previously been made. Examination revealed limited flexion of the lumbar spine and tenderness over L2 vertebra. CT scan demonstrated an abnormal bone texture of the body of L2, plus an associated soft tissue mass, whilst a bone scan revealed uptake of radioisotope in L2 and multiple hot spots in the rest of the skeleton. ESR was 15 mm/h but a full blood count and film was normal.

Diagnosis — Ewing sarcoma

Clinical features of bone tumours

	Osteosarcoma	Ewing's tumour
Age (years) at greatest risk Sex ratio boys : girls	Girls:10–14; Boys: 15–18 1.5–2 : 1	Boys and girls: 10–15 1.5 : 1
Anatomical distribution	Femur — 53% Tibia — 26% Humerus — 11% Fibula — 4% Scapula — 2% Pelvis, vertebrae, scapula, ribs, skull, radius, ulna, digits — 1% or less	Pelvis — 28% Scapula — 17% Femur — 13% Tibia — 12% Fibula — 11% Ribs — 9% Humerus — 6% Vertebrae — 6% Digits, radius, ulna, sternum, clavicle, mandible — 3% or less
Special presentations	Previous radiotherapy field Previous retinoblastoma Part of family cancer syndrome (Li Fraumeni) Osteogenesis imperfecta Maffuci syndrome (endochondroma, haemangioma and skin pigmentation)	Chest wall soft tissue tumours may be extra-osseous (neuroepithelioma/Askin's tumour)
Radiological appearances	Metaphyseal May be lytic or with new bone formation Lifts or breaches periosteum Sunburst appearance	Diaphyseal Destructive lesion 'Onion skin' periosteal lamellation Extension to soft tissues
Sites of metastases	10–15% are metastatic at presentation Chest Bones Skin Brain	20% are metastatic at presentation Chest Bone Lungs Lymph nodes
Biological factors	Mutation of p53 gene (loss of heterozygosity for 13q14 (Retinoblastoma gene) and 17p13.	Elevated serum LDH t(11;22)

Problem

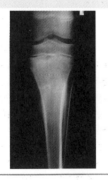

- A 14-year-old boy with no significant history of trauma presents with a month's history of persistent knee pain, which is worse at night. Swelling and limitation of movement of the knee had developed in the past week. X-rays reveal a lytic lesion with surrounding sclerosis of the metaphasis of the femur. A bone scan shows increased uptake in the knee but none elsewhere in the skeleton.

Diagnosis — Osteosarcoma

Bone tumours commonly present with pain or swelling and so mimic more common conditions such as structural backache, osteomyelitis or arthritis. Significant features in the history include pain being worse at night, a previous tumour (e.g. retinoblastoma), or previous radiation or a cancer-family history. Delays in diagnosis are common, insidious onset of bone pain in the absence of physical findings may even lead to psychiatric referral when initial physical treatments fail to produce an improvement. Careful review of repeated imaging should lead to the diagnosis of malignancy.

Modern surgical techniques aim to avoid amputation of limbs by the use of extendable prostheses. In such cases subsequent limb function is heavily dependent upon effective physical rehabilitation in both the short and long term. Some tumours in the axial skeleton often reach a large size or have metastasised by the time of diagnosis, leading to a poorer prognosis. Although chest metastases can occur after completion of treatment, a proportion of patients may be cured by surgical resection of these.

Rarely, bone tumours with other histologies may be identified. Bone lymphoma may present with an isolated lesion without evidence of leukaemia.

Langerhans cell histiocytosis

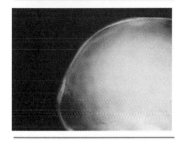

Langerhans cell histiocytosis (LCH) may also mimic the symptomatology and radiology of malignant bone tumours. This is an important differential diagnosis as treatment should be the least possible to eradicate the symptoms and not follow the intensive approaches adopted in malignant tumours. Careful staging of the patient to identify disease in organs, bone and soft tissues assists with the selection of the optimal treatment. Isolated bone disease may respond to curettage biopsy, whilst more extensive involvement may respond to intralesional or systemic steroids. Multisystem involvement may require systemic chemotherapy in rare cases. When presenting in infancy, the illness can be life threatening due to organ failures. The disease may run a remitting and relapsing course with the severity of symptoms reducing over time and often burning itself out in adolescence.

SARCOMA

Problem

- A 4-year-old boy presented with a week's history of periorbital swelling, displacement of the globe laterally and the appearance of pink tissue at the medial canthus of his right eye.

Rhabdomyosarcoma in the orbit

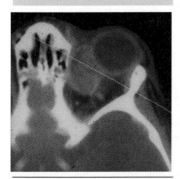

Diagnosis — Soft tissue sarcoma
Rhabdomyosarcoma accounts for the majority of soft tissue sarcomas (STS) in childhood. They can arise anywhere within connective tissue even in structures lacking striated muscle. In childhood (<10 years) they most commonly occur in the head and neck region or in association with the genitourinary tract. In adolescence they more commonly arise in the trunk or limbs. Certain sites are associated with a low risk of metastatic spread (e.g. orbit, bladder and prostate), whilst other sites have a high risk (e.g. parameningeal sites, paratesticular and retroperitoneal tumours). Local extension of primary tumours is common and requires careful evaluation when planning local therapy. Histological grading of tumours identifies two main variants — embryonal and alveolar — with the former providing a more

favourable prognosis. Treatment is with a combination of chemo-therapy, surgery and radiotherapy. Gaining local control of the primary tumour is the main focus of therapy as metastatic tumours are rarely curable. Prognosis is linked to the site of the primary and its amenability to surgical removal or adequate irradiation. Metastatic, parameningeal and CNS tumours have very poor prognoses.

TREATMENT PROBLEMS

Children with malignant disease present many specific problems during treatment and effective management involves anticipating these difficulties.

Anaemia is a common complication of chemotherapy. Spontaneous correction does take place with time although symptomatic anaemia during chemotherapy is best treated with blood transfusion. This is important if anaesthesia is planned or there are signs of spontaneous bleeding. Neutropenia (neutrophils count $1.0 \times 10^9/l$) places the child at increased risk of overwhelming bacterial infection. If there is fever, blood cultures should be taken and broad spectrum antibiotics commenced to cover gram-positive and gram-negative organisms including *Pseudomonas aeruginosa*. Viral infections are not usually life threatening at presentation unless there has been a prolonged prodrome or there is a low lymphocyte count ($< 1 \times 10^9/l$) or im-munoglobulin level. Bleeding due to thrombocytopenia or dissemi-nated intravascular coagulation (DIC) is common as a presenting feature and should be actively sought. Covert sites for bleeding include the retinae, brain, renal tract and gastro-intestinal tract. If the platelet count is low ($< 20 \times 10^9/l$) and there is spontaneous bleed-ing or a planned invasive procedure, then platelets should be given to raise the count above $50 \times 10^9/l$, and time to consider the invasive procedure.

Coagulopathy. When DIC complicates the presentation of a malig-nancy, it may be mild or severe. Treatment of mild forms is dependent upon giving platelets and clotting concentrates, whilst severe cases may tax even the most experienced haematologist and laboratory. Treating any infection and the cancer vigorously whilst providing maximum clotting factor and platelet support as well as applying effective local treatment to sites of bleeding is necessary in such situa-tions. Acute promyelocytic leukaemia is notorious for severe DIC at presentation. This type of leukaemia is now known to be sensitive to treatment with trans retinoic acid which promotes cellular differen-tiation of the blast cell without concomitant tumour lysis and severe DIC.

Problem

Blood levels

Na	129 mmol/L
K+	6.3 mmol/L
HCO3	27 mmol/L
Urea	9 mmol/L
Creatinine	175 umol/L
Ca^{2+}	1.9 mmol/L
PO_4	–6 mmol/L
Mg^{2+}	0.9 mmol/L
Albumen	30 g/L

Pathways from the DNA purines to uric acid

adenosine		guanosine
⇩		⇩
inosine		guanine
⇩		⇩
hypoxanthine	⇨	xanthine
		⇩
		uric acid

• A 7-year-old girl with high count ALL has been started on treatment with vincristine and prednisolone. She received 3 litres/24 hours of 4% dextrose and 0.18% saline, along with allopurinol. She weighs 30 kg. She developed a positive fluid balance of 2 litres and oedema 12 hours after starting chemotherapy. Her renal function tests are in the margin!

Diagnosis — Metabolic disturbances (tumour lysis syndrome)

High count T cell ALL and B cell lymphoblastic lymphoma more commonly present with metabolic disturbances either before or during remission induction therapy. Occasionally patients with low count common ALL, CML and hepatoblastoma may develop the syndrome. The syndrome is thought to result from rapid breakdown of tumour cells leading to a urate nephropathy. This complication further compounds the difficulties of excreting intracellular electrolytes (K and PO_4) released by the dying cells. The principles of treatment are:

— Anticipate the problem, consult the nephrologist.
— Prepare the patient prior to commencing treatment.
— Minimise the rate of initial cell kill and block uric acid production.
— Increase the solubility of urates in the urine by alkalinisation of urine, and maximise the output of urine by forced diuresis.
— Intensively monitor renal function, electrolytes and fluid balance.
— Treat rising [K+] urgently with calcium resonium, glucose and insulin and salbutamol.

All newly diagnosed patients with ALL and B cell lymphoma as well as patients with AML with evidence of renal impairment at diagnosis, should be treated to minimise the effects of tumour lysis. If there is evidence of the syndrome being established before commencing antileukaemia treatment, preparation for dialysis should be discussed with nephrologists prior to commencement of leukaemia therapy. Hyperkalaemia and hyperphosphataemia can develop rapidly and be indications for dialysis, even in the absence of levels of creatinine suggesting renal failure. Monitoring fluid balance is particularly important with the forced alkaline diuresis. This aspect of treatment is aimed at maximising urine output and maintaining a urine pH > 8.0. The bicarbonate required for successful alkalinisation may require significant amounts of sodium to be given which may aggravate the development of a significant positive fluid balance. If this occurs, the first step should be to reduce fluid input to a level where the patient is capable of excreting the water load. The use of osmotic or loop diuretics to encourage urine output in patients with impaired renal function should be used cautiously as they may cause further renal damage. The process of cell lysis is often active at presentation but is rapidly accelerated by initiation of treatment. It is important to remember that the cells in the above leukaemias and lymphomas are often very sensitive to steroids and consequently the ill-thought use of such agents — often as part of the treatment of urticarial reactions to blood products

— may precipitate an unexpected biochemical emergency for the child.

Cancer pain. Children with malignant disease often have pain either at presentation or during their treatment. Understanding the cause of pain can assist with planning optimum treatment approaches. Successful management of symptoms requires a combination of careful ongoing assessment of pain severity, a supportive multi-disciplinary clinical team, flexibility of prescribing practices devolved to those responsible for control of symptoms and a commitment to individualise approaches.

Causes of cancer pain and treatment strategies

Nerve compression/transection (phantom limb pain)	Regional local anaesthetic block/nerve transection, transcutaneous electrical nerve stimulation (TENS), carbamazepine, non-opioid/opioid analgesia
Raised intracranial pressure	Operative relief of raised intracranial pressure, dexamethasone, non-opioid/opioid analgesia
Inflammation	Non-steroidal anti-flammatories, non-opioid/opioid analgesia
Bone pain	Non-steroidal anti-inflammatories, palliative chemotherapy/radiotherapy, non-opioid/opioid analgesia
Visceral pain	Non-opioid / opioid analgesia, palliative chemotherapy/radiotherapy
Injections/procedures/treatments or activities	Assessment of benefits, explanation and distraction techniques, planned local analgesia/topical/general anaesthesia
Anxiety, depression, coping difficulties	Explanation and emotional support, antidepressants, anxiolytics, massage, relaxation techniques, deversionary activities, hypnosis
Unknown causes	Child and family assessment, trial of non-opioid/opioid analgesia, trial of steroids

Central venous lines. The use of permanent central venous catheters has revolutionised the treatment and support of children with malignant disease and, in some cases, allowed the intensification of treatment which would have previously been impossible. Almost all children now have one of these inserted. The choice of an external (Hickman, Broviac) or internal (Ports) line must be tailored to individual requirements, giving the child choice where possible. These catheters are associated with a range of problems which can cause significant difficulties with treatment. About 25% are taken out early, the commonest reason being that they become dislodged. In addition, they can become infected, blocked, fractured or punctured. Close attention to their ongoing care is essential, with clear guidelines and policies being maintained by all staff using them.

'Cure'. Overall 5-year survival rates for childhood cancer stand at about 65%. This represents cure in the majority although the definition of cure for children with these diseases has not been formally defined. Such figures give no indication of the burden of morbidity borne by the survivors as a result of their cancer or its treatment.

Survival figures

Five year survival against year of diagnosis

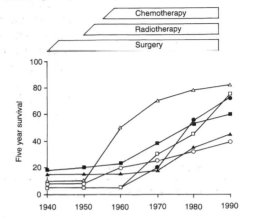

- ● ALL
- □ Non-Hodgkins lymphoma
- △ Wilms tumour
- ■ Rhabdomyosarcoma
- ▲ CNS tumours
- ○ Neuroblastoma

LATE EFFECTS

Problem

- A 3-year-old girl was treated for a medulloblastoma with surgical resection, chemotherapy and cranio-spinal radiotherapy. At the age of 8, she presents with early signs of puberty, pubic hair development, breast development and monthly lower abdominal pain. Her height and weight lie on the 50 centile for her age, her bone age is 11.3 years. Investigations reveal a normal T4 with a raised TSH, poor response to GH stimulation and pelvic ultrasound demonstrates large ovaries with many follicles.

Diagnosis — Growth disorder following radiotherapy

Prior craniospinal radiotherapy is now one of the commonest reasons for initiating growth hormone therapy in childhood. Irradiation of the pineal gland and the hypothalamus leads to damage of GHRF secreting cells. GH deficiency leads to reduced growth velocity and delayed bone age develops. Assessing such children requires great care as the combination of precocious puberty in girls and early thyroid failure secondary to scatter doses of radiation, may co-exist. Irradiation of testes or ovaries will prevent puberty developing and lead to infertility.

Problem

- A 12-year-old boy was treated for acute leukaemia at the age of 4 years and retreated for an isolated CNS relapse at the age of 7 years. As a result of this he received an initial course of cranial radiotherapy during his first treatment and a subsequent course of cranio-spinal radiotherapy to treat the CNS relapse. He presents to the school doctor with a history of disruptive behaviour. He is in the remedial class and seems to have difficulty in following instructions. He has a reading age of 6 years and performs poorly at mathematics.

Diagnosis — Radiation induced intellectual damage

The difficulty here is deciding whether the disturbed behaviour is learnt during the extensive prior treatments or is organic, secondary to the combined effects of two courses of radiation. Cranial irradiation at an early age is recognised to lead to deterioration in intellectual performance particularly affecting short term memory, mental arithmetic and the ability to concentrate. Early psychometric assessment permits the identification of those predisposed to these learning difficulties and can be used to advise teachers on optimal learning strategies.

Problem

- A 19-year-old woman develops signs of congestive cardiac failure during the second trimester of pregnancy. She has a previous medical history of treatment for rhabdomyosarcoma early in childhood for which she received a cumulative dose of 300 mg/m^2 of doxorubicin. Echocardiography demonstrates a reduced left ventricular ejection fraction of 15%.

Diagnosis — Anthracycline congestive cardiomyopathy

Anthracylines, high dose cyclophosphamide and cardiac irradiation can all predispose to congestive cardiomyopathy. There are also early disturbing reports of early coronary artery disease in young adulthood.

Problem

- A 10-year-old girl presents with extreme lethargy, muscle weakness, dehydration and bone pains. She was previously treated for facial rhabdomyosarcoma with ifosfamide, actinomycin and vincristine. During treatment she was noted to require extensive electrolyte replacement with potassium and magnesium. Investigations demonstrated a metabolic acidosis, hypocalcaemia, hypophosphataemia, hypokalaemia, a raised creatinine and alkaline phosphatase.

Diagnosis — Acquired renal tubular acidosis secondary to ifosfamide

Ifosfamide and cisplatin can damage both glomerular and tubular function in the kidney. Cisplatin also damages hearing leading to high tone deafness. The renal problems may manifest themselves during

Acquired renal tubular defect

Na	128
K	2.2
HCO$_3$	12
Urea	2.3
Ca	2.3
Phosphate	0.4
Glucose	4.5
Alk. phos.	5080 iu/L
ALT	35 iu/L
Bilirubin	12 umol/L

Note: Generalised aminoaciduria and glycosuria were detected.

therapy with signs of excessive electrolyte loss (H^+, K^+, Mg^{2+}, Ca^{2+} or PO_4). These abnormalities may resolve once therapy is completed, although they may persist and lead to chronic metabolic disturbances of the sort described in the above problem. Treatment is directed at replacing the electrolytes.

Infertility is frequently cited as a possible side effect of cancer therapy. The use of sterilising chemotherapy prior to the commencement of pubertal development seems to be associated with normal fertility in both boys and girls. Sterilising chemotherapy given after puberty is more likely to affect boys than girls. Irradiation of gonads in both sexes will lead to sterility. There is little evidence that there is a higher incidence of congenital abnormalities amongst children of cancer survivors, although those with a cancer predisposition may pass on that tendency to their children.

FURTHER READING

Chessels JM, Hann IM Leukemia and lymphoma. In: Balliere's Clinical Paediatrics
Peckham M, Pinedo HM, Veeronesi U, Rare tumours in childhood. In: Oxford Textbook of Oncology. Oxford Medical Publications, Oxford
Pinkerton CR, Cutting P, Sefion B Chilhood cancer management. Chapman and Hall, London
Plowman N, Pinkerton CR Paediatric oncology. Chapman and Hall, London

16 Growth and glands

Normal growth and development depends on a delicately poised regulatory system. Endocrinology is the study of this system and by convention it has focused on hormonal pathways. Progress in molecular biology is shifting this emphasis towards the complex interrelationships between endocrine and paracrine messengers, their cellular receptors and the response mechanisms which determine expression of the genome. However we should not lose sight of the wealth of information which can be gathered from careful observation and measurement of children.

SHORT STATURE

Short stature describes the lower end of the height distribution for a given population and it is not necessarily indicative of abnormality. Reference height charts should illustrate action levels outside of which a child's height warrants more detailed evaluation. In the UK, recently revised growth charts have corrected the cross-sectional reference ranges for secular trend, and have also introduced more specific action thresholds, namely the 0.4 and 99.6 centiles. The 0.4 centile equates to a standard deviation score of −2.67; in other words only one normal child in 260 has a height below this line.

Growth monitoring is an essential component of child health surveillance programmes. Poor growth is a marker of chronic health disorders and deprivation. The recognition of abnormal short stature may identify previously unrecognised problems, and longitudinal measurement is an essential parameter by which to judge the success of health or social interventions. Current recommendations are that height and weight should be measured and plotted on a reference chart at the following ages:

— 18–24 months   — At school entry
— 39–42 months   — 7–8 years.

Later measurements should be included for children and adolescents in whom there is concern about health or growth.

Causes of growth failure

Antenatal	Chromosomal and genetic
	Autosomal chromosome disorders, e.g. trisomies, deletions
	Sex chromosome disorders, e.g. 45XO and variants
	Syndromatic intrauterine growth retardation, e.g. Russell–Silver, Prader–Willi
	Congenital infections
	Skeletal disorders
	Uteroplacental disorders
	Maternal disorders
Postnatal	Organ and systemic disorders
	Malnutrition
Childhood	Familial short stature
	Social and environmental problems
	Organ and systemic disorders
	Conspicuous, e.g. severe asthma
	Inconspicuous, e.g. coeliac or Crohn disease
	Endocrine disorders
	Growth hormone (GH) deficiency
	Congenital
	Familial, e.g. gene deletion
	Idiopathic
	Multiple pituitary hormone deficiency
	Acquired
	Tumours, e.g. craniopharyngioma, dysgerminoma, optic nerve glioma
	Irradiation
	Trauma
	Inflammation
	GH receptor defects, e.g. Laron syndrome
	Insulin-like growth factor (IGF) receptor defects
	Hypothyroidism
	Adrenal failure
Adolescence	
	Constitutional delay of growth and puberty
	Hypogonadism

Referral for specialist advice on short stature is appropriate when:

— A single height measurement falls below 0.4 centile.
— The height trajectory crosses a complete channel on the 9 centile growth chart between any pair of the above measurements.
— The child's growth causes family concern.
— Associated signs or symptoms suggest a health disorder.

Diagnosis — Short stature ? Cause

A careful history includes details of pregnancy, birth and early health, current general health and nutritional status. Ideally the parent-held health record will incorporate a growth record. Environmental and emotional deprivation always need consideration. Parental heights and age of onset of puberty need to be documented, and the former incorporated on the child's growth chart.

Measurement

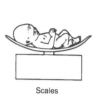

Scales

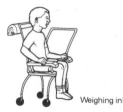

Weighing in!

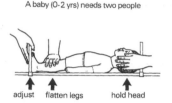

A baby (0-2 yrs) needs two people

adjust   flatten legs   hold head

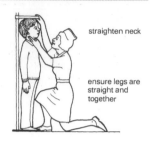

straighten neck

ensure legs are straight and together

Examination

Accurate height, sitting height, head circumference and weight measurements are essential. These require standard procedures and access to reliable equipment. Pubertal staging by the Tanner method, and testicular volume measurement with an orchidometer are needed to assess adolescent growth. General review must incorporate fundoscopy, visual acuity and field assessment.

Disproportionate growth indicative of a skeletal dysplasia is usually evident on inspection and may be confirmed by comparing sitting with standing height. Dysmorphic or asymmetrical growth provide clues to syndromes, for example, *Turner syndrome* and *Russell–Silver syndrome*. Midline facial defects or nystagmus point to developmental anomalies such as septo-optic dysplasia. Despite the extensive list of disorders causing growth failure, the majority of children can be satisfactorily assessed with the minimum of investigation. *Growth hormone (GH) deficiency* is relatively easy to confirm when it is severe, one component of multiple pituitary hormone deficiency or secondary to a structural lesion. However the majority of short children who benefit from biosynthetic GH therapy have isolated, partial deficiency without an obvious anatomical basis, and they are not easily differentiated from children with normal variant short stature. In practice GH deficiency is confirmed by the exclusion of other growth restraints,

Initial investigation of short stature

Investigation	Interpretation
Full blood count	Anaemia, malnutrition
ESR	Chronic inflammatory bowel disease
Calcium, phosphate, alkaline phosphatase	Malnutrition, hypophosphataemic rickets
Electrolytes, urea, creatinine	Renal failure, adrenal failure
Thyroxine, TSH	Hypothyroidism
09.00h or postexercise cortisol	Adrenal failure
Gliadin antibodies	Coeliac disease
Chromosome analysis	Turner syndrome
Urinalysis	Renal tract disorder

Optional investigation of short stature — guided by preliminary findings

Investigation	Interpretation
Blood	
Insulin-like growth factor-1 (IGF-1)	GH deficiency
IGF-binding protein -3	
Dynamic hormone tests	
Glucagon test, Clonidine test, Arginine test	GH deficiency (see text)
TRH test	TSH/thyroxine deficiency
LHRH test	Gonadotrophin deficiency
Tetracosactrin test	ACTH/cortisol deficiency
ACTH measurements	
Urine	
Osmolality (second sample after overnight fluid restriction)	Diabetes insipidus
GH in overnight collection	GH deficiency
Imaging	
Pituitary area imaging (MRI better than CT scan)	Congenital or acquired structural disorder
Ovarian and uterine ultrasound	Pubertal assessment, gonadal dysgenesis
Skeletal survey	Definition of skeletal dysplasia

subnormal height velocity over at least 6–12 months, and a measure of GH secretion. Unfortunately the standard GH provocation tests have a number of pitfalls, particularly when used in late childhood.

Detailed pituitary assessment is required in only a small minority of children presenting with short stature. The combination of additional presenting features (e.g. visual impairment), a confirmed subnormal height velocity, initial investigations (e.g. low TSH and low thyroxine) and pituitary area imaging will identify those who need comprehensive assessment of pituitary function. Insulin induced hypoglycaemia is the traditional and most standardised stimulus of GH and ACTH/cortisol production, but it is potentially hazardous in children and is not recommended other than under strictly monitored conditions. Glucagon, clonidine and arginine in combination with TRH and LHRH are now more widely used alternatives, but glucagon carries the risk of delayed hypoglycaemia and clonidine may produce symptomatic hypotension. No single provocation test is entirely reliable in establishing whether a child is GH deficient. Thyroxine and cortisol deficiencies should be corrected before assessing GH secretory capacity, and those with delayed puberty may require short term sex steroid priming before testing.

The failings of pharmacological tests have generated interest in measurement of physiological secretion. Blood sampling needs to be frequent and overnight to capture the pulsatile pattern associated with stage 3 and 4 sleep. Urinary growth hormone has the attraction of being non-invasive and potentially capable of providing an integrated measure of the pulsatile production. However only a minute fraction of GH can be recovered in urine, and there is an overlap between normally growing and deficient children. Insulin-like growth factor-1 (IGF-1) and IGF-binding protein-3 (IGFBP3) blood levels reflect GH sufficiency and may provide a useful single blood sample investigation.

The following are common presentations in the growth service.

Problem

- A healthy short child.
- Short parent(s).
- Bone age close to chronological age.
- Normal height velocity.

Diagnosis — Familial short stature

Explain and reassure. The family may have read that GH therapy can improve the final height of normal short children. The scientific evidence is still being collected and it is debatable whether this is an appropriate use of an expensive and still relatively untested health resource.

Problem

- Boys in the majority.
- Normal general health.
- Delayed puberty confirmed by orchidometer.
- Family history of delayed puberty.
- Bone age delayed.
- Subnormal height velocity but spontaneous catch up growth in the second half of puberty.

Diagnosis — Constitutional delay of growth and puberty (CDGP)

This usually reflects a genetically determined slow tempo of growth and may present in late childhood when height deviates across centiles, or in adolescence because of both short stature and delayed puberty. The resultant loss of self-esteem commonly produces behavioural problems. A family history confirms the diagnosis, but when this is absent it is essential to exclude acquired growth restraints such as Crohn disease or underlying hypogonadism.

Management. Explanation and reassurance satisfy most adolescents. Endocrine manipulation of the tempo of puberty and the allied growth spurt can be offered to a carefully selected minority. In boys low dose androgen therapy, for example oxandrolone 2.5 mg daily for 3–6 months, accelerates height velocity without subtracting from adult height. This is more effective in boys poised on the second half of puberty, that is with testicular volumes above 8–10 ml. Others are more focused on sexual maturation and welcome the effects of a short course of either intramuscular depot testosterone or oral testosterone undecanoate.

Problem

- Height deviation in a preschool child.
- Immature facial appearance.
- Truncal obesity.
- No detectable growth restraints on initial health assessment.
- Delayed bone age.
- Subnormal clonidine and glucagon induced GH responses.

Diagnosis — Isolated GH deficiency (IGHD)

Further steps in evaluation include checking that there are no coexistent pituitary hormone deficiencies. Remember that the underlying lesion may be evolving and that other deficiencies may arise later. Detailed and possibly repeated pituitary area MRI scans may identify an anatomical explanation. Acceleration of the height velocity from a baseline of less than 4–5 cm/year to at least 7–8 cm/year on replacement biosynthetic GH is confirmation of genuine deficiency. A poor response requires review of the diagnosis or compliance.

Problem

- Abnormal behaviour manifested by unusual affection towards strangers, and rapid acceptance of hospital admission.
- Rapid catch up growth following change to an improved environment.

Diagnosis — Deprivation with secondary hypothalamic dysfunction

This disorder highlights the need for comprehensive evaluation of a child's background before embarking on endocrine investigations. Such a patient can fulfil the criteria for GH deficiency because of secondary alteration in the normal regulation of pulsatile GH secretion. If multidisciplinary review supports the risk of deprivation, then the growth rate needs to be reassessed in a supervised setting.

Problem

- Severe growth failure starting in infancy.
- Neonatal or later hypoglycaemia.
- Prolonged neonatal jaundice.
- Micropenis and/or cryptorchidism.
- Collapse in association with hyponatraemia.
- Thirst, polyuria and hypernatraemia.

Diagnosis — Congenital hypopituitarism (multiple pituitary hormone deficiency)

These infants present with a spectrum of problems dependent on the range and severity of hormone deficiencies. Persistent hypoglycaemia reflects both GH and ACTH/cortisol deficiency. Hypothyroidism and cortisol deficiency can result in either unconjugated or conjugated hyperbilirubinaemia. GH and gonadotrophin deficiency accounts for micropenis. ACTH/cortisol deficiency manifests as poor weight gain or as hyponatraemic collapse, possibly precipitated by coincidental illness. Diabetes insipidus is readily overlooked in infancy and may come to light because of fits secondary to hypernatraemia.

A child with these features and signs of visual impairment, e.g. nystagmus, might have *septo-optic dysplasia*. Others have manifestations of a midline developmental anomaly, e.g. central cleft palate, frontal encephalocele or single central incisor. High resolution MRI imaging not only establishes the anatomical basis of the hypopituitarism but also predicts the likelihood of emerging multiple hormone deficiency.

Pituitary hormone replacement programme

Hormone	Dose range	Monitoring schedule
Biosynthetic GH (Somatropin)	12–15 U/m² SA/week s.c.	3–6 monthly height 1–2 yearly bone age
Thyroxine	100 µg/m² SA/day oral	6–12 monthly free T4
Hydrocortisone	10–12 mg/m² SA/day oral	Clinical criteria, e.g. energy level
Desmopressin	5–20 µg/day nasal or 50–300 µg/day oral	Thirst, polyuria plasma E&U, osmolality
Testosterone	i.m. depot injection 100–250 mg/month escalating dose	From age 12–14 years
Ethinyloestradiol	2–20 µg/day escalating dose (progestogen introduced after 1–2 years)	From age 12–14 years

SA = surface area.

Problem

- Visual problems; asymmetrical bitemporal field loss and optic atrophy (some first present to ophthalmology).
- Headache and signs of raised intracranial pressure.
- Growth failure and delayed puberty.

Diagnosis — Craniopharyngioma or dysgerminoma

Priorities are to arrange urgent neurosurgical management directed at controlling raised intracranial pressure, preserving vision and defining the nature of the pituitary area tumour. Endocrine assessment before neurosurgery can be limited to checking height, pubertal status, thyroid function and excluding diabetes insipidus which may be unmasked by the use of dexamethasone to prevent cerebral oedema. The early postoperative period requires precise fluid management because ADH requirement is difficult to predict; a low dose vasopressin infusion may be useful before conversion to more regular nasal or oral desmopressin replacement. The majority of patients will require a staged introduction of a full pituitary replacement programme.

Modern regimens of cytotoxic and radiotherapy have substantially improved survival from childhood malignancy. Radiotherapy directed at the brain, spine, thyroid or gonads is likely to interfere with endocrine function and spinal growth. Long term monitoring programmes must encompass careful measurement of height, pubertal development, skeletal maturation and thyroid function.

Problem

- A girl whose height at age 7 years is inappropriately low for parental stature.
- Past history of recurrent otitis media.
- Low hair line.
- Multiple cutaneous pigmented naevi.
- Narrow nail beds.

Diagnosis — Turner syndrome

Turner syndrome is a relatively common disorder, around one in 2000 female births. About 60% have 45X karyotype, the remainder having mosaicism, X deletions, isochromosomes or ring forms. A small but important group have Y chromosome material and are at risk of gonadal neoplasia. A common misconception is that Turner syndrome girls are easily recognisable with conspicuous dysmorphic features. The reality is that many girls are overlooked until discrepant short stature and more subtle features are looked for. A karyotype needs to be performed whenever the diagnosis is possible.

The mean birth weight is reduced by 500 g and length by 3 cm. The growth rate is normal for the first 1–2 years and then deviates through childhood without spontaneous pubertal acceleration, giving a mean final height of 143 cm (UK data). Turner girls are not usually GH deficient but are potentially amenable to height improvement if treated with high dosage GH therapy, 25–30 U/m^2 SA /week given as a daily subcutaneous injection. There is still debate as to the preferred age span for treatment but it is likely to be between age 3–5 years and 12–14 years. There is an increased incidence of autoimmune disorders so that growth failure may be exacerbated by hypothyroidism. The girls will also require a graded escalation of oestrogen replacement from age 12 to 15 years.

DELAYED PUBERTY

Testicular growth

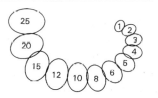

Ninety-seven per cent of girls have reached Tanner breast or pubic hair stage 2 by age 13.2 years, and 97 per cent of 14.2 year-old boys have testicular volumes of 4 ml or more. The majority of healthy children who enter puberty late have constitutional delay, and a positive family history provides confirmation. Longitudinal growth records may also establish that the child has had a slow tempo of maturation with gradually deviating height from mid to late childhood. An interrupted or unusually prolonged puberty, over 5 years, does require investigation.

Problem

- 15-year-old boy concerned by lack of pubertal progress.
- Associated behavioural problems including aggression.
- Normal general health and keen footballer.
- Height in 2–9th centile channel.
- Normal prepubertal sized penis.
- Testicular volumes 6–8 ml.

Diagnosis — Constitutional delay of growth and puberty (CDGP)

Therapeutic intervention is justified when loss of self-esteem and reactive behavioural problems disrupt life and education. A 3–6 month course of testosterone depot injections, e.g. Sustanon 100 monthly, is usually adequate to trigger acceptable sexual development.

Causes of delayed puberty

Both sexes	Constitutional delay of growth and puberty (CDGP) familial and non-familial
	Hypogonadotrophic hypogonadism (defective LHRH release)
	Isolated gonadotrophin deficiency (associated hyposmia in Kallman syndrome)
	Multiple pituitary hormone deficiency
	Brain disorders, e.g. congenital, tumours, irradiation
	Syndromatic e.g. – Prader–Willi
	Chronic systemic disease and malnutrition
	Anorexia nervosa, exercise amenorrhoea
	Hypergonadotrophic hypogonadism (defective gonads)
Girls	Gonadal dysgenesis including Tumer syndrome
	Ovarian damage, e.g. irradiation, chemotherapy
Boys	Seminiferous tubular dysgenesis including Klinefelter syndrome and Noonan syndrome
	Testicular damage, e.g. irradiation, chemotherapy, ischaemia
	Anorchia

Problem

- 12-year-old boy with an infantile penis and testicular volumes 1 ml.
- Normal height growth.
- Bilateral orchidopexy at age 2 years.
- Family history of infertility.
- Prepubertal levels of plasma testosterone, LH, FSH.
- Absent LH, FSH response to LHRH stimulation.

LHRH 2.5 µg/kg body weight by i.v. bolus to a maximum 100 µg. Plasma for LH, FSH at 0, 30, 60, (optional 90, 120) minutes. Stimulated LH, FSH levels relate to pubertal stage.

Diagnosis — Familial gonadotrophin deficiency

An anatomically normal but small penis suggests that the gonads had sufficient Leydig cell activity to generate adequate testosterone during male genital differentiation. The endocrine control of testicular descent is complex but bilateral undescended and persistently small testes are consistent with gonadotrophin, LH deficiency. Baseline and LHRH stimulated LH and FSH levels will be low but are not indicative of pathology in the pre-adolescent.

Hyposmia points towards *Kallman syndrome* (X-linked dominant with frequency of one in 10 000 males and one in 50 000 females), and may be further confirmed by detailed coronal plane MRI imaging of the olfactory stalk area.

The aim in patients with confirmed or suspected hypogonadism is to provide a gradually escalating dosage of exogenous testosterone in an attempt to create as normal a puberty as is possible. From age 12 years testosterone depot injections are commenced at a dosage of 50–100 mg 4–6 weekly, and over 3–4 years increased to an adult requirement of 250 mg 2–4 weekly. This regimen alone cannot promote testicular development and fertility. In anticipation of fertility hCG injections are used to promote testicular growth, and combined hCG and FSH to induce spermatogenesis. Pulsatile subcutaneous administration of gonadotrophin-releasing hormone is a more physiological but currently less available approach.

Problem

- A 1-year-old with impalpable testes since birth but a normal penis.
- High baseline plasma gonadotrophin, LH and FSH levels.
- Normal male karyotype.
- Absent plasma testosterone response to hCG stimulation.

Short version hCG 1000 units i.m. daily for 3 days. Long version hCG 2000 units i.m. twice weekly for 3 weeks. Plasma testosterone at baseline and 24–48 h after last injection. Testosterone should increase by greater than 2–3 fold.

Diagnosis — Vanishing testes syndrome

This is an example of anticipating delayed puberty and working with a paediatric surgeon to unravel the cause of bilateral cryptorchidism when biochemical investigation suggests absent functional gonads. Normal male differentiation points to testicular damage in late fetal life, possibly intrauterine torsion and ischaemia. The endocrine assessment may not be clear-cut and any testosterone response justifies imaging procedures and surgical exploration either to salvage potentially viable testes or remove dysgenic gonads. The family needs sensitive counselling and details of a strategy for later endocrine replacement and prosthetic gonad insertion.

Problem

- A 14-year-old girl with breast stage 2 but no additional pubertal features.
- Height 156 cm (25th centile), weight 45 kg (10th centile).
- Healthy, competitive swimmer.
- Pelvic ultrasound showing multicystic changes of ovaries and uterus of length 3.5 cm.
- Prepubertal baseline levels of oestradiol, LH, FSH, prolactin.
- Normal thyroxine, TSH levels.
- Normal female karyotype.

Diagnosis — Constitutional or exercise induced delay of puberty

Pelvic ultrasound is valuable for confirming ovarian maturation, in which multicystic changes are normal, and changing uterine size and shape as an index of oestrogen activity. LHRH tests seldom help.

This presentation is consistent with delay possibly accentuated by intensive physical training. It is useful to document maternal menarche to see if there is a discrepancy favouring either exercise as a factor, or an associated eating disorder. Explanation rather than endocrine intervention is likely to suffice.

Problem	• A 12-year-old girl with pubic hair stage 3 but no breast development. • Height 127 cm (below 0.4th centile), weight 28 kg (2nd centile). • Pelvic ultrasound unable to demonstrate ovaries and showing prepubertal uterus. • Elevated LH, FSH. • Karyotype 46, X Xp- (deletion of short arm of an X).

Diagnosis — Turner syndrome

The growth aspects are discussed above. There is a wide variation in the rate at which girls with Turner syndrome lose ovarian function, 20–30% may have early breast changes but very few reach menarche. Sex hormone replacement should be planned from age 12 to 14 years, starting with low dose ethinyloestradiol 2 μg daily and escalating through 6–12-monthly steps of 5 and 10 μg daily up to a usual requirement of 20 μg. A cyclical progestogen needs to be added when daily oestrogen dose exceeds 10 μg, and longer term replacement may be provided with a combined oral or transcutaneous product. Sex hormone replacement benefits skeletal structure, lipid profile and uterine growth which may in due course be a consideration for ovum donation techniques.

PRECOCIOUS PUBERTY

True sexual precocity refers to an abnormally early puberty in which physical changes follow a normal progression and lead to full sexual maturity. It results from either normal or abnormal activation of the hypothalamic-pituitary-gonadal axis. False sexual precocity is suggested by an unusual progression of sexual maturation, and is likely to be due to an abnormal hormonal pathway or gonadal autonomy.

The age range of normal puberty is wide but the following are generally accepted as indicating precocious puberty: girls commencing sexual development under the age of 6 years or having menarche under 8 years; boys commencing sexual development under 9 years. More important is the impact of sexual maturation on the individual child and family. Height acceleration, skeletal advance and the potential impact on final height are also factors in evaluating early puberty and the place for drug intervention.

Problem	• Girl aged 6.5 years. • Height 126 cm (> 91st centile — midparental height at 50th centile). • Breast and pubic hair stage 2–3. • Bone age 8.2 years. • Pelvic ultrasound: ovarian volumes 1 ml each with three to four cysts of 4 mm or more, uterine length 35 mm.

LHRH 2.5 μg/kg body weight to a maximum 100 μg i.v. with samples at baseline, 20 and 60 minutes, baseline oestradiol 80 pmol/l, baseline LH 1.5 U/l increasing to 8 U/l, baseline FSH 2.0 U/l increasing to 5 U/l.

Causes of precocious puberty

Complete isosexual or true precocious puberty, LHRH pulse generator dependent

Constitutional
Organic brain disease: tumours, trauma, post-infectious, irradiation

Incomplete or false precocious puberty, LHRH pulse generator independent

Girls	Ovarian cysts and tumours
	Adrenal oestrogen producing tumours
Boys	hCG secreting tumours
	Congenital adrenal hyperplasia
	21α-hydroxylase deficiency
	11β-hydroxylase deficiency
	Adrenal tumours
	Leydig cell tumours
	Familial testotoxicosis
Both sexes	McCune–Albright syndrome
	Primary hypothyroidism
	Exogenous sex steroid exposure

Partial forms of precocious puberty

Premature thelarche
Premature adrenarche
Premature isolated menarche

Diagnosis — Complete isosexual precocious puberty — presumed constitutional

The majority of girls have no apparent pathology underlying their early puberty. Assessment includes a family history of age of puberty, potential drug exposure and symptoms of intracranial disorders. Abnormal skin pigmentation may indicate neurofibromatosis or McCune–Albright syndrome, the latter being associated with autonomous ovarian activity and cyst formation. A normal pattern of puberty accompanied by ultrasound evidence of bilateral ovarian maturation through the multicystic phase supports gonadotrophin dependent puberty, and has reduced the need for LHRH tests, which are not always easily interpretable. Ovarian ultrasound is also useful in excluding rare ovarian tumours; unilateral large ovarian cysts can be monitored in anticipation of spontaneous resolution. In girls cranial imaging has a lower priority unless there are additional clinical indications.

The family requires sensitive explanation and continued support while the cause and pace of puberty are reviewed. The puberty may progress slowly or subside. Advancing physical changes and the threat of inappropriately early menses merit intervention. Current approaches include the use of subcutaneous depot formulations of gonadorelin analogues, goserelin or leuprorelin, which are effective in suppressing gonadotrophin dependent puberty. The impact of precocious puberty on final height is largely determined by the extent of bone age advance at presentation.

Problem	• Girl aged 4 years. • Asymmetrical fluctuating breast enlargement. • No other pubertal findings. • Height appropriate to age and family. • Bone age equivalent to chronological age. • Pelvic ultrasound: ovarian volumes under 1 ml with only micro-cysts, uterus infantile.

Diagnosis — Premature thelarche

Girls with isolated breast development have increased pulsatile FSH production rather than LH which predominates in true precocious puberty. There may be resultant ovarian cysts. Premature thelarche commonly subsides but there is an overlap with progressive puberty, the so-called thelarche variant.

Problem	• Boy or girl age 5–7 years. • Pubic hair growth. • Associated increase in apocrine activity. • Modest height acceleration and bone age advance. • Gonads prepubertal on palpation or imaging. • Plasma androgens in normal pubertal range.

Diagnosis — Premature adrenarche (pubarche)

Increased zona reticularis production of androgens, dehydro-epi-androsterone and androstenedione, is a normal and usually inconspicuous event from age 6 to 8 years. It may be paralleled by the above clinical features, particularly in dark haired and in Mediterranean and Asian children. Phallic enlargement, more extreme bone age advance, and high androgen levels suggest late presenting forms of congenital adrenal hyperplasia. Adrenal tumours usually exhibit faster progression and a mixed pattern of androgen and cortisol excess.

Problem	• Boy age 3 years. • Penile and pubic hair growth (stage 3). • Testicular volumes 6–8 ml. • Height record demonstrates abnormally fast growth. • Bone age 5 years. • Plasma testosterone 5 nmol/l (prepubertal <0.5).

Diagnosis — Male central precocious puberty (presumed intracranial tumour)

Boys are 20 times less likely to present with precocious puberty and the underlying cause is likely to be pathological. High priority must be given to cranial CT or MRI scans. Dysgerminomas may be suspected if tumour markers, hCG or AFP, are raised in blood or CSF.

AMBIGUOUS GENITALIA

An understanding of the embryology of sexual differentiation is essential in developing strategies for the investigation of sexual ambiguity and in the counselling of families. Molecular genetic studies have localised the regulatory switch gene determining male gender to a highly conserved 14-kb fragment of the short arm of the Y chromosome, termed SRY (sex-determining region of the human Y chromosome). Expression of SRY in somatic cells occurs during a critical phase in the differentiation of the germinal ridge, between 7 and 8 weeks' gestation. The resultant testicular tissue contains seminiferous and Sertoli cells, the latter producing müllerian inhibitory factor (MIF). The gene for MIF is coded on chromosome 19 and determines the regression of the müllerian ducts, while testosterone promotes the differentiation of the wolffian system into the male internal genitalia. A double dose effect of an Xp locus appears to play a role in determining ovarian differentiation, and it is less certain that ovarian development represents merely a default programme. Functional ovaries are not however required for female internal genitalia formation.

Male differentiation of the urogenital sinus and external genitalia is dependent on testosterone and specifically dihydrotestosterone (DHT) in the first 14 weeks. Production of DHT by the enzyme 5α-reductase is coded on chromosome 2, and tissue response on androgen receptors on Xq. The practical implications are that gender has four main components:

A classification of ambiguous genitalia

Virilised female (no palpable gonads), XX karyotype
Congenital adrenal hyperplasia
Adrenal adenoma
Nodular adrenal hyperplasia
Transplacental androgen excess
    Maternal adrenal or ovarian tumour
    Maternal virilising adrenal hyperplasia
    Maternal androgen therapy

Undervirilised male (gonads may or may not be palpable), XY karyotype
Disorders of testicular differentiation
    Leydig cell hypoplasia (gonadotrophin unresponsiveness)
    Pure or mixed gonadal dysgenesis
    Drash anomalad (associated glomerulonephritis and Wilms tumour)
Disorders of testicular function
    Enzyme defects in testosterone and/or corticosteroid synthesis
    Defects in MIF synthesis or action
Disorders of androgen dependent target tissues
    5α-reductase deficiency
    Complete and partial androgen insensitivity

Varied karyotypes with malformed, streak or mixed gonads

Malformation syndromes associated with gonadal and genital anomalies
e.g. clitoromegaly due to neurofibromatosis

— Genetic: usually signified by karyotype but there are exceptions, e.g. XX males.
— Gonadal: testes, ovaries or incompletely differentiated gonads.
— Phenotypic: complete male differentiation being dependent on intact testosterone and MIF pathways.
— Psychological: the end-result of prenatal and postnatal influences.

Expert multidisciplinary appraisal is required so that not only is a specific diagnosis made, but also the most appropriate functional gender is selected for the child. Potential life-threatening complications, for example hypoglycaemia or a salt-losing crisis, must also be anticipated. Confirmation of the underlying disorder is necessary for genetic counselling.

Problem

- Newborn with phallic enlargement and a partially enclosed urethra.
- Partial labioscrotal fusion.
- Impalpable gonads.
- Pelvic ultrasound — uterus visible.
- Chromosome analysis — 46XX normal.
- Plasma 17-OH progesterone at 48 hours = 400 nmol/l.

Diagnosis — Congenital adrenal hyperplasia (21-hydroxylase deficiency)

This girl's parents need to be counselled that the virilisation is limited to the external genitalia, and that the upper vagina, uterus, fallopian ducts and ovaries are normal. A salt-losing problem may be anticipated by monitoring for a rise in plasma potassium. Long-term management is largely successful in providing for a near normal female sexual identity. A corrective genitoplasty is performed in the first months of life although later procedures may be required to ensure vaginal patency.

Maternal dexamethasone administration in the critical 6–14-week period of fetal differentiation may reduce virilisation of future affected female infants.

Problem

- Newborn with phallic enlargement and a partially enclosed urethra.
- Incomplete labioscrotal fusion.
- Bilateral palpable gonads.
- Pelvic ultrasound — no uterus visible.
- Chromosome analysis — 46XY normal.
- Plasma 17-OH progesterone at 48 hours = 5 nmol/l (normal).

Diagnosis — Partial androgen insensitivity

This diagnosis requires confirmation that the testes are morphologically normal on imaging or biopsy, that they are capable of testosterone synthesis and that the 5α-reductase step is intact. hCG stimulation with androgen analysis in plasma and urine samples is used to assess the Leydig cell reserve and the integrity of the testosterone/DHT pathway.

Short version hCG 1000 units daily for 3 days i.m. Long version hCG 2000 units twice weekly for 3 weeks i.m. Plasma and urine collection at baseline and 24–48 h after last injection. Normal infant boys: testosterone increases by greater than 2–3 fold (peak >2 nmol/l).

Partial androgen insensitivity encompasses a spectrum from almost complete feminisation of the external genitalia to an apparently normal male with oligospermia. In the more severe forms the key decision is whether the phallus has sufficient erectile tissue to allow for growth and a satisfactory male role. A trial of exogenous testosterone depot injections 25 mg monthly for 3 months can be used to judge whether there is an adequate increase in stretched penile length. It is obviously preferable to be able to give clear guidance on preferred gender without this delay. If a female role is agreed, the management includes genitoplasty with construction of a vagina (the uterus and fallopian tubes are absent), removal of the testes to avoid masculinisation in puberty, and an unequivocal commitment to raising the child as a girl. Genital skin fibroblast culture can be used to study androgen receptor defects. Oestrogen replacement is introduced from age 12 years.

Complete androgen insensitivity may present as an infant girl with inguinal hernias containing testes, or in adolescence because of primary amenorrhoea in a girl with complete breast development. Apart from the challenge of explanation and support, gonadectomy must be planned to avoid the risk of germ-cell cancer.

Problem

- Newborn with phallic enlargement and a partially enclosed urethra.
- Incomplete labioscrotal fusion.
- Unilateral right palpable gonad.
- Abdominal and pelvic ultrasound — left gonad not visualised, uterine derivative visible.
- Chromosome analysis — 46 XY/45 X.
- Plasma 17-OH progesterone at 48 hours = 10 nmol/l (normal).

Diagnosis — Partial gonadal dysgenesis

Partial gonadal dysgenesis refers to gonads which contain both ovarian and testicular elements, and complete gonadal dysgenesis to streak gonads. There is commonly asymmetry with one streak and one dysplastic testis or ovotestis. The presence of Y chromosome material in peripheral blood or gonadal tissue increases the risk of malignancy, and justifies gonadectomy where there is doubt about the functional role of the gonads. The clinical spectrum of gonadal dysgenesis is broad, and should be considered in boys with micropenis or cryptorchidism. Serial testicular imaging and biopsy may be required because of the malignancy risk. Some children have Turner syndrome features and others have associated renal malformations as in Drash syndrome or the WAGR complex (Wilms tumour, aniridia, genital anomalies and mental retardation) linked to chromosome 11 deletion.

ADRENAL DISORDERS

Congenital adrenal hyperplasia (CAH) is due to defects of the enzyme sequence converting cholesterol to cortisol, aldosterone and sex steroids may manifest as:

— Masculinisation of females (see above).
— Undermasculinisation of males.
— Salt-loss, either as an acute crisis or as failure to thrive.
— Hypertension (salt retention).
— Postnatal virilisation with growth acceleration.

Over 90% of cases of CAH have 21-hydroxylase deficiency and this is associated with salt loss in around 75%. The incidence in most populations is in the region of one in 5–15 000 live births.

Problem

- A 3-week-old male infant presented with 7–10-day history of vomiting initially interpreted as gastro-oesophageal reflux.
- Poor peripheral perfusion and more than 10% dehydrated.
- Normal genitalia (increased pigmentation).
- Plasma electrolytes: Na 118 mmol/l, K 7.4 mmol/l, bicarbonate 12 mmol/l, urea 16 mmol/l.
- Urine microscopy normal.
- Microbiology samples, no growth.
- Plasma 17-OH progesterone 650 nmol/l (elevated).
- Plasma testosterone 15 nmol/l (elevated).

Diagnosis — 21-hydroxylase deficiency (salt-loser)
The clinical and biochemical picture is indicative of an adrenal crisis. The differential includes renal tract infection particularly in an infant with underlying severe vesicoureteric reflux or obstructive uropathy. An equivocally raised 17-OH progesterone level collected at a time of fluid depletion should be repeated after circulatory and salt replacement. In the face of life-threatening illness the infant needs urgent intravenous treatment with hydrocortisone 25 mg followed by 5 mg/kg/day before reduction to a maintenance dose. It is possible to confirm or refute the diagnosis later in management despite starting corticosteroids. Urine steroid analysis is reserved for cases with atypical presentations.

Typical maintenance treatment consists of hydrocortisone 20 mg/m² SA/day in divided dosage and fludrocortisone 50–200 µg/day (150 µg/m² SA/day). Infants with more severe salt loss require added sodium chloride 5–15 mmol/kg/day. Longer term monitoring of both sexes consists of careful growth measurement; an active child with a normal height velocity is likely to be appropriately treated. The hydrocortisone dosage should be sufficient to suppress plasma testosterone and androstenedione levels to the normal prepubertal range. Salivary or capillary blood 17-OH progesterone profiles are optional tools for further refinement of dosage. The fludrocortisone dose is initially guided by plasma electrolyte levels but later by control of salt-craving, blood pressure and, if problematical, plasma renin activity measurement.

Families must have clear written guidance on increasing hydrocortisone dose at the onset of coincidental illness, and should be provided with injection hydrocortisone for emergencies. Young children with congenital adrenal hyperplasia are also vulnerable to hypoglycaemia.

Problem	• A 3-year old boy with penile and pubic hair growth. • Height increase from the 50th centile at age 18 months to > 90th centile. • Testes infantile, volumes 1 ml. • Left hand bone age equivalent to age 5.5 years. • Blood pressure normal. • Plasma 17-OH progesterone 200 nmol/l (elevated).

Diagnosis — 21-hydroxylase deficiency (non-salt-loser)

There is a wide spectrum of this disorder ranging from newborn female infants with severe masculinisation, to young children with partial precocious puberty and growth acceleration, to young women with hirsutism, acne and ovulatory problems. The last group is referred to as having non-classical CAH. The range of gene mutations

Differential diagnosis of adrenal failure

Infancy	Adrenal
	Congenital adrenal hyperplasia
	Congenital adrenal hypoplasia
	Sporadic in association with pituitary hypoplasia
	Autosomal recessive
	X-linked cytomegalic form
	X-linked with glycerol kinase deficiency
	Familial glucocorticoid deficiency (with achalasia and alacrima)
	Infarction
Children	Adrenal
	Autoimmune
	Isolated
	Polyglandular
	Type 1 — hypoparathyroidism, mucocutaneous candidiasis
	Type 2 — thyroid disease, IDDM
	Adrenoleucodystrophies
	Infarction, haemorrhage
	Infective — tuberculosis, fungal, AIDS related
	Infiltrative — lymphoma
	Drug induced
	Pituitary
	Panhypopituitarism
	Isolated ACTH deficiency
	Hypothalamic

responsible for CAH accounts for the variable relationship between clinical and molecular genetic findings; apparent non-salt-losers may benefit from mineralocorticoids, and discordance may exist between siblings despite the same mutation. A similar clinical presentation but accompanied by hypertension and less impressive 17-OH progesterone elevation would suggest *11β-hydroxylase deficiency* which is the second most common variety of CAH. This is confirmed by finding an increased plasma 11-deoxycortisol and matching urinary steroid profile.

Problem

- Insidious onset of weakness.
- Weight loss.
- Constipation.
- Abnormal pigmentation, notably palmar creases and buccal mucosa.
- Plasma electrolytes Na 124 mmol/l, K 5.6 mmol/l, urea 8 mmol/l.
- Fasting blood glucose 3.6 mmol/l.
- 0900h cortisol 50 nmol/l (normal 150–700 nmol/l).
- ACTH >200 ng/l (normal 20–80 ng/l).
- Subnormal short synacthen (tetracosactrin) test 250 µg or 35 µg/kg body weight i.m. or i.v. Normal response: cortisol increase ≥ 200 nmol/l, cortisol peak ≥ 500 nmol/l.

Diagnosis — Addison disease

Primary adrenal failure is rare in childhood and is therefore readily overlooked until it becomes an emergency due to circulatory collapse. Additional clues may be provided by a family history of autoimmune disease or by finding vitiligo. A low plasma sodium merits a cortisol measurement, and if possible a sample promptly separated and frozen for ACTH assay. Hyperkalaemia is less evident but if present points to primary adrenal pathology rather than the secondary or hypopituitary failure. Positive adrenal cytoplasmic antibodies suggest an autoimmune cause and raise the possibility of associated disorders, for example hypothyroidism and insulin-dependent diabetes.

Emergency treatment includes intravenous hydrocortisone 50 mg followed by 5 mg/kg/day before reduction to a maintenance dose of 15 mg/m² SA/day. The presenting extracellular depletion and hypoglycaemia may require intravenous replacement. Fludrocortisone 100–200 µg/day is the usual aldosterone substitution. Monitoring therapy places more emphasis on energy and quality of life rather than blood cortisol and ACTH levels. Families must have written guidelines on dosage increase at the onset of coincidental illness and for surgery.

Adrenoleucodystrophies are rare inherited peroxisomal disorders of either X-linkage or autosomal recessive inheritance, and in some families adrenal failure may be the presenting problem. Elevated very long chain fatty acids (VLCFA) and phytanic levels provide biochemical confirmation.

Primary hypoaldosteronism (corticosterone 18-methyl oxidase deficiencies, types I and II) results in salt-wasting and hyperkalaemia without cortisol deficiency, and is suggested by raised plasma renin activity with low aldosterone levels but elevated 18-hydroxycorticosterone. Urine steroid HPLC confirms elevated tetrahydro-18-hydroxy-11-dehydrocorticosterone and reduced tetrahydroaldosterone.

Pseudohypoaldosteronism is distinguished by elevated plasma aldosterone and urinary tetrahydroaldosterone levels. Measured renal salt loss continues despite the administration of fludrocortisone and the diagnosis may be further refined by monocyte mineralocorticoid receptor studies.

Problem

- A 4-year-old girl with a 6-month history of increasing obesity.
- Pubic and body hair growth.
- Aggressive behaviour.
- Hypertension.
- Plasma testosterone 6 nmol/l (normal prepubertal <0.5 nmol/l).
- Abdominal ultrasound — no detectable abnormality.
- Abdominal MRI (or CT scan) — consistent with adrenal tumour, diameter less than 5 cm.

Diagnosis — Adrenal adenoma or carcinoma

Adrenal cortex tumours are usually manifest by features of both cortisol and androgen excess. Cortisol excess results in reduced height growth, but central obesity combined with limb muscle wasting, heightened facial colouring, skin striae and bruising, hypertension and mood changes. Androgen effects may be superimposed on this picture or occur separately. Adrenal tumours are more common in girls and result in virilisation with hirsutism, acne and clitoromegaly. Boys present with false precocious puberty, the testes remaining inappropriately small.

Modern imaging procedures have largely displaced endocrine manoeuvres in the differentiation of adrenal tumours from pituitary or, even more rarely, ectopic sources of ACTH production. Neither of the latter options would result in virilisation. Good prognosis in adrenal tumours is determined by small size, absence of capsular invasion and no metastases; histological criteria are less secure.

Management. Unilateral adrenalectomy is the appropriate management but the unaffected adrenal cortex will be atrophied and prolonged hydrocortisone replacement will be necessary.

ACTH-dependent Cushing syndrome (Cushing disease) is very rare before age 10 years, and is readily dismissed in the majority of young patients who present with obesity linked to diet; the latter usually have increased height growth. Increasing obesity accompanied by growth failure merits investigation for an endocrine or syndromatic disorder. The confirmation of sustained hypercortisolism linked to inappropriately elevated ACTH production can be a demanding exercise because of equivocal results from basal (plasma and urinary cortisol, plasma ACTH) and dynamic function (low and high dose dexamethasone suppression) tests. The picture may not be resolved even with high resolution pituitary imaging, and such patients must be evaluated in partnership with experienced centres. Preferred treatment is trans-sphenoidal removal of an identified pituitary adenoma but MRI may be unsuccessful in defining a lesion in around 40%.

Adrenal steroid mediated hypertension is usually recognised following presentation with features of cortisol or androgen excess. It may however occur as the presenting problem as in *glucocorticoid suppressible hyperaldosteronism* (GSH). GSH can cause severe hypertension in young children resulting in renal failure and cerebrovascular accidents. It is inherited as an autosomal dominant and suggested by hypokalaemia, suppressed plasma renin activity, and increased plasma aldosterone. The molecular basis is a chimaeric gene for 11β-hydroxylase/aldosterone synthase. The importance of this diagnosis is that life-threatening hypertension is reversed by dexamethasone.

DIABETES

Diabetes management has shifted away from hospital inpatient and outpatient practice towards better support in home and community. Specialist diabetes nurses play a crucial role in reducing hospital episodes, and in generating the education and motivation which provide the foundations of long term target control. The majority of hospital staff have few opportunities to manage diabetes, and the focus tends to be on newly diagnosed children with ketoacidosis, or on existing diabetics who present with sudden poor control or hypoglycaemia. Public awareness, professional alertness and prompt referral can reduce the incidence of ketoacidosis to less than 10% of newly diagnosed cases. Despite this, children still die from ketoacidosis mainly as a result of hypokalaemia or cerebral oedema, and there is a powerful case for following practice guidelines.

The recognition of the sick diabetic child is based on:

— Dehydration greater than 5% (an initial body weight is useful for calculating fluid replacement).
— Drowsiness.
— Hyperventilation and ketosis indicative of acidosis (plasma bicarbonate usually <15 mmol/l, pH < 7.2).

Diagnosis — Diabetic ketoacidosis

Severe collapse necessitates general resuscitation (airway, breathing and circulation). An initial blood sample is collected for blood glucose, plasma electrolytes and urea, PCV and full blood count (optional arterial blood gas and microbiological samples) and a reliable intravenous infusion is established. Oral fluids should be delayed until the risk of vomiting has receded. Careful documentation of observations and fluid administration is essential, and must be seamless between emergency reception and in-patient departments.

Management

The main components of subsequent management are:

Fluids
1. Initial re-expansion of circulating volume 10–20 ml/kg over 1 hour as 0.9% saline or 4.5% human albumin solution.
2. Early rehydration 0.9% saline plus KCl, volume calculated to provide deficit and maintenance evenly over 48 hours. The deficit should not be assumed to be greater than 10% in order to avoid the risk of overhydration. When blood glucose falls below 12–14 mmol/l, the fluid is changed to 0.18% saline with 4% dextrose plus KCl (serial plasma sodium should normally show a rise as the hyperglycaemia is corrected. A falling sodium is an indication for using 0.45% rather than 0.18% saline as a precaution against osmotic decompensation and cerebral oedema.) Bicarbonate infusion is seldom required and should only be considered if the child is profoundly acidotic, pH less than 7.0, and shocked. Bicarbonate infusion accentuates the risk of hypokalaemia and produces a paradoxical fall in intracellular and CSF pH.
3. Continued rehydration, 0.18% saline with 4% dextrose plus KCl until oral fluid intake adequate

Insulin
1. Human soluble insulin infusion, initial rate 0.1 units/kg/h via an infusion pump into the main intravenous line titrated to produce a gradual fall in blood glucose not exceeding 5 mmol/l/h. When the level falls below 12–14 mmol/l, the infusion is unlikely to exceed 0.025–0.05 units/kg/h. Blood glucose values less than 5 mmol/l may justify a 30-minute pause in infusion followed by increased frequency of blood glucose checks. However prolonged cessation of insulin should be avoided as it is required to correct ketogenesis; the strength of dextrose infusion may have to be increased to compensate. The infusion should be continued until 30 minutes after the first subcutaneous insulin injection.
2. Initial subcutaneous insulin regimen. Patients able to eat snacks, and free of abdominal symptoms, can transfer to a regimen close to that on which they will be discharged, for example a premixed formulation comprising soluble 30% plus isophane 70%, total daily dose 0.5–0.7 units/kg/day divided into two-thirds before breakfast and one-third before evening meal. Additional doses of soluble insulin, 1–4 units, may be added before midday meal or bedtime snack if hyperglycaemia, e.g. above 15 mmol/l, recurs.

Problem	• Falling level of consciousness (confirmed by Glasgow Coma Scale).
	• Headache.
	• Fits not due to hypoglycaemia.
	• Small pupils.

Diagnosis — Cerebral oedema

This is a rare, severe and unpredictable complication of diabetic ketoacidosis; newly diagnosed children under age 5 years are at greatest risk. The mechanism remains unknown but evidence favours a link to the rate and type of fluid replacement, and cellular inability to adjust to rapid shifts in osmolality. Serial cranial imaging has demonstrated subclinical brain swelling during treatment. Management includes steps to reduce, monitor and control intracranial pressure preferably in a unit with intensive care and neurosurgical resources.

| Problem | • Adolescent diabetic with deteriorating metabolic control and repeated hospital admission with ketoacidosis. |

Diagnosis — So-called Brittle Diabetes (or Brittle Diabetic!)

There are physiological and behavioural reasons why diabetic control deteriorates in adolescence. Increasing growth hormone and sex hormone production requires a matching increase in insulin availability but this is difficult to provide without adding to the risk from nocturnal hypoglycaemia. Compliance is an unnatural state in this age group, and rebellion or dispair may fuel eating disorders, as well as omission or manipulation of the insulin dose. It is important not to neglect coincidental disorders such as infection or allied autoimmune disease, for example hypothyroidism and coeliac disease. The insulin regimen should be reviewed in parallel with a sensitive approach to dietary advice. There may be scope for converting the insulin injections to a more intensive system based on soluble insulin before meals and isophane at bedtime. A large proportion of young diabetics are using pen injector devices which promote a more flexible approach. In the absence of an easily identifiable or amenable solution for disappointing control, carers must remain supportive and avoid judgmental conflict.

HYPOGLYCAEMIA

Other than in diabetics, hypoglycaemia is uncommon after the newborn period but blood glucose estimation should be part of the immediate assessment of children presenting with coma, collapse, convulsions or sudden behavioural change. A blood stick test suggesting a level below 4 mmol/l must be supported by a laboratory measurement;

the current definition of hypoglycaemia being a value under 2.6 mmol/l. Samples of the initial blood collected during hypoglycaemia need to be collected into the following containers.

The right bottle!

Blood glucose	fluoride
Intermediary metabolites: lactate, acetoacetate, 3-hydroxybutyrate, free fatty acids, alanine	heparin
Hormones: insulin, C-peptide, proinsulin, growth hormone, cortisol, ACTH	heparin
Ammonia, LFTs	heparin
Save sample for additional specialist assays, e.g. carnitine analysis	

The first urine passed should also be retained for:
ketones, non-glucose reducing substances, organic and amino acids, toxicology.

The first urine passed should also be retained for: ketones, non-glucose reducing substances, organic and amino acids, and toxicology.

Initial management in the symptomatic child may require intravenous glucose but it is important to calculate and regulate administration so as to avoid potential problems due to hyperosmolar overload. The initial bolus should be limited to Dextrose 25% 0.25–0.5 g/kg (10–20 ml/10 kg) over 5 minutes and it may be sufficient to use Dextrose 10% 0.2 g/kg (2 ml/kg). This is followed by an infusion of Dextrose 10% titrated to provide 5–8 mg/kg/min and maintain a normal blood glucose, ensuring that the total fluid intake is not excessive.

Causes of hypoglycaemia

Endocrine causes of hypoglycaemia
Deficiency
    Growth hormone — hypopituitarism
    ACTH/cortisol — hypopituitarism
    Cortisol — adrenal failure
Excess (glucose utilisation rate > 10–12 mg/kg/min)
    Insulin mediated
        Endogenous — transient
            Infants of diabetic mothers
            SGA infants
            Beckwith syndrome
        Endogenous — persistent
            Nesidioblastosis
            Insulinoma
        Exogenous
    Non-insulin mediated (tumour producing IGF-I, IGF-II)

Metabolic causes of hypoglycaemia
Carbohydrate
    Glycogen storage diseases (types I, III, VI, IX)
    Defects of gluconeogenesis
    Fructosaemia
    Galactosaemia
Fatty acid
    Fatty acid oxidation defects
    Ketone-body utilisation defects
    Respiratory-chain defects
Organic acid
    Maple syrup urine disease
    Methylmalonic and proprionic aciduria
Amino acid
    Tyrosinaemia

Other causes of hypoglycaemia
Systemic
    Liver failure
    Toxins, alcohol

Calculation of glucose requirement may assist in the diagnosis, normal infants having a fasting hepatic glucose production rate of 5–8 mg/kg/min falling during childhood to 1–2 mg/kg/min. Glucose utilisation exceeding 10–12 mg/kg/min suggests hyperinsulinism.

Investigative priorities will be guided by detailed history and examination. A family history of consanguinity or infant deaths favours a metabolic disorder. The duration of fasting or a requirement for coincidental illness to provoke hypoglycaemia should be documented. Hypoglycaemia shortly after feeding points to fructosaemia or poisoning. The availability of insulin, oral hypoglycaemic drugs or salicylates in the household may be relevant. Alcohol is a potential hypoglycaemic agent in children.

Examination may reveal growth failure, other signs of potential endocrine deficiency e.g. micropenis, or abnormal pigmentation. Hepatomegaly suggests glycogen storage disease, disorders of gluconeogenesis or fatty acid oxidation.

Ketonuria accompanying hypoglycaemia is useful in decidin which investigative pathway to follow. Ketonuria or a plasma β-hydroxbutyrate greater than 1.0 mmol/l is consistent with most metabolic disorders and endocrine deficiencies. Absent ketonuria suggests hyperinsulinism, fatty acid oxidation or respiratory-chain defects.

A carefully monitored overnight or more prolonged fast to induce hypoglycaemia, with serial hormone and metabolite measurement, may be required for further definition of the underlying cause.

Problem

- Full-term infant with persistent hypoglycaemia.
- Glucose requirement exceeds 12 mg/kg/min.
- Metabolite profile at age 5 days: lactate 1.1 mmol/l (1.1–2.3), β-hydroxybutyrate 0.1 mmol/l (0.1–1.0), free-fatty acids 0.2 mmol/l (0.5–1.6).
- Insulin corresponding to glucose <3 mmol/l, insulin 15 mU/l (<10).

Diagnosis — Hyperinsulinism, presumed nesidioblastosis

The combination of high glucose requirement, low metabolites and an inappropriately elevated insulin in an infant without other at-risk factors suggests nesidioblastosis, a developmental disorganisation of the endocrine pancreas in which hyperplastic β-cells are abnormally dispersed. It is usually sporadic but may recur in families as an autosomal recessive disorder. The hypoglycaemia may not be recognised until later in infancy, and there is a spectrum of severity with milder cases resolving during medical management. Endogenous hyperinsulinism in childhood or adolescence is more in keeping with a discrete islet cell adenoma amenable to localised resection.

The priority is to avoid brain-threatening hypoglycaemia with dextrose infusion, frequent oral feeds, and an escalating strategy of drugs; diazoxide 5–20 mg/kg/day combined with a thiazide diuretic, followed by octreotide 1–15 µg/kg/day. Failed medical management necessitates prompt surgery, usually subtotal pancreatectomy. In an older patient with suspected hyperinsulinism, parallel measurement of insulin, C-peptide and proinsulin at the time of hypoglycaemia is valuable in confirming a likely insulinoma.

THYROID DISORDERS

Problem

- 42-week gestation newborn aged 16 days.
- Notification of elevated Thyroid Stimulating Hormone level (TSH >200 mU/l) on 6 day capillary blood sample.
- Repeat TSH 400 mU/l, free thyroxine 8 pmol/l (12–24).

Diagnosis — Congenital hypothyroidism

Systematic population screening of TSH detects an incidence of congenital hypothyroidism of one in 3500–4500. Around 90% are sporadic failures of differentiation (agenesis, hypoplasia) or migration (ectopic). In most populations errors of thyroid hormone synthesis account for less than 5–10%. There does not appear to be a link with maternal autoimmune thyroid disease.

Careful history and examination often detects features consistent with the diagnosis, e.g. prolonged jaundice, but experience has established that these findings do not reliably alert professionals to the need for thyroid function tests. It also has to be emphasised that screening programmes vary in efficiency, and as many as one in 10–30 affected infants will not be detected by a threshold of TSH 20–30 mU/l. TSH based screening will not detect hypopituitary based hypothyroidism, a rarer problem which will usually manifest in other ways. Screening based on thyroxine is less reliable, 10–20% of infants with congenital hypothyroidism having values in the low normal range.

The need for radio-isotopic imaging of the thyroid at diagnosis is debatable. Advocates claim that a normal configuration of thyroid tissue suggests a biosynthetic defect, and that the size of residual tissue is a guide to prognosis. In severe hypothyroidism the knee X-ray demonstrates incomplete maturation of the epiphyses; however surveys have shown that the initial level of thyroxine is a more reliable marker of future intelligence.

A successful screening programme must be linked to fast track referral, confirmation and counselling, with immediate commencement of replacement thyroxine, usual starting dose 25 µg/day. This is titrated upwards to suppress the TSH to the normal range, with longer term dosage in the range 100 µg/m^2 SA/day. As in any endocrine replacement programme, clinical monitoring includes growth, development and general well-being. A large UK study demonstrated that mean IQ at age 5 years was 106 compared to an expected 112 (adjusted for secular trend), and that there was a threshold effect between learning difficulty and an initial thyroxine below 40 nmol/l (60–150).

Problem

- Equivocal screening TSH result, 20–50 mU/l.

Diagnosis — Suspected congenital hypothyroidism

The success and relative simplicity of early thyroxine replacement should not detract from the life-long concern that it causes and commitment that it requires. It is important to question the underlying diagnosis, and to confirm persistence in equivocal cases. In doubtful cases it is reasonable to commence thyroxine replacement but with an agenda to stop and re-evaluate with repeat TSH measurement and thyroid imaging.

The picture in extremely premature and sick infants is further complicated by the occurrence of normal TSH in parallel with low thyroxine levels. The levels should be judged against gestation matched standards but there is an entity of temporary hypothalamic-hypopituitary hypothyroidism. It is uncertain whether low thyroxine levels in sick preterm infants are of functional significance. The fetal brain has a specific deiodinase which preferentially converts thyroxine to T3 so that cerebral tissue is relatively protected. The place for intervening with TRH to promote lung maturation is being assessed.

Problem

- Older child with increasing weight gain but subnormal height growth.
- Easily fatigued.
- Ill-defined limb pains.
- Modest symmetrical thyroid enlargement.
- TSH elevation.
- Free thyroxine low or borderline.
- High titre antimicrosomal thyroid antibodies.
- Delayed bone age.

Diagnosis — Acquired autoimmune hypothyroidism

Autoimmune hypothyroidism is the most common cause of acquired hypothyroidism in non-endemic goitre regions. It is commoner in girls and there is likely to be a family history. Recognition may be delayed by its insidious evolution or because of less familiar presentations. A minority have an initial thyrotoxic phase. There is also an uncommon self-limiting or subacute thyroiditis, usually linked to upper respiratory symptoms, a painful goitre and cervical lymphadenopathy. The thyroiditis may result in a transient biochemical hyper- or hypothyroidism.

Management is based on thyroxine replacement, young persons normally tolerating a rapid dose escalation to 100 µg/m^2 SA/day. The resulting physical and behavioural changes are often dramatic and usually well received, but the sudden emergence of an active adolescent may need parental preparation. There have been reports of benign raised intracranial pressure during introduction.

Other presentations of acquired hypothyroidism

Hormone overlap (TSH with FSH, prolactin)
    Premature thelarche
    Premature menarche
    Premature testicular enlargement
    Galactorrhoea
    Ovarian cysts
Enlarged pituitary sella
Non-sexual hirsutism
Creatinine and creatinine phosphokinase elevation
Factor IX deficiency and epistaxes
Muscular hypertrophy and dysfunction, Kocher–Debré–Semelagne syndrome
Epiphyseal dysgenesis, slipped upper femoral epiphysis
Deteriorating diabetic control
Impaired performance or growth in Down, Turner and Klinefelter syndromes

The natural history of autoimmune thyroid disease is variable; initially obvious cases are likely to persist but children with borderline findings such as a minimal goitre and marginal TSH elevation need reassessment before commitment to lifelong therapy. It is probable that so-called adolescent 'colloid goitre' is at the mild end of this spectrum with the girls at greater risk of nodular goitre in later life.

Problem

- Concentration problems and sleep disturbance.
- Heat intolerance.
- Accelerated height growth but weight loss.
- Proptosis.
- Symmetrical smooth goitre.
- Tremor and tachycardia.
- Free thyroxine elevated, TSH suppressed.
- High titre TSH receptor antibodies.

Diagnosis — Juvenile hyperthyroidism (Graves disease)

Juvenile hyperthyroidism is part of the spectrum of autoimmune thyroid disease related to the action of thyroid-stimulating immunoglobulins. Seldom seen in young children it becomes increasingly common during adolescence notably in girls. The onset may be insidious or abrupt; the latter may represent a transient hyperthyroid phase in an autoimmune thyroiditis. Thyroid ultrasound examination helps to exclude the low risk of autonomous nodules.

Medical management with carbimazole, initial dose 0.4–0.6 mg/kg/day up to a maximum of 30 mg/day and maintenance 0.1–0.3 mg/kg/day is the favoured option in young patients even for long term control. Prominent autonomic symptoms merit additional β-adrenergic blocking agents, propranolol 0.75–2 mg/kg/day. There is still debate as to whether more aggressive higher dose carbimazole regimens coupled to replacement thyroxine promote a higher remission of the disease. A reasonable strategy is to provide biochemical control for 1–2 years before attempting carbimazole withdrawal. The size of the residual goitre is some guide to the likelihood of relapse. Approximately 60% enter permanent remission. Active disease persisting for more than 4–5 years, inability to tolerate anti-thyroid drugs, or major compliance problems are indications for either partial thyroidectomy or radioactive iodine. In expert hands surgery has the advantage of short hospitalisation followed by a good chance of sustained freedom from medication. Radioactive iodine is increasingly favoured in US centres because of its safety and effectiveness. The risk of late neoplasia is negligible but there is likelihood of eventual hypothyroidism and a requirement for long term supervision.

Problem

- Pregnancy in a woman with controlled thyrotoxicosis (low dose propylthiouracil and thyroxine replacement).
- Maternal blood contains high titre of thyroid stimulating immunoglobulins (TSI; approximately one in 70 at risk pregnancies).

Diagnosis — Potential fetal and neonatal thyrotoxicosis

This is a rare problem given that there is a low risk of maternal thyrotoxicosis, one to two per 1000 pregnancies, and an even lower risk of transfer of functionally significant TSI across the placenta. It is however potentially lethal to the fetus and dangerous to the newborn. The time and pattern of presentation varies according to the functional impact of mixed stimulatory and inhibitory populations of TSH receptor antibodies. Maternal antithyroid therapy may suppress fetal and early neonatal thyroid activity so that problems do not emerge until 7–10 days. TSI assays are not widely available and a practical alternative is to remain alert to persistent fetal tachycardia and poor fetal growth as warning signs, and to instruct midwifery staff to be alert to postnatal signs. Features include tachycardia, irritability, poor weight gain, diarrhoea, a staring gaze and a palpable thyroid enlargement. Late problems include heart failure, hepatosplenomegaly and thrombocytopenia. The diagnosis is confirmed by increased plasma free thyroxine and a low TSH; levels at 2–5 days being more discriminatory than at birth.

Treatment is based on one or more of the following: Lugol's iodine 1 drop three times daily, propranolol 1–2 mg/kg/day and carbimazole 0.5–1.0 mg/kg/day. Symptoms should settle over 2–3 days, and treatment needs to be continued for 3–12 weeks.

PARATHYROID DISORDERS

Problem
- Dysmorphic SGA infant.
- Failure to thrive with recurrent infections.
- Outflow tract cardiac anomaly.
- Hypoplastic thymus with reduced T cell sets.
- Borderline hypocalcaemia.
- Chromosome 22q11 deletion confirmed on FISH analysis.

Diagnosis — Early recognition parathyroid hormone deficient hypoparathyroidism: DiGeorge syndrome

Several phenotypes have been linked to 22q11 deletion and a collective acronym, CATCH 22, has been proposed to encompass Cardiac abnormality, Abnormal facies, T cell deficit due to thymic hypoplasia, Cleft palate, and Hypocalcaemia. The hypocalcaemia is not always symptomatic and often resolves.

Problem
- 6-year-old with longstanding poorly controlled seizures.
- Deteriorating school performance.
- Dental enamel hypoplasia.
- Positive Chvostek and Trousseau signs.
- Plasma calcium 1.7 mmol/l (2.1–2.7) phosphate 1.6 mmol/l (0.7–1.4).
- Plasma parathyroid hormone <10 ng/l (10–65).
- Cranial CT — basal ganglia calcification.

Diagnosis — Late recognition parathyroid hormone deficient hypoparathyroidism

The spectrum of hypoparathyroidism varies from acute hypocalcaemic convulsions in the newborn, through tetanic manifestations such as laryngospasm in infancy, to delayed recognition in children erroneously labelled as having primary epilepsy. Muscle cramps, weakness and an elevated creatinine kinase may be other presentations. Dry skin, brittle nails, poor dentition and cataracts are additional features. Hypoparathyroidism is confirmed by hypocalcaemia, hyperphosphataemia and normal renal function, together with low PTH levels using a sensitive assay. Associated findings include an elevated urinary phosphate and low serum 1, 25(OH)$_2$D levels. Hypomagnesaemia should also be excluded.

Problem
- 8-year-old with short stature and relative obesity.
- Round facies and brachydactyly.
- Borderline learning difficulties.
- Plasma calcium 1.9 mmol/l (2.1–2.7), phosphate 1.4 mmol/l (0.7–1.4).
- Plasma parathyroid hormone 80 ng/l (10–65).
- Free thyroxine 8 pmol/l (12–24), TSH 8 mU/l (1.5–3.5).
- Hand X-ray shortened 4th metacarpals.

Diagnosis — Pseudohypoparathyroidism and borderline hypothyroidism

PTH resistance is a heterogeneous group of disorders with several patterns of inheritance; autosomal dominant, autosomal recessive and X-linked. The molecular basis lies at several points in the PTH receptor–Gs protein–adenylate cyclase complex. Components of this complex are shared with other peptide hormones and hence the association with TSH and gonadotrophin resistance. By convention patients with somatic features but no readily apparent biochemical abnormality are classified as having *pseudopseudo-hypoparathyroidism*. Detailed family studies have suggested an overlap with for example delayed development of hypocalcaemia.

The clinical and radiological signs together with sensitive plasma PTH measurement normally distinguish PTH deficiency and resistance. Further classification of PTH resistance is based on cyclic-AMP response to PTH infusion, Gs-protein assay and molecular genetic studies.

Management of hypocalcaemic patients consists of alfacalcidol 40–50 ng/kg/day aiming for relief from neuromuscular symptoms and plasma calcium in the range 2.0–2.2 mmol/l. Ensuring that urinary calcium/creatinine ratios remain below 0.7 mmol/mmol reduces the risk of nephrocalcinosis.

Differential diagnosis of childhood hypercalcaemia

Hyperparathyroidism
Primary
   Sporadic adenoma, hyperplasia
   Familial multiple endocrine neoplasia (MEN-1, 2)
   Familial hypocalciuric hypercalcaemia (FHH)
   Neonatal primary hyperparathyroidism
Secondary
   Chronic renal failure, ectopic

Non-parathyroid
Syndromatic (William's syndrome)
Vitamin A, D excess
Malignancy
Sarcoidosis
Other endocrine, e.g. Thyrotoxicosis, Adrenal insufficiency

Problem

- Polyuria and polydipsia.
- Renal colic due to calculi.
- Plasma calcium elevated (repeated measurement), phosphate reduced.
- PTH inappropriately high for calcium levels.
- Urinary calcium, Uca/Ucreatinine ratio, increased in proportion to hypercalcaemia.

Diagnosis — Hyperparathyroidism

Primary hyperparathyroidism is rare in childhood, two to five per 100 000, and may be sporadic or familial. It has to be differentiated from non-endocrine causes of hypercalcaemia, and from *familial hypocalciuric hypercalcaemia* (FHH), an autosomal dominant in which hypercalcaemia occurs in the first decade and is associated with an inappropriately normal PTH secretion but low renal calcium clearance. FHH is seldom symptomatic but some cases of *neonatal primary hyperparathyroidism*, a life threatening condition, appear to be homozygous FHH with generalised parathyroid hyperplasia.

FURTHER READING

Brook CGD 1995 Clinical paediatric endocrinology, 3rd edn. Blackwell, Oxford
Buckler JMH 1994 Growth disorders in children, BMJ Publishing Group, London
Kappy MS, Blizzard RM, Migeon CJ, Wilkins The diagnosis and treatment of endocrine disorders in childhood and adolescence, 4th edn. Charles C Thomas, Springfield
Kelnar CJH 1995 Childhood and adolescent diabetes. Chapman & Hall, London
Wilson JD, Foster, DW 1992 Williams textbook of endocrinology, 8th edn. WB Saunders, Philadelphia

17 Bones and Joints

The usual presenting symptoms of joint pain and bone pathology are pain, swelling, limitations of movement and deformity, either singly or in combination. To any of these may be added systemic disturbance. The presentation and age of a child can help with narrowing diagnostic possibilities. In the acutely ill child, investigation and management must occur immediately. If sepsis is suspected blood cultures must always be sent before antibiotics are started. Delay in diagnosis and the institution of the proper treatment may lead to severe limb deformities, bone necrosis, discharging sinuses and pathological fractures. Giving intravenous antibiotics to a child with acute bone pain of unknown cause is not likely to do much harm, whereas withholding antibiotics in order to be absolutely sure of the right diagnosis or organism sensitivity may result in permanent disability and deformity. An apparently healthy child may present with an acute joint problem which unmasks a congenital anomaly, a bleeding disorder or an acquired condition such as a nutritional deficiency.

History. A carefully obtained history is important. It is useful to clarify in the well child the reason for referral. It may be that it is either the child or the parent who has worries, but not both. There may be a family or social history of disability heightening anxiety within the child or parent who are keen to have a specific diagnosis excluded. On the other hand, the family might be seeking practical advice for the child's symptoms when they already know the diagnosis. History taking will follow the normal pattern. A history of trauma may mislead in two ways. The possibility of a pathological fracture may not be considered because there does not seem to have been significant trauma (and pain may not be a major complaint) and, conversely, since all children sustain frequent minor falls and bumps, a painful swelling may be considered to be entirely traumatic when in fact there is an additional underlying problem. A history of pain in the knee raises the possibility of hip pathology, and pain in the thigh or hip of back pathology.

Observation. In the more acutely presenting conditions with pain and muscle spasm, observation is extremely important since it is the only part of the examination likely to be entirely pain free for the child. The general appearance and demeanour of the child will indicate whether he/she is ill or well. The child's position and attitude, if in bed, and gait and posture, if ambulant, are important. Acute joint

Positions of comfort

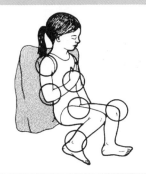

pathology will cause the child to adopt the position of maximum synovial capacity of that joint, i.e. minimum tension. Protective muscle spasm, or muscle wasting may be obvious, and swelling may be present.

Palpation includes firstly that of the pulse, and of the skin for fever and sweating. Skin temperature, swelling and redness at the site of pain is assessed and compared with that of skin at a distance. Skin temperature is best assessed using the backs of one's fingers rather than the palmar aspect. Areas of tenderness need to be accurately pinpointed; this is especially important in acute osteitis, since this is the means by which the child's progress is monitored. To slide the pulp of one's finger down the subcutaneous border of the tibia in a toddler may be the only way to diagnose a hairline spiral fracture (often initially undetectable radiographically).

Percussion is sometimes useful, especially in the spine, or over areas of doubtful bone tenderness.

Assessment of function must always be left until the end since it is likely to be the most upsetting part of the examination for the child. One can usually determine how to proceed by first asking the child how much he/she can move, or how well he/she can walk. If some movement is possible and not too painful, then a full careful comparative examination of all movements of the normal and affected limb must be carried out, making accurate notes on the degree of limitation. If the child cannot or will not move at all, any assessment has to be carried out extremely gently and slowly. It is important to note constancy in functional ability. A child may be unable to bend the knee during formal testing but easily climb onto the examination couch. It is wise to perform any investigations requiring the child's co-operation (like X-rays) before rather than after taking blood or putting up a drip, except where sepsis needs immediate treatment. Where movement is extremely painful, it may not be possible to obtain technically perfect X-rays.

THE ACUTELY ILL CHILD WITH JOINT INVOLVEMENT

The acutely ill child with joint involvement

Septic arthritis	Leukaemia
Acute osteomyelitis	Polyarteritis nodosa
Systemic JCA	Systemic lupus erythematosus
Reiter syndrome	Parvovirus B19
Kawasaki	HIV
Streptococcal disease	Henoch–Schönlein purpura

Problem

- In the older child severe throbbing bone pain.
- Inability to move due to pain and muscle spasm.
- Associated abdominal pain and vomiting.
- Swelling and warmth with acute local bony tenderness.

Diagnosis — Acute osteitis

There may be a history of minor trauma, skin sepsis or throat infection a few days before presentation. Examination shows a very sick child with a high fever, possibly with delirium and dehydration. If the history of initial limb pain becomes lost in the more recent acute symptoms, the child is quite likely to be sent in as a case of acute meningitis, or as an acute surgical abdominal emergency.

Problem

- Child who resists all movement.
- Looks toxic and has a fever (in the neonatal period the temperature may be subnormal).
- Has one or more painful joints, the child lying with the affected joint in the position of maximum relaxation.
- With swollen, hot, red and very tender joints.

Diagnosis — Septic arthritis

This serious condition occurs in young children, usually under 5 and neonates. This diagnosis should always be considered in any child with a swollen or painful joint as prompt diagnosis can prevent serious destruction. Any joint can be affected, in neonates several joints can be involved. Relevant investigations include blood culture, WBC, CRP (C-reactive protein) and X-rays. This diagnosis should not be discounted if initial investigations are normal. If the clinical picture suggests sepsis, treatment should be commenced and investigations repeated after 24 hours. Joint aspiration will relieve pain, confirm the diagnosis and will provide pus for bacteriology.

Careful examination should reveal the site of most acute bone tenderness, but this can be very difficult to determine in a delirious child. Blood culture, full blood count and X-rays must be carried out. The latter are likely to show soft tissue swelling only initially, with no obvious abnormality.

Immediate investigation

Full blood count and ESR
Blood culture
CRP
Blood electrolytes
X-rays

Common organisms in childhood septic arthritis

Staphylococcus aureus
Haemophilus influenzae
Escherichia coli
Streptococcus
Salmonella

Septic arthritis

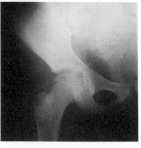

presenting with pain

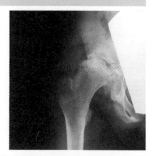

2½ years later

Treatment. Intravenous flucloxacillin should be commenced urgently (within an hour or so of admission) as soon as a blood culture has been taken. The antibiotic may be modified later in the light of Gram stain, culture results and clinical progress. Pain relief is largely secured by providing efficient immobilisation by traction or splintage of a joint into a good functional position. The efficacy of treatment is assessed clinically. Continuing pain and fever 24 hours after admission with a hot swollen joint, suggests that repeat aspiration or open drainage is necessary, together with a review of the antibiotic regimen. An infected hyperaemic limb is at risk of pathological fracture, so splintage needs to be maintained for some time. Physiotherapy may be started as soon as all the general and local signs have settled. Night splintage may be necessary for a time to correct persisting degrees of deformity.

Prognosis is usually excellent unless, as can occur in the neonate, extensive bone destruction has occurred by the time of presentation (this is most common at the hip), in which case the joint may be permanently damaged. Early osteoarthritis will then result.

Immediate and review management of the ill child with joint involvement

Immediate	Review
Intravenous fluids	Repeated clinical reassessment
Blood and plasma if septicaemic	Daily haemoglobin estimation (pus produces anaemia)
Nasogastric aspiration	
Immobilisation of joints in a functional position	Reconsider blood transfusion
Traction — for hip — to relieve pain	Reconsider dose, type and route of antibiotic
Antipyrexial measures	Assess nutritional, including iron status
Antibiotic (where necessary)	
Anti-inflammatory medication	
Pain control	

Problem

- Newborn with the clinical features of septicaemia, i.e. lethargy, food refusal, hypothermia, ileus and possibly peripheral circulatory collapse.
- Localised tenderness of limb with varying degrees of swelling and redness. These are often multifocal.
- Sometimes a recognised source of infection in the form of umbilical cord sepsis.

Diagnosis (1) — Diffuse neonatal osteitis

The initial X-ray in a neonate may well already show evidence of bone destruction, indicating that in this age group the primary site of infection is usually bone with very rapid spread to the joints because of the blood supply. The X-ray may be apparently normal at the time of initial presentation but bone destruction will be evident rapidly, and always within 2 weeks.

Treatment. It is urgent to commence intravenous antibiotics. Flucloxacillin/ampicillin are the drugs of choice, since the likeliest organism is *Staphylococcus aureus*. Other possibilities are *E.coli*, streptococcus and haemophilus, and the antibiotic regimen must be reviewed as soon as the culture/sensitivity results are available. The baby may develop a paralytic ileus secondary to septicaemia. Neonates rapidly develop anaemia with pyogenic infection. The baby is nursed in whatever position seems most comfortable, supporting the limb with rolled towels; formal splintage or traction is not advisable because skin breakdown occurs so readily, especially in a swollen hyperaemic area.

The outcome is good except in a late-presenting case of osteitis of the upper femoral metaphysis; this lesion is intra-articular and if pus is already present in the hip joint severe bone and cartilage destruction of the epiphysis and metaphysis will result, and be irrecoverable, leading to severe permanent crippling.

The acutely ill baby with joint involvement

Neonatal osteitis
Infantile cortical hyperostosis
Infantile polyarteritis nodosa
Kawasaki

Diagnosis (2) — Infantile cortical hyperostosis (Caffey disease)

This is a puzzling condition, occurring in babies normally under 3 months of age. It has many of the clinical features of diffuse neonatal osteitis. The ribs, mandible, maxilla, bones of the shoulder region and the lower limbs can be involved. The ESR and WBC are usually raised and there is some anaemia. X-rays will eventually show the classical cortical thickening with sub-periosteal new bone but in the very early stages diagnosis may be difficult. Acute infective lesions have to be excluded. Treatment is then with anti-inflammatory drugs. The symptoms and signs resolve spontaneously over several weeks or months. There are no long-term problems.

Problem

- A history of a recent sore throat.
- The child is ill with a high fever, and
- A hot swollen painful joint.

Diagnosis — Streptococcal disease — ? Rheumatic fever

The streptococcus is responsible for many acute illnesses with joint involvement. It can produce a reactive effusion which is sterile. Children may have single or repeated episodes of joint pain, particularly at the hip. ESR, ASO titre, throat swab, chest X-ray for heart size and ECG will help define the condition. Nowadays, rheumatic fever with skin rash, cardiac signs and rheumatic nodules is rare in Britain. If the diagnosis still remains doubtful one should proceed to joint aspiration immediately to exclude sepsis.

Treatment. Anti-inflammatories and penicillin should be given if the streptococcus is identified. Recurring episodes should be treated with long term penicillin. Rheumatic fever is treated with aspirin (levels monitored) and penicillin which must be started immediately and continued indefinitely. Full recovery of joint function should occur but cardiac problems may persist.

Problem

- Arthralgia.
- Conjunctivitis.
- Urethritis.

Diagnosis — Reiter syndrome

Following a gastro-intestinal infection, i.e. yersinia or campylobacter. Treat the initial infection where appropriate and give an anti-inflammatory drug until fully mobile.

Problem

- 'Slapped cheek' redness on face.
- Myalgia and arthralgia.
- Mild febrile illness.

Diagnosis — Parvovirus B19 (Fifth disease)

Often mistaken for rubella. Some children continue to have constitutional features for 6–12 months, which is hard to differentiate from systemic arthritis. Treat with anti-inflammatory drug.

Problem

- One acutely warm swollen joint and nothing else initially, but other symptoms and signs rapidly follow.

Diagnosis — Henoch–Schönlein purpura (HSP)

Abdominal pain, melaena, haematemesis, pain in other large joints, a purpuric rash especially on the limbs and buttocks, and oedema of the hands, feet, face and scrotum.

Treatment is symptomatic only. The condition will eventually resolve spontaneously. Rarely renal disease follows.

Problem

- Fever, persistent over at least 5 days.
- Changes in the extremities (red palms and soles, oedema then membranous desquamation).
- Conjunctival injection.
- Polymorphic rash.
- Red lips, strawberry tongue.
- Lymphadenopathy.

Diagnosis — Kawasaki disease

Investigations should look for multiple system involvement including ECG, cardiac echo, abdominal ultrasound and urinalysis. Aspirin and high dose intravenous gammaglobulin are recommended. Dipyridamole and prostacyclin can be considered, while the use of corticosteroids is controversial. Death either early or late is from myocardial infarction.

Problem

- A child may present with malaise, fever, skin rash, abdominal pain and arthropathy. There may be myalgia, ischaemic heart disease, renal and neurological complications.

Diagnosis — Polyarteritis nodosa (PAN)

It is more common in boys. The plasma characteristically has a green tinge. Antineutrophil cytoplasmic antibodies can be detected but are not diagnostic. Technetium 99, renal DMSA (dimercaptosuccinic acid) scanning may show renal vasculitis. The most valuable test is renal and hepatic angiography.

Treatment is with steroids, cyclophosphamide and dipyridamole. Mortality is over 20%, in spite of intensive therapy.

Problem

- A teenage girl may present with fever, arthralgia, rashes, myalgia, lethargy, abdominal pain and weight loss. She may also have mouth ulcers, headaches, alopecia and sun sensitivity, whilst intellectual and personality changes may have occurred.

Diagnosis — Systemic lupus erythematosus (SLE)

Pancytopenia can occur with a raised ESR. Antinuclear antibodies and anti-DNA antibodies can be detected with low complement levels and high complement turnover. The CRP only rises with active infection. Multisystem examination clinically and diagnostically should be undertaken. Anti-phospholipid syndrome should be considered. Antiplatelet drugs, anti-inflammatory drugs, corticosteroids (oral or pulse), azathiopine or cyclophosphamide can be used. Mortality and morbidity remains high.

Problem

- A young child presents with spiking fever, malaise, anorexia, weight loss and progressive anaemia.
- Flitting polyarthritis.
- Rash prominent on trunk — can be itchy.

Diagnosis — Systemic juvenile chronic arthritis (systemic JCA)

Polyserositis can occur. Infection and reticuloendothelial disorders have to be excluded. Immunodeficiency disorders including HIV have to be considered. High dose ibuprofen 40–60 mg/kg/day in 6 doses can settle the symptoms. Persistent arthritis can occur when the systemic features are controlled. Methotrexate or steroids may be needed. Deflazacort can be used to reduce bone thinning, but seems to control systemic features less well. Some children will have an unremitting destructive disease, while others have a good long term outcome.

THE WELL CHILD WITH AN ACUTE JOINT PROBLEM

The well child with an acute joint problem

Haemarthrosis ± bleeding disorder
Intra-articular fracture
Pulled elbow
Perthes disease
Monarthritis
Irritable hip

Problem

- A boy with swollen tender joint with limited movement.
- No systemic disturbance.
- May have a previously diagnosed bleeding disorder.

Diagnosis — haemarthrosis with haemophilia or Christmas disease
A joint bleed, uncommon under the age of 2 years, may be the presenting symptom of a blood disorder. Septic or traumatic arthritis will need to be excluded.

Treatment. Intravenous cryoprecipitate 2 units/kg body weight. This should raise the Factor VIII level by about 20%. In a severe haemarthrosis joint aspiration can then be performed under very strictly aseptic conditions, and bedrest and traction instituted. Cryoprecipitate is repeated 12 hourly for a further 48 hours. Physiotherapy and protected weight bearing should be started as soon as the joint swelling has subsided. A packed-cell blood transfusion may be given, if necessary, after the cryoprecipitate replacement therapy. If the child's family have a freezer, and an individual able to give intravenous injections, treatment with cryoprecipitate can be started at home at the first sign of a bleed. Rapid treatment with cryoprecipitate and immobilisation prevents the gross joint damage which used to occur.

Problem

- History of trauma.
- Warm, swollen, painful joint with restriction of movement.

Diagnosis — Intra-articular fracture
Carefully taken X-rays of good quality should demonstrate the fracture, but the presence of blood in the joint and the nature of some intra-articular fractures may make them difficult to diagnose. If in doubt, joint aspiration will confirm the nature of the intra-articular fluid. Joint aspiration, reduction and immobilisation will relieve pain and aid healing. The progress depends on the severity of any articular damage, which may result in later osteo-arthritis.

Problem

- A hot swollen painful joint, usually the knee, with muscle spasm.

Diagnosis — Monarticular juvenile chronic arthritis (JCA)

The monarticular presentation of juvenile chronic arthritis is usually relatively insidious and without much pain. In a few children, however, the presenting symptoms and signs may be relatively acute. Muscle wasting and widening of the tibial plateau may suggest that the disease has actually been present for over 3 months. A family history of HLA B27 associated disease may be present in the older child whilst the younger child, especially the girl, may have a positive antinuclear antibody and evidence of chronic iridocyclitis on slit-lamp examination of the eye. An arthroscopic synovial biopsy is rarely necessary.

Treatment. Anti-inflammatory medication should be commenced, e.g. Naprosyn 20 mg/kg/day in 2 doses, and intra-articular steroids considered. A home physiotherapy regimen should be started. Splints can be provided to obtain the best functioning position.

Problem

- Onset of a limp and pain in one hip or knee.
- No other evidence of illness.
- No swelling but restriction of movement at the hip joint, especially of internal rotation, abduction and extension, sometimes with tenderness of the hip joint anteriorly.

Diagnosis — Irritable hip (observation hip, transient synovitis, coxalgia fugax)

An X-ray may show slight widening of the joint space. Ultrasound, bone scan or MRI can be considered. Full blood count and ESR are normal.

Treatment. Initiate bed rest and traction until all movements are full and free, which is usually about 7–10 days. Should the pain not settle within 24 hours on rest and traction, another diagnosis should be sought, joint aspiration done and blood culture repeated. Most children recover completely but a small proportion (2% or so) go on to Perthes disease or some other hip joint pathology. All such children therefore should be re-examined and re-X-rayed if necessary 3 months later.

Problem

- Painless limp in a well boy (aged 4–8 years).
- Limitation of internal rotation, abduction and hip extension.

Diagnosis — Perthes disease

A cause of avascular necrosis of the femoral head. Initial X-rays may show a widened joint space. Early isotope bone scans may show a photopenic area in the femoral head. Later increased uptake around the ischaemic area suggests repair.

Treatment depends upon the extent of involvement and phase in the disease on diagnosis. Bed rest and traction may be adequate, but some children need a surgical containment procedure, such as femoral osteotomy. Two-thirds will have a good clinical result. Osteoarthrosis is a late complication.

Perthes disease

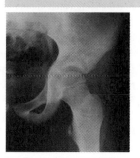

presenting with
pain

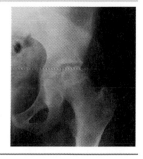

1 year
later

Problem

- A young toddler presents with a history of a sudden jolt to the arm from an adult who was holding his/her hand (usually pulling the child away from danger).
- A painful arm which the child is reluctant to move.
- Pseudo-paralysis and restriction of all elbow movements especially supination, often with no obvious tenderness and poor pain localisation.

Diagnosis — Pulled elbow

A pulled elbow is a distal dislocation of the immature radial head through the annular ligament. Radiographs are normal.

Treatment. Manipulative reduction is required. Hold the flexed elbow firmly in one hand and the forearm in the other hand, slightly distract the forearm, fully supinate and push it gently, but firmly, towards the elbow. This manoeuvre, if carried out expeditiously, usually straight after the initial examination, does not require anaesthesia. Cure is immediate and gratifyingly obvious!

THE CHILD WITH A SUBACUTE JOINT PROBLEM AND ADDITIONAL FEATURES

The child with chronic joint involvement and other problems

Tuberculous arthritis
Scurvy
Skeletal dysplasia
   i.e. Stickler syndrome
Syndrome
   i.e. William syndrome

Problem

- Persistent stiff joint, particularly knee or wrist.
- Possible night sweats and low grade fever.

Diagnosis — Tuberculous arthritis

Clinically, the joint is swollen with deep tethering of the overlying skin. There may not be a history of foreign travel or TB contact. The child may not complain of systemic disturbance. Full blood count, Heaf test, early morning urines for microscopy and culture and chest X-ray may help. The joint X-ray may remain normal for 3 months. A synovial biopsy may be necessary. Children with AIDS may have an atypical organism.

Treatment. Rest with local traction may be necessary initially to reduce muscle spasm. Anti-tuberculous therapy should be continued for 9–12 months. Early treatment will lessen joint destruction. Late surgery may be needed for ankylosis or osteoarthrosis.

Problem

- Bruising and bleeding from the gums.
- Nutritional deficits, i.e. vitamin D and iron, where the whole diet is inadequate.
- Very rarely this may produce painful warm swellings of the limbs due to subperiosteal bleeds or even pathological fractures.

Diagnosis — Scurvy

X-rays will confirm the presence of periosteal elevation with new bone formation, and may show minor fractures at different stages of healing. Carefully questioning about diet and the nutritional state will help differentiate it from non-accidental injury. Give vitamin C orally in large doses (200 mg per day plus fresh orange and lemon juice). The start of treatment can be combined with 24-hour urine collections to confirm the diagnosis. Symptoms are relieved within a day or two, but bone structures take several months to become normal. Weight bearing should be restricted until some recovery has occurred. The prognosis is excellent as long as the basic dietary problem is resolved.

A non-inflammatory arthropathy may occur in association with a syndrome or skeletal dysplasia. Pointers to this are moderate or severe learning difficulties or a sensorineural hearing loss or visual impairment. These conditions often have a genetic basis. The practical management of the arthropathy is often symptomatic treatment, which fails to prevent progressive deformity and disability, e.g. Stickler syndrome, tricho-rhino-phalangeal syndrome.

THE WELL CHILD WITH A CHRONIC JOINT OR BONE PROBLEM

Problem

- Joint pains — particularly knees.
- Night waking with pain.
- Pain worse after exercise.
- Girls aged 2–5, 10–13.
- Boys aged 4–7.

The well child with a chronic joint problem

Osgood–Schlatter	Polyarticular hypermobility
Osteoid osteoma	syndrome
Slipped upper femoral	Congenital dislocation of
epiphysis	the hip
Pauciarticular — JCA	Lyme disease

Diagnosis — Hypermobility

A typical story often with a family history of 'growing pains' and familial hypermobility. Reassurance, wedged footwear, anti-inflammatory treatment and maintenance of muscle power help these children. There are no long term complications.

Problem

- Pain in the hip, thigh or knee in an otherwise healthy child.
- Limited internal rotation, abduction and extension of the hip.
- Careful measurement may show a little true shortening.
- X-rays of hip joint showing the capital epiphysis sliding downwards and backwards.

Diagnosis — Slipped upper femoral epiphysis (adolescent coxa vara, acute epiphysiolysis)

This condition is due to an imbalance of growth hormone/sex hormone ratio; two differing physical types of child may be affected; the overweight, gonadally immature child with a normal growth hormone level and a reduced sex hormone level, or the thin, lanky, rapidly growing child with an increased growth hormone level and a normal sex hormone level. Most of the girls fall into this latter group. The age range is 10–16 years, the girls presenting younger than boys. It is eventually bilateral in 25% of cases. The symptoms may be chronic or acute-on-chronic following unusual physical activity or minor trauma. X-ray the hip joints with both lateral projections.

Slipped femoral epiphysis

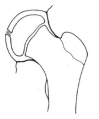 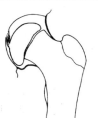 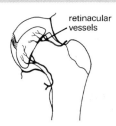

retinacular vessels

Normal   Slipped   May compromise blood supply

Slipped femoral epiphysis presenting with pain (A), 4 weeks later (B) and 2 years later (C)

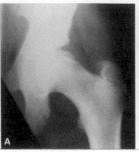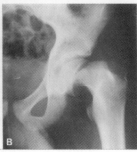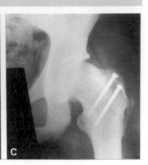

Treatment. This depends on the degree of slip at the time of diagnosis. In mild cases, pins may prevent further slip. In severe cases, pinning increases the risk of avascular necrosis. It may be necessary to allow fusion to occur spontaneously and then correct any persisting deformity. The other hip must be carefully watched until the epiphysis has fused. Early osteoarthrosis is common.

Problem
- A pain free limp.

Congenital dislocation of the hips—bilateral

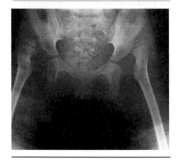

Diagnosis — Congenital dislocation of the hip

In spite of hip screening programmes, a small number will be detected between the ages of 1 and 4 years because of an abnormality of gait. Typically the parents say that either the child is reluctant to walk independently or that she (it is six times more common in girls) is doing so but is noticed to have an uneven gait. Bilateral cases are likely to be missed for longer than unilateral for although the gait is abnormal it is symmetrically so. Examination of the child shows an apparent shortening of the leg, additional posterior thigh creases and limitation of abduction of the hip in flexion. X-ray or ultrasound confirms the diagnosis.

Treatment. Skin traction should be applied for a period of at least 3 weeks. This can be done nursing the child either on a 40° inclined mattress, on gallows traction or on a frame. After 3 weeks, an adductor tenotomy is carried out, and the adequacy of reduction assessed clinically and radiologically. If this is satisfactory, maintenance of the reduction, usually in the 'frog' position, is achieved using a plaster of Paris hip spica. A Salter or a femoral osteotomy may be necessary, to contain the head. Major surgery is much more likely when the child presents after 1 year with complete dislocation. Early osteoarthrosis is a complication.

Problem
- A common complaint is of a 10–15-year-old boy who has pain in one or both knees particularly on exercise. The site of the tibial tubercle is warm, tender and painful.

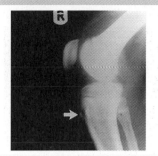

Osgood–Schlatter disease

Diagnosis — Osgood–Schlatter disease

A history of discomfort on climbing stairs is very typical. The knee joint itself is entirely normal. Quadriceps contraction against resistance will reproduce the pain. X-rays will eventually show irregularity and fragmentation of the epiphyses with overlying soft tissue swelling. It is considered to be a traction apophysitis.

Treatment depends on the severity of the symptoms, since the condition will eventually resolve spontaneously. If symptoms are severe, a plaster of Paris cylinder for 4–6 weeks may be necessary; if not so severe, restriction of physical activities, such as running, football and excessive stair climbing, may be all that is necessary. There are no long term problems after fusion has occurred (at 17–19 years).

Problem

- Less frequently there is a history of acute bone pain which is worse at night. Local bone tenderness with warmth, and muscle wasting may become obvious only after several months.
- X-ray shows a central lucent area surrounded by a more dense area and periosteal new bone giving rise to cortical thickening.
- Blood investigations are normal.

Diagnosis — Osteoid osteoma

Anti-inflammatory drugs relieve the pain in this benign and eventually self-limiting condition. Excision of the central nidus of rarefaction is so immediately curative that it is normally considered the treatment of choice. Bone pain of increasing persistence, particularly if associated with local tenderness, striking muscle wasting and general systemic disturbance, should alert one to the possibility of a malignant lesion. These include *osteosarcomas* which occur mostly between the ages of 12 and 20 years, *Ewing tumour* arising especially in long bone diaphyses and *secondary neuroblastomas* in those under the age of 4 years.

Problem

- Flitting polyarthralgia.
- Later large-joint arthritis (rarely small-joint).

Diagnosis — Lyme disease

Borrelia burgdorferi is the causative spirochaete. Diagnosis is by antibody detection.

Treatment. Amoxycillin should be given for 1 month at least.

Problem

- A limp, and
- Joint swelling.

Diagnosis — Juvenile chronic arthritis (JCA) and juvenile rheumatoid arthritis (JRA)

This is a heterogeneous group of diseases with arthritis as a common feature. The younger girl may have a history of a recurrent stiff neck.

On examination there is often peri-articular joint swelling with effusion. Limitation of movement occurs and in the lower limb weight is often borne on the opposite leg. ANA and slit-lamp examinations can help with the diagnosis.

The older boy may have a single swollen knee and a family history of HLA B27 related disease. Sacro-iliac changes are not seen until late adolescence.

Management. With the use of splints, joints should be kept in a good functional position both during rest and use. Physiotherapy and hydrotherapy should help maintain both a full range of movements and muscle strength. Anti-inflammatory treatment should be started: Naprosyn 20 mg/kg/day in 2 doses, or ibuprofen 20–40 mg/kg/day in 4 doses.

Prognosis

Polyarticular onset. Most children will have a good long-term outlook:

Pauciarticular onset:

1. The majority of these will have a good outcome but rarely they may develop blindness or severe joint problems.
2. Many of the boys will have continuous disease in adulthood and may develop juvenile ankylosing spondylitis.

Juvenile rheumatoid arthritis. Rapid progression can occur. Second line drugs are often started at diagnosis, i.e. gold, sulphasalazine or methotrexate.

SINGLE OR MULTIPLE FRACTURES — PATHOLOGICAL OR IN UNUSUAL POSITIONS

Problem

- Many fractures of different ages in a pre-mobile infant.

Diagnosis — Child abuse

Fractures as a manifestation of child abuse most frequently occur in pre-school children, particularly in those under the age of 18 months. Frequently, more than one fracture is found and therefore skeletal surveys should be undertaken to identify any asymptomatic fractures. Fractures may appear to be of varying age, implying repeated abuse. Burns and significant bruising often around the head and neck can be seen along with fractures. Rib fractures without known chest trauma suggest child abuse. Gripping and twisting injuries frequently produce spiral or oblique fractures of the long bones or subperiosteal new bone formation. Spiral fractures of the humeral shaft are frequently caused by such abuse. Traction injuries seem to produce metaphyseal chip fractures. Child abuse may be suggested from the clinical presentation and fracture pattern. Other causes of pathological fracture always need to be considered. Involvement of other statutory agencies is mandatory if child abuse is considered. This should lead to prompt interdisciplinary discussion leading to an overall management plan. This must occur along with appropriate medical care.

Problem

- Child who has abnormally fragile bones.
- Fractures occurring in utero or in early childhood.
- Abnormally blue sclerae.
- Hyperextensible joints.

Diagnosis — Osteogenesis imperfecta

There are different degrees of severity of bone density. Type II is always lethal from multiple prenatal fractures giving a stillborn child. Others may be born with multiple fractures and obvious deformities (often with palpable callus at the site of the fractures) and there may be evidence of brain damage sustained during delivery due to the extreme fragility of the vault of the skull. The other forms of the condition present at some time during childhood. Where there is a family history of the condition, it may be recognised in the child before a fracture has occurred by certain other features, including blue sclerae, hyperextensible joints, ocular defects, fine hair, growth retardation and translucent hypoplastic milk teeth. These features, however, may not be obvious (or necessarily present), and the condition may be brought to light by a pathological fracture occurring with minimal trauma.

Osteogenesis imperfecta

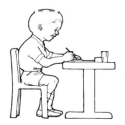

Skeletal deformities
  due to multiple fractures
Blue sclera—
  of no significance
Malformation—
  in temporal bone ?deafness
Misformed—
  pointed teeth

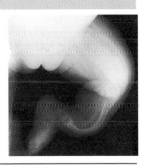

Investigation. X-rays show slender, fragile-looking osteoporotic bones with evidence of bending due to the physiological stresses of weight bearing (in the pelvis, femora and tibiae) and breathing (in the ribs).

Treatment. Immobilisation of fractures for any length of time increases the degree of osteoporosis, and therefore the risk of further fractures. The varus deformity of the femur and tibia also predisposes to fracture. Intramedullary nailing for fracture reduction and correction of varus deformity has many advantages. After healing has occurred, the nail adds some strength to the bone in the long term but will need to be replaced as growth occurs. It is not a technique suitable for very severely affected children.

The prognosis. This is extremely poor in the prenatally occurring condition, but better in the later onset form, in whom a reasonably normal life span may be predicted. One must aim to prevent deformity during childhood; the tendency to fracture with minimal trauma lessens after puberty. Severe kyphoscoliosis may eventually occur.

Problem

- The pathological fracture is associated with highly dense bone on X-ray, often with loss of the marrow cavity.

Diagnosis — Osteopetrosis

This is a sclerosing bone dysplasia. The bones are very brittle, although less likely to fracture than in osteogenesis imperfecta. The condition may be diagnosed at any age from the prenatal period but usually during adolescence. Clinically there is aplastic anaemia, hepatosplenomegaly and lymphadenopathy. Various bony foramina may become narrowed, leading to cranial nerve palsies and hydrocephalus. Some growth retardation is likely and dental caries is common. X-rays show a dense structureless appearance to all bones.

Treatment is that of fractures, anaemia and bone infection. Fracture healing tends to be delayed (unlike osteogenesis imperfecta in which healing is a relatively normal process).

Prognosis depends very largely on the degree of anaemia. Severely affected children are likely to die during childhood; the less severely affected survive, but may develop hydrocephalus, blindness, deafness, fractures and deformities. The anaemia may recur in later life.

DEFORMITY — CONGENITAL AND ACQUIRED

Deformity or skeletal disproportion may be the principal reason for a child's initial referral. It is likely to be non-urgent (except in a neonate) and the cause may be a congenital anomaly although occasionally acquired. Growth retardation may or may not be present.

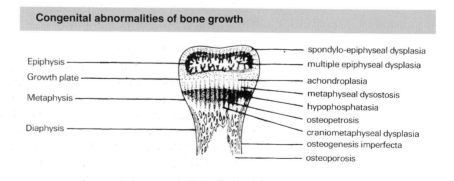

Congenital abnormalities of bone growth

Epiphysis
Growth plate
Metaphysis
Diaphysis

spondylo-epiphyseal dysplasia
multiple epiphyseal dysplasia
achondroplasia
metaphyseal dysostosis
hypophosphatasia
osteopetrosis
craniometaphyseal dysplasia
osteogenesis imperfecta
osteoporosis

Problem 1st Pattern

Features of achondroplasia

Normal size trunk
Frontal, parietal and occipital bossing
Short cranial base
Bridge of nose wide and flattened
Hydrocephalus may develop
Short limbs, especially proximally
Broad palm of hands
Short fingers
Broad shoulders
Narrow rib cage
Lumbar lordosis
Waddling gait

- The first cause of restricted growth and deformity is readily recognised. The marked lordosis is due to lumbar vertebral wedging while the resultant forward tilt of the pelvis produces prominence of the abdomen and the buttocks. There is a typical waddling gait. Hydrocephalus may be present.

Diagnosis — Achondroplasia

This condition is quite common and is usually recognised at or shortly after birth. It is the most common form of adult dwarfism, with no associated learning difficulties, the adult height usually being about 130 cm. There are some lethal forms of dwarfism, i.e. thanatophoric dwarf. X-rays show abrupt flaring of the metaphyseal ends of the long bones, with a narrow growth plate and a relatively large broad epiphysis. The metaphysis may be wedged and partially invest the epiphysis. The pedicles of the vertebrae are shorter and thicker than normal, sometimes resulting in narrowing of the spinal canal sufficient to produce cord compression.

Treatment. This is symptomatic, i.e. osteotomy for severe bow leg. Bone lengthening procedures can give useful additional height.

Problem 2nd Pattern

- The typical features become obvious as the child starts to walk. A severe degree of kyphosis and lordosis develops, with hypermobile enlarged joints, knock-knee and flat foot deformities and a waddling gait. Dwarfism is marked.

Diagnosis — MPS Morquio

This is a storage disorder with no associated intellectual impairment. X-rays show flattened vertebral bodies (with an irregular contour and a central anterior projection. The femoral capital epiphyses are irregular, flattened and fragmented, and there is coxa vara.) Treatment is symptomatic.

Problem 3rd Pattern

In early childhood the coarse facial appearance develops with a big tongue, large head and a short neck. A protruding abdomen with large liver and spleen; fixed flexion deformities of the hips and knees which, with the gross kyphosis of the spine and general growth retardation, result in restricted growth.

Diagnosis — MPS Hurler

This is another mucopolysaccharide disorder. X-rays of the spine will distinguish Hurlers from Morquios. In Hurlers the anterior projection from the vertebral body is from the lower border, not centrally. Hip X-rays show a greatly increased neck/shaft angle (coxa valga) which, together with acetabular dysplasia, may result in hip dislocation. Urine assay will show dermatan sulphate and heparin sulphate.

Treatment. Up to now treatment has not been indicated, except occasionally to make nursing easier.

Hurler syndrome

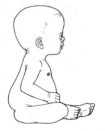

coarse facies

clouding of cornea

macroglossia

skeletal deformity

physical and mental retardation

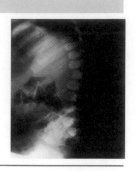

Problem 4th Pattern

- A further condition, more common in boys and starting during early childhood, may be more marked on one side of the body. Failure of endochondral ossification results in persistence of cartilage in the metaphyses producing expansion, usually initially in the region of the major joints, but also in the facial bones, pelvis and most strikingly in the small long bones of the hands. Limb length may be affected, and gross deformity may occur especially of the hands. The cartilaginous expansions in the hand bones frequently result in pathological fractures.

Diagnosis — Ollier disease

X-rays of the hands show globular lesions expanding the bones and thinning or even transgressing the cortex. In the long bones the meta-physeal lesions extend down into the diaphysis giving areas of alternating lucent and less lucent longitudinal striations. If one of the metaphyseal lesions reaches the surface of the bone, it grows towards the epiphysis rather than the diaphysis (the reverse of diaphyseal aclasis).

Treatment. Hand lesions that are seriously affecting function should be trimmed and curetted, with grafting if necessary. Only the most troublesome lesions must be selected, since it is impossible to deal with them all. Leg length inequality may be improved by a leg lengthening or shortening procedure. Intellect and life expectancy are normal, but the degree of disability, especially of hand function, may be considerable.

Problem 5th Pattern

- Other children present with hard bony outgrowths, usually near the epiphyses.

Diagnosis — Diaphyseal aclasis

This is a relatively common disorder, again more common in boys, and usually presenting because of deformity in middle childhood. Often the initial lumps may be in the region of the knee, shoulder or wrist, i.e. the most actively growing ends of the long bones. They can also occur in the scapula, iliac, clavicle and even in the base of the skull. A patient may have up to 20 separate exostoses. The cartilage-capped exostoses arise as a result of failure of proper modelling at the metaphysis, but with further growth the lesions migrate away from the epiphysis towards the diaphysis, becoming elongated or even pedunculated. They may cause local retardation of growth, or even cessation of growth and deformity. Sometimes joint movement is affected. X-rays are diagnostic. The lesions may be symmetrical on the two sides of the body.

Treatment. This is essentially symptomatic, the lesions that are causing trouble should be removed, but the need for osteotomy or limb inequality procedures is likely to be much less than in dyschondroplasia. Sarcomatous change can occur in adolescence, but the risk is probably not great. However, if a lesion which has remained unchanged for years suddenly starts to grow rapidly again, the possibility of malignant change should be seriously considered.

Problem

- A group of particularly distressing children are born with gross distortion of their limbs not due to underlying fractures.

Diagnosis — Arthrogryposis multiplex congenita (amyoplasia, myodystrophica fetalis)

This rare and ill-understood condition may be a congenital failure of muscle development, or a prenatal degeneration of normally developed muscles due to some neuromuscular disease process. Whatever the cause, the result is severe multiple joint deformities, of both arms and legs, and sometimes also of the spine, with normal skin sensation.

Treatment. Passive stretching, manipulation and splintage should be started from birth. Surgery may be needed to improve function.

Problem

- A frequent congenital abnormality involves the foot and ankle, with varying degrees of equinus or calcaneus and varus or valgus deformity.

Diagnosis — Clubfoot

The incidence of this condition in the otherwise normal child is 1.2 per 1000 live births, more commonly in boys. Most of the clubfoot deformities are a talipes equinovarus; 1% are a talipes calcaneovalgus with vertical talus. In talipes equinovarus ankle joint movement is reduced by 50% and the tendo Achilles, tibialis posterior and flexor hallucis longus tendons are all shortened.

Treatment is urgent and should start on the day of birth. It may include not only serial plasters, but also soft tissue and bone surgery. Serial weekly plaster of Paris plasters are applied for 6 weeks, when an open operation may be done if necessary on the tendo Achilles to correct the equinus. Manipulation and Robert Jones strapping is then continued to correct the varus. Further soft tissue procedures such as tendon transplant may be necessary later. Persistent deformity in early childhood may necessitate bony procedures such as a triple arth-rodesis after most of the growth of the foot has taken place. Talipes calcaneovalgus with vertical talus is considerably more difficult to treat, and surgery is always necessary.

Manipulation of clubfoot

① Hold   Move ➡   ② Hold   Move

Prognosis is very variable. Some clubfeet correct to almost complete normality and size, others are very difficult to correct, require multiple surgery and will always be smaller than normal.

Problem

Some children, particularly infants or adolescents of Asian origin, present with:

- Swollen wrists and ankles.
- Distortion of the legs with bowing of the tibia and femur.
- A rickety rosary (enlargement of the anterior ends of the ribs).
- Raised alkaline phosphatase, low serum phosphate and normal or reduced serum calcium.

Disordered bone growth in rickets

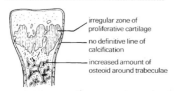

irregular zone of proliferative cartilage

no definitive line of calcification

increased amount of osteoid around trabeculae

Diagnosis — Rickets

Classically this was the name given to the infantile condition, formerly so common, caused by an inadequate dietary intake of vitamin D. Similar clinical and radiographic features may be seen however in children whose dietary intake of vitamin D is adequate, but in whom there are other problems of calcium and phosphorus uptake, retention or utilisation due to renal or gut problems.

Rickets due to inadequate oral intake of vitamin D is now uncommon in its florid form. It occurs in the young infant but the deformities may not be recognised by the parents until the child is walking, by which time there is likely to be gross femoral and tibial bowing with bowleg, or less commonly a severe knock-knee deformity due to muscle weakness and lax ligaments. The other classical features are delayed closure of the anterior fontanelle, frontal skull bossing, a rickety rosary, swollen wrists and ankles and a pot belly. Growth retardation is present but not severe. X-rays of the wrists will confirm the diagnosis. The growth plate is wide, the metaphysis expanded and cupped, calcification is diminished producing an osteoporotic appearance, and the appearance of the secondary centre of ossification in the epiphyses is delayed.

Treatment. This is oral vitamin D supplementation together with correction of the diet. A dosage of 1500–5000 IU/day will produce rapid clinical improvement and evidence of X-ray healing in 2–4 weeks. The prognosis for complete resolution of the deformities is good in the very young child, but obviously becomes less so with increasing age of presentation.

Problem

Some children have the clinical features of rickets with:

- Adequate oral intake of vitamin D.
- Renal failure.

Diagnosis — Renal osteodystrophy

The clinical features are similar to those of vitamin D deficiency rickets, but the child is older. Growth retardation is much more marked and knock-knee more common than bowleg. There will usually be other evidence of renal disease, i.e. thirst, polyuria and general debility. Factors which may be implicated are the diminished gut absorption of calcium seen in chronic renal disease, stimulation of the parathyroids by the resultant low serum calcium to mobilise skeletal calcium excessively, impaired glomerular filtration of phosphates resulting in hyperphosphatasia and the possible presence of vitamin D antagonists in the blood in chronic azotaemic states. Investigations will show evidence of renal disease, with anaemia and acidosis and a high phosphorous and low calcium in the blood. X-rays may show evidence of hyperparathyroidism as well as those of classical rickets.

Treatment. Large doses of vitamin D will improve calcium absorption from the gut and will therefore improve or heal the skeletal changes. Great care needs to be taken however, since any tendency to hypercalcaemia will obviously be highly dangerous. The oral dosage recommended is in the order of 25 000–250 000 IU/day initially, going on to a maintenance dosage of 10 000 IU/day. The serum calcium must be monitored very regularly to avoid the risk of further renal damage.

Problem

- Adequate intake of vitamin D.
- No renal failure but a renal tubular defect(s).

Diagnosis — Either (a) Vitamin D resistant or phosphaturic rickets or (b) Fanconi syndrome

Again, the clinical features are similar to vitamin D deficiency rickets but are usually not noticed until the child is walking, and the child may not present medically until 3 or 4 years old. Bowleg or knock-knee may occur, sometimes unilaterally. There is always retardation of growth. The underlying abnormality in the renal tubules may be a defect of phosphate reabsorption alone (phosphaturic rickets) or it may be a more complex primary or secondary defect in the reabsorption of phosphate, glucose and amino acid (Fanconi syndrome).

Treatment of phosphaturic rickets is by oral vitamin D 50 000–100 000 IU/day depending on age, with extremely careful monitoring of the serum calcium. It may be impossible to give a dose of vitamin D high enough to restore normal growth and prevent further deformity, without producing hypercalcaemia. There is a place for external splintage and intramedullary nailing to try to diminish deformity.

Treatment of Fanconi syndrome depends on the exact nature of the multiple tubular defect, and of the underlying causative disorder. Oral vitamin D in a dosage similar to that for phosphaturic rickets is usually appropriate (with the same proviso about serum calcium monitoring), except where the underlying pathology is cystinosis. In this case the best treatment for the bone disease is phosphate administration, vitamin D being used only with extreme care.

Rickets may also occur due to malabsorptive states resulting in impaired absorption or utilisation of vitamin D.

SPINAL DEFORMITY — CONGENITAL OR ACQUIRED

Problem

- Deformity of the spine (often picked up on routine medical examination).

Causes of scoliosis

Idiopathic
Congenital vertebral anomalies
Neurofibromatosis
Unilateral muscle paralysis
Unilateral irradiation damage to vertebral

Diagnosis — Scoliosis

This may be postural (secondary to leg length inequality, pain or muscle weakness, in which case there is no spinal rotation) or structural where there is curvature of the spine with rotation of the vertebrae bodies towards the convexity of the curve. In a structural scoliosis the curve persists when the child is asked to touch his/her toes, and the ribs will be humped on the convex side of the curve. Structural scoliosis is always important, postural never (except to find and treat the cause). Any curvature of the spine noted in an infant must be followed up until the age of at least 1 year. The majority of these idiopathic infantile scolioses will have resolved completely by the time the child walks, but if they do not, they go on to a relatively severe form with a poor prognosis. Various patterns of the disease process are seen with

Spinal curvature

Kyphosis   Lordosis   Scoliosis (Rt)   Scoliosis (Lt)

differing ages of onset and levels of spinal involvement. X-rays of the spine are done with careful measurement of the angle of the primary curve.

Treatment. In general if the curvature is less than 20°, one can watch and wait, if 20–40° a Milwaukee brace will hold 70% of cases, and if greater than 50° fusion is likely to be necessary with or without a Harrington rod. Prognosis will depend on the age of onset, the spinal level and the age at which treatment starts. The younger the child at onset and the higher the curve the worse the prognosis. Timely preventative surgery is infinitely preferable to later corrective surgery.

| **Problem** | • Less commonly children have a posterior curve of the spine. |

Diagnosis — Kyphosis, lordosis

This occurs sometimes in young infants with Morquio–Brailsford syndrome, achondroplasia, and juvenile osteoporosis, and of course is normal in all babies when they first start to sit. *Adolescent kyphosis (Scheuermann disease, vertebral osteochondritis)* is very common mainly in boys over 12 years and usually presents because of the round-shouldered appearance and backache. On examination forward spinal flexion and straight leg raising are limited. X-rays show anterior wedging of the vertebral bodies of the lower thoracic and upper lumbar spine, with increased density and later fragmentation of the ring epiphyses especially anteriorly. The disc spaces may be narrow. The adjacent metaphyseal regions are less dense than normal especially anteriorly.

Treatment is symptomatic, i.e. short periods of rest and restriction of activities for episodes of severe backache. It is doubtful whether it is possible to influence the natural history of the disease or the final degree of kyphosis by other measures, except in very rapidly progressive cases. Backache may recur in adult life due to secondary osteoarthritic change

BACK PAIN

Back pain in young people	
Tumours	Cushing disease
Infection	Spondylolisthesis
Disc protrusion	Osteochondritis
Discitis	Injury
Osteoporosis	Posture
idiopathic	Psychologica
iatrogenic (steroid)	
immobility	

Problem

- Back pain.
- Unwillingness to stand or walk.

Diagnosis — Back pain ?Seek a cause

Children under the age of 10 rarely complain of persistent back pain and should not be accepted as being psychological. If there is muscle spasm and loss of movement then there is invariably serious underlying pathology. A full history and examination should be taken thinking of underlying malignancy. Full neurological examination must be included. Spinal X-rays should include many levels higher than the perceived area of pain, spinal MRI is often needed. In older children (10 years and over) there may be structural problems or sports injuries. It is always important to know if there is a friend or family member with backache and if it has followed an injury, whether there is any ongoing compensation claim and disability. Psychological back pain may hurt all over. Structural causes need to be excluded and the depth of investigation balanced by the amount of psychosocial pathology.

Problem

- Pain in back and leg.

Diagnosis (1) — Adolescent disc protrusion

Examination of the teenager with a disc protrusion reveals an abnormal gait and tilted posture, together with lumbar muscle spasm and restricted straight leg raising. X-rays of the lumbar spine may show some disc narrowing. Bed rest in the acute stage, followed by mobilisation with a plaster of Paris jacket or corset support, and exercises are usually adequate. Surgery will ultimately be necessary in about 30%.

Disorders of gait

Hysterical gait
Fibromyalgia
Postviral syndrome
Sympathetic reflex algodystrophy
Chronic fatigue syndrome

Diagnosis (2) — Spondylolisthesis

Examination of the teenager with spondylolisthesis shows limitation of forward flexion of the spine with asymmetry, limited straight leg raising and local tenderness. In severe cases one can palpate the step caused by the forward slip of L5 or S1 with resultant prominence of the spine of L5 and sacrum, with a hollow above. X-rays, AP, lateral and oblique, of the lumbosacral spine will confirm the diagnosis. If the presentation is acute and especially if there is evidence of root pressure, surgery is likely to be necessary, that is a decompression procedure ± fusion. If the presentation is not acute, conservative management by a corset support may be sufficient, but the child must be X-rayed regularly until growth has ceased to determine if the degree of slip is increasing. The incidental finding of a child with an asymptomatic spondylolisthesis requires follow up until growth has ceased but function may remain full and symptom free. Back problems in adult life may persist in either disc protrusion or spondylolisthesis if the degree of slip has been severe.

Problem

- Tiredness.
- Disturbed sleep pattern.
- Muscle aching.
- Inability to attend school.
- Laboured gait.
- Joint pains.
- Depression.

Diagnosis — Possibly chronic fatigue syndrome

Management. An intense physiotherapy mobilisation regimen. Many children and young people present with a combination of these problems. They either require a diagnosis or are already labelled by a doctor or the family. Terms used are post viral syndrome, chronic fatigue syndrome, ME, fibromyalgia or school refuser. Serious treatable pathology needs to be excluded. When it is decided that this diagnostic fatigue spectrum is relevant then further opinions and investigations should be stopped immediately. Currently there are no useful routine investigations helpful, so many children referred for a second opinion may need no laboratory investigations. It is important to know why a young person has been referred and what expectations both they and the family have from the consultation. Debating the diagnostic label is not worth starting but management is.

First these young people and their families need to be reassured that this illness pattern has been seen before and that with their commitment to work with professionals then there is every reason why they should be able to return, in time, to full function and health. The process may be long, with retrograde steps, and is invariably hard work for everyone, not only the patient.

These young people need to re-educate their sleep pattern, which requires a structured programme that does not include watching the television until midnight. Co-operation of the young person and all family members in adhering to a daily timetable is what will lead to successful rehabilitation. Anti-depressants, sleeping tablets or a psychiatric referral are occasionally needed, particularly if there is ongoing psychodynamic triggers. The physiotherapist and teachers are the key personnel in mobilisation. Daily attendance at a hospital school with an integrated programme of a sickness to a well behaviour programme is often needed. Occasionally hospital admission will be required because of geography. It is important that the young person negotiates the programme with the staff and that the parents are not involved in the implementation of the work during school hours.

There needs to be objective ways of monitoring progress with clear documentation in part to show the young person their recovery. Some children need to be able to get better without losing face. It may be important to offer a treatment not given before to allow them to improve initially. The concept of a downward spiral of ill health moving to an upward spiral of well being is often worth discussing, but making the transition depends on their confidence in the rehabilitation team.

FURTHER READING

Cassidy JT 1994 Textbook of pediatric rheumatology, 3rd edn Saunders, London

Jacobs JC 1993 Pediatric rheumatology for the practitioner, 2nd edn. Springer-Verlag, Berlin

Schaller JG 1994 Pediatric and heritable disorders. Current Opinion in Rheumatology 6: 509–546

Schaller JG 1995 Pediatric and heritable disorders. Current Opinion in Rheumatology 7: 417–458

Tachdjian MO 1997 Clinical pediatric orthopedics. The art of diagnosis and principles of management. Appleton & Large, New York

Woo P 1990 Paediatric rheumatology update. Oxford University Press Oxford

Worlock P 1986 Patterns of fractures in accidental and non-accidental injury in children: a comparative study, British Medical Journal 293 (6539): 100–102

Wynne-Davies R 1995 Atlas of skeletal dysplasias. Churchill Livingstone, Edinburgh

18 Muscle and movement

All movements are produced by muscle contraction, but there are four main systems which contribute to that activity.

The pyramidal system is involved in conscious voluntary motor acts. Axons from pyramidal cells in the motor cortex of the frontal lobes travel varying distances to synapse in the motor nuclei in the brainstem (cortico-bulbar tracts) and anterior horns of the spinal cord (cortico-spinal tracts). Malfunction of this system causes spastic weakness.

The extrapyramidal system includes the basal ganglia and their various connections. It is involved in the unconscious adjustment and maintenance of postural tone. Malfunction of this system causes abnormal movements or postures.

The two proprioceptive systems are the cerebellum and its connections and the posterior columns of the spinal cord and their connections. The former is involved in the unconscious and the latter in the conscious monitoring of ongoing movement and motor activity. Malfunction of either system causes ataxia.

Each lower motor neurone unit comprises an anterior horn cell with an axon running in a peripheral nerve to supply neuromuscular junctions on several muscle fibres. One lower motor unit will serve three to six muscle fibres in a small muscle in the hand but about 2000 in a large muscle like the gastrocnemius. This is the final common path used in the generation of all movement. Malfunction of this system causes flaccid weakness.

The primary motor cortex, basal ganglia and lower motor neurone

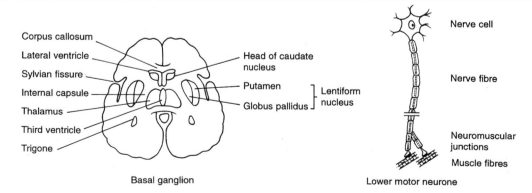

Corpus callosum
Lateral ventricle
Sylvian fissure
Internal capsule
Thalamus
Third ventricle
Trigone

Head of caudate nucleus
Putamen ⎤ Lentiform
Globus pallidus ⎦ nucleus

Basal ganglion

Nerve cell

Nerve fibre

Neuromuscular junctions
Muscle fibres

Lower motor neurone

Disorders of the motor systems may be acute (includes relapsing-remitting), chronic non-progressive or chronic progressive.

SPASTIC WEAKNESS

Spasticity is characterised by increased muscle tone of a 'clasp-knife' type, abnormally brisk tendon reflexes, loss of superficial reflexes (e.g. abdominals and cremasterics) and extensor plantar responses. It is thought to be due to the reduced central inhibition of the gamma motor system secondary to pyramidal system malfunction. When there is an *acute* lesion involving the motor cortex or pyramidal tracts in brain or spinal cord, there is often a period during which muscle tone is actually reduced in the paralysed limbs. This phenomenon is called cranial or spinal shock and may be confused with acute flaccid weakness of lower motor unit type. However tendon reflexes are usually retained, plantar reflexes are usually extensor and the limb is usually seen to withdraw reflexly to painful stimuli. Hypotonia due to cranial or spinal shock wears off after a few days and is replaced by increased tone of the clasp-knife type.

Problem

• Sudden weakness down one side.

Diagnosis — Acute hemiplegia ? Cause
Although an acute hemiplegia might theoretically result from a localised lesion of the pyramidal tract in the brainstem or spinal cord, in practice it is almost always caused by a lesion in one or other cerebral hemisphere. The arm is usually more affected than the leg. A visual field defect of the homonymous hemianopia type may be present and implies involvement of the lateral geniculate body, optic radiation or visual cortex on the opposite side of the brain. Dysphasia can be associated if the speech centres in the dominant hemisphere are affected.

The pathogenesis may be that of infarction from arterial or venous occlusion, infarction without occlusion (e.g. hypoxic-ischaemic insult), temporary ischaemia, haemorrhage into the brain, inflammatory damage to brain or blood vessels, or post-ictal.

— A family history of *hemiplegic migraine* would suggest this diagnosis, especially if the hemiparesis recovered within 24 hours and was associated with headache and vomiting at the onset.
— A preceding convulsion may suggest a *Todd paralysis*, especially if the hemiplegia recovers within 24 hours. Permanent hemiplegia may follow generalised or focal status epilepticus.
— A Negro child with an acute hemiplegia should be suspected of having *sickle cell disease* (Hb S-S) or *sickle-C disease* (HbS-C).
— A history of trauma to the neck or pharynx ('the pencil-in-the-mouth fall') may indicate *traumatic thrombosis* of one carotid artery.

— Preceding head trauma would suggest an *epidural* or *subdural haematoma*.
— Cranial bruits are often physiological in infancy but a loud one, especially if unilateral, would suggest an intracranial *arteriovenous malformation*.
— If the hemiplegia is due to haemorrhage from an arteriovenous malformation, neck stiffness may be present due to blood in the subarachnoid spaces. Neck stiffness might also suggest *purulent* or *tuberculous meningitis* (causing inflammatory intracranial arterial or venous thrombosis) or *herpes simplex encephalitis*.
— The finding of otitis especially if associated with mastoiditis suggests *cerebral venous thrombosis*.
— A history of learning difficulties and epilepsy with arachnodactyly, genu valgum, malar erythema and dislocated lenses would suggest *homocystinuria* in which thromboembolic episodes occur in about half the patients.
— Multiple *café-au-lait* patches and subcutaneous neurofibromata suggest *neurofibromatosis* which may be associated with stenosis or occlusion of the supraclinoid segment of the internal carotid artery.
— *Dehydration* (especially hypernatraemic) and the *thrombophilias* (e.g. protein S or C deficiency, anti-thrombin III deficiency) may predispose to venous or arterial thrombosis.
— The presence of cyanotic congenital heart disease (right to left shunt) suggests either cerebral arterial or venous thrombosis due to *polycythaemia* or *cerebral abscess*.
— Bacterial endocarditis or cardiac arrhythmia may produce *cerebral embolisation*, although this is rare in childhood.
— Acute hemiplegia is sometimes seen as a complication of *cardiac surgery* (especially open heart operations).
— *Clotting disorders* (e.g. haemophilia, thrombocytopenia) can underlie acute hemiplegia due to intracerebral bleeding.

Investigations. Certain investigations may be suggested by the initial assessment, e.g. ECG, echocardiogram, blood culture, haemoglobin electrophoresis and amino acid chromatography. CSF will help rule out suspected encephalitis or meningitis and might show evidence of subarachnoid haemorrhage. Lumbar puncture would, of course, be deferred if there was evidence of raised intracranial pressure. CT or MRI scan will diagnose cerebral infarction, arterial venous malformations with or without bleeding, epidural and subdural haemangiomas and cerebral abscess. The child with an acute hemiplegia of unknown cause whose scan is normal or shows cerebral infarction will require MR angiography or conventional catheter angiography. Such children may show:

— Stenosis of the supraclinoid part of the internal carotid artery and proximal parts of the anterior and middle cerebral arteries with telangiectatic collaterals in the region of the basal ganglia ('moya-moya disease').

— Stenosis of the origin of one internal carotid artery.
— Occlusion of the supraclinoid part of the internal carotid artery or one or more branch of the middle cerebral artery.
— Fibromuscular dysplasia or dissecting aneurysm of the intracranial arteries.
— Evidence of arteritic inflammation.
— A normal angiogram.

Carotid angiography is required pre-operatively in a child who has been shown to have an arterio-venous malformation on CT or MRI scan.

Right carotid angiogram showing frontal arteriovenous malformation

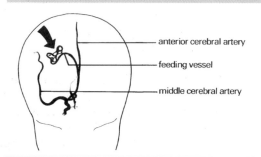
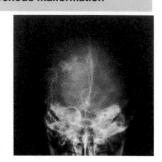

anterior cerebral artery

feeding vessel

middle cerebral artery

Management. Surgery would be required for children with arterio-venous malformations, cerebral abscesses, and epidural or subdural haematomas. Surgery might also be considered for the child with stenosis of the origin of one internal carotid artery or the child with moya-moya disease. Hemispherectomy may be required for children with intractable seizures following an acute hemiplegia in infancy. Venesection will reduce symptomatic polycythaemia in cyanotic congenital heart disease. Antiepileptic drugs would be required for epilepsy. Homo-cystinuria is treated with pyridoxine or a low methenamine diet. Low dosage aspirin may reduce the risk of recurrence in those children with abnormalities on angiography. Physiotherapy should be aimed at increasing use of the affected limbs and preventing contractures.

Prognosis is very variable. When associated with generalised or focal status epilepticus at the onset, the prognosis for recovery of the hemiplegia is usually very poor and epilepsy may be difficult to control. Even when infarction is shown on scanning and arterial occlusion on angiography, a proportion of children make a full recovery and have no relapses. The finding of the 'moya-moya' appearance on angiography makes a relapsing-remitting course likely but not inevitable.

Problem   • Sudden weakness in both legs.

Diagnosis — Acute spastic paraplegia or quadriplegia ? Cause

Rapid development of weakness in both legs with inability to stand and walk is a paediatric emergency. In the early stages there is reduced muscle tone but a lower motor neurone lesion such as *Guillain–Barre syndrome* is usually excluded clinically by the finding of preserved tendon reflexes, extensor plantar responses and sensory loss with an upper level corresponding to the motor deficit.

— Neck stiffness suggests subarachnoid haemorrhage from a spinal angioma, meningitis secondary to a spinal epidural abscess, a post-infectious myelitis or atlanto-axial dislocation.
— A history of trauma is usual with a fracture-dislocation of the spine but this might not be forthcoming in non-accidental injury.
— Severe back pain or fever suggests spinal epidural abscess or post-infectious myelitis.
— A history of preceding viral illness (particularly chickenpox, mumps or measles) is common in children with a post-infectious myelitis.
— Hysterical paraplegia can cause diagnostic difficulties. Contraction of antagonists may be noted during attempted movement. There is no alteration in muscle tone or reflexes and no retention of urine. Apparent sensory loss is common but the sensory level does not usually comply with the dermatome map and it may be possible to show that it changes considerably during the course of the examination. History may reveal some obvious recent emotional upset but often this is not the case.

Prompt investigation is required for all cases of acute paraplegia with the possible exception of hysterical paraplegia. In the latter case it may be possible to be sufficiently certain of the diagnosis on clinical grounds to be able to avoid investigations which can sometimes serve to reinforce the symptoms.

Investigation

Plain spinal X-rays may show vertebral osteomyelitis in the case of an epidural abscess and should demonstrate an atlanto-axial dislocation if lateral cervical views are taken in flexion and extension.

Spinal MRI scan is the emergency imaging method of choice if available, but if not, *myelography* would be required. Both would be expected to demonstrate a haematomyelia associated with a spinal angioma or a spinal epidural abscess and show cord swelling associated with post-infectious myelitis, but only the MRI scan would show high signal in that area in the absence of cord swelling.

CSF would be sampled if myelography is carried out. The fluid is usually blood stained in the presence of a haematomyelia. A mild pleocytosis is common in both spinal epidural abscess and in post-infectious myelitis. Changes of a frankly purulent meningitis may occur if an epidural abscess has burst into the subarachnoid space. If spinal MRI scanning is carried out, it may not be necessary to do a diagnostic lumbar puncture which carries a risk of aggravating the paraplegia at least temporarily.

MRI spinal scan —postinfectious myelitis. High signal and swelling in the cervical region

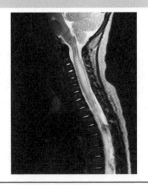

Spinal angiography may be required pre-operatively to demonstrate the extent of a spinal angioma.

Management

Children with acute paraplegia associated with a spinal angioma require neurosurgery to evacuate any haematomyelia and ligate the arteries feeding the angioma. In skilled hands a few children make a fair recovery. Post-infectious myelitis is managed medically. Dexamethasone probably aids recovery particularly when there is marked cord swelling. About 60% of children will have a good return of function and only 15% fail to show any improvement. Spinal epidural abscess represents a surgical emergency treated by laminectomy, decompression and drainage. Antibiotic therapy is given for at least 6 weeks to treat the underlying vertebral osteomyelitis. The prognosis for full recovery is good if treatment is prompt. Hysterical paraplegia is best treated by a doctor who is sufficiently confident of the diagnosis to be able to suggest to the child and parents that such conditions are not uncommon and that full recovery is to be expected within a short time. 'No-nonsense' physiotherapy with incremental goals may have a part to play. Usually the child is back to normal in a few days or weeks and has no permanent psychiatric disorder. Occasionally psychiatric referral is required in the presence of overt emotional disturbance or if invalidism seems to be a danger.

Problem

• Longstanding, non-progressive spastic weakness.

Hemiplegia

Posture

Posture in left hemiplegia

Spastic hand

Diagnosis — Cerebral palsy ? Cause

Cerebral palsy is usually the cause and implies damage to or malformation of the motor areas of the brain occurring before birth or during the first few years of life. The pathology is permanent and non-progressive, although the clinical picture may change during life. The disabilities produced interfere with normal motor development and there may be other complicating neurological or mental features. Very rarely a chronic non-progressive spastic paraplegia or quadriplegia may be due to damage to the spinal cord occurring before or during birth.

Hemiplegic cerebral palsy is not usually diagnosed until a baby is 6–8 months old when it is noted that one hand is being used to reach out to grasp much more than the other which is kept fisted. Later it becomes more obvious that there is little spontaneous movement of the affected arm which is held flexed at the elbow, adducted at the shoulder and shows increased muscle tone and reflexes. The leg on the same side is also found to be affected but less severely so than the arm. Congenital hemiplegic cerebral palsy is usually due to damage to one hemisphere some time during pregnancy. The commonest finding on scanning is that of a porencephalic cyst in the distribution of the middle cerebral artery suggesting old infarction in that area.

Quadriplegic cerebral palsy. Infants with this condition tend to keep both hands fisted most of the time and the arms adducted at the shoulders. They fail to reach out to grasp with either hand at the usual time despite normal visual following and sitting is usually delayed. Posture in ventral suspension is almost too good with the back straight and the head above the plane of the body. However there is still marked head lag when the infant is pulled from the lying to sitting position. Muscle tone and reflexes are increased more in the arms than in the legs. Later on walking is delayed and feeding and speech may be affected if there is spasticity of the tongue, lips and palate. Causes include cerebral malformation syndromes, autosomal recessive inheritance, hypoxic-ischaemic insults, encephalitis, meningitis and trauma.

Diplegic cerebral palsy. This affects the legs much more than the arms which only may be minimally affected. It commonly occurs in preterm babies and is considered to be due to hypoxic-ischaemic damage occurring before 36 weeks' gestation. The white matter near the lateral aspects of the lateral ventricles is particularly vulnerable at this time because of the immature circulation. Damage in this area is called periventricular leukomalacia. Occasionally this can happen in utero without the baby being born prematurely and this probably explains the few children with spastic diplegia who are born at term. Pulling to stand and walking is usually delayed. Both legs are noted to become rigidly extended and scissor in vertical suspension. Tone is particularly increased in the calf muscles and there may be ankle clonus. When supported the baby can bear the full body weight on the legs but 'goes up onto the toes'. When independent walking is achieved it tends to be with the help of aids and there is a tendency to be flexed and scissor at the hips, flexed at the knees and up on the toes.

Associated problems

Children with cerebral palsy often have associated handicaps, this is one of the reasons why such children require very careful assessment if all the problems are going to be managed optimally. The following are some of the more frequent associated handicaps:

Learning difficulties. Some degree of learning difficulty is seen in about 60% of children with cerebral palsy. It tends to be more common amongst children with spastic quadriplegia than hemiplegia or diplegia. It should never be forgotten that children with very severe cerebral palsy may sometimes have normal learning skills.

Epilepsy occurs in about a third of patients. Generalised tonic clonic seizures are the commonest seizure type but any kind may occur including simple and complex partial seizures, absence seizures, drop attacks and infantile spasms.

Visual impairment is due to errors of refraction, disuse amblyopia or optic atrophy and is seen in some 20% of children with cerebral palsy. Squint due to external ocular muscle imbalance or a paralysis occurs in about a third of these children.

Perceptual defects largely involve visual perception and occur in a high proportion of children with cerebral palsy. This is one reason why some cerebral palsied children do less well in school than might be expected by their assessed abilities.

Shortening of Achilles tendon

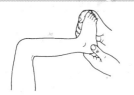

passive dorsiflexion; knee flexed tests contracture of soleus

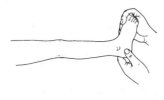

passive dorsiflexion; knee extended tests gastrocnemius contracture

Hearing loss occurs to some degree in about 10%. This used to be a bigger problem in the past when more children were seen with choreoathetosis following kernicturus.

Speech disorders are common and due to a variety of causes, including hearing loss, specific language disorders, learning difficulties, and inco-ordination of tongue, palate and lip movements used in speech production.

Behaviour disorders may be due to the frustrations of being handicapped, to strained family life brought on by the presence of a handicapped child or to the hyperactive distractable type of behaviour disorder which may be more fundamentally associated with brain damage.

Orthopaedic deformities tend to arise because of longstanding muscle weakness and spasticity. Scoliosis and dislocation of the hips may develop. Fixed contractures are liable to produce flexion and adduction at the hips, flexion at the knees and equinus deformity at the ankles.

Social problems are common. The presence of a handicapped child in the family is liable to accentuate many of the everyday stresses to which a family is exposed. The way in which a family copes with these stresses has an important bearing on the outcome for a child with cerebral palsy.

Assessment & management

Care needs to be planned from the beginning, as soon as the diagnosis is suspected. It is probably best carried out by a team which includes a paediatrician, an orthopaedic surgeon, a community paediatrician, an ophthalmologist, an audiologist, an occupational therapist, a physiotherapist, a speech therapist, a psychologist and a social worker. From an early age it should be possible to identify and anticipate medical, psychological, social and educational problems so that plans can be made to try and minimise or avoid these. One very important initial step is to help the parents to accept emotionally as well as intellectually the reality of their situation so that they will then be more likely to encourage their child in a positive way to make use of his/her abilities rather than to overprotect or reject the child. Placement of such children in day nurseries or nursery schools with special provision for the handicapped child can be very helpful in encouraging socialisation and opportunity for creative play. It also helps the parents with the very definite physical and emotional strain of looking after a handicapped child.

Most children with cerebral palsy benefit from regular physiotherapy which aims to encourage motor development, to inhibit abnormal motor activity and to prevent the development of contractures from impaired muscle growth. The best results, as judged by improving independence, are obtained by enrolling the parents as therapists and giving them a programme to follow at home between visits to the department so that treatment is carried out on a daily basis. Splinting or callipering may be required if contractures threaten or to increase stability for a temporary period. Injection of botulinum toxin into over-acting spastic muscles is a promising new treatment for dynamic contractures. Even with adequate physiotherapy, longstanding muscle weakness or spasticity can produce fixed contractures. Surgical correction by muscle slides or transplants or tendon lengthening may be required for such fixed deformities.

The associated disorders that may require treatment are numerous. Strabismus may require orthoptic therapy or correction by operation. Epileptic seizures are treated by appropriate antiepileptic drugs. Some patients with behaviour disorder and specific learning difficulties may be helped by psychiatric treatment or remedial teaching. As the age of school entry approaches, help is required from the community paediatrician and educational psychologist members of the team to decide the most appropriate educational placement. This may be in a school for physically handicapped children, in an ordinary mainstream school, in a school for children with learning disabilities, or in a residential school catering for children with special needs which cannot be met otherwise.

The next major hurdle faced by a family with a child with cerebral palsy is that which occurs at the end of the school period when decisions have to be made about employment. Between a third and a half of patients with cerebral palsy may be expected to be gainfully employed on leaving school. An individual patient's chances of obtaining work will depend chiefly on the severity of the physical disabilities and any associated learning difficulties. Facilities for handicapped children leaving school who cannot find suitable work are not very extensive. There is room for more co-ordinated professional help for families with a handicapped child facing this hurdle. There is evidence that early diagnosis and sound management in early childhood is more likely to produce a school leaver who is realistic about the extent of his/her handicaps, determined to achieve as much independence as possible and therefore more likely to gain employment.

Problem	• Chronic progressive spastic weakness.

Although brain diseases may cause chronic progressive hemiplegia (hemispheric tumours, chronic unilateral encephalitis) or quadriparesis (leukodystrophies, cerebral SLE, brainstem tumours), these conditions are usually associated with dementia, changes in level of consciousness or seizures and are discussed elsewhere.

Problem	• Progressive weakness in legs with or without arm involvement.

Diagnosis — Chronic progressive spinal paraparesis or quadriparesis
Depending whether the lesion is below or above the cervical cord, the presentation is that of a progressive paraparesis or quadriparesis. The main concern is the possibility of a spinal tumour. Backache with root pains suggests an extramedullary or extradural tumour rather than an intramedullary tumour. The most common spinal tumours in childhood in order of frequency are: (1) *'developmental' tumours* (lipomas, dermoid cysts and teratomas); (2) *gliomas* (astrocytomas and ependymomas); (3) *metastatic tumours* (neuroblastoma, ependymoblastoma

and medulloblastoma), *lymphomas* or *leukaemias* which would usually occur during the later stages of these diseases so that the diagnosis would be suspected on clinical grounds; (4) *sarcomas*; (5) *neurofibromas* which might be suggested by the finding of multiple *café au lait* skin patches. A family history of chronic progressive paraplegia would make the diagnosis of *hereditary spastic paraplegia* likely. Sensory loss or early bladder involvement would be against this diagnosis. Cutaneous anomalies overlying the spine (hairy patch, vascular or pigmented naevi, dermal sinus or subcutaneous lipoma) would suggest *spinal dysraphism* with cord tethering or a 'developmental tumour'.

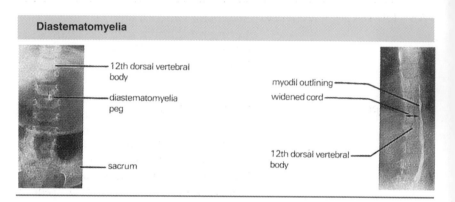

Diastematomyelia

12th dorsal vertebral body

diastematomyelia peg

sacrum

myodil outlining

widened cord

12th dorsal vertebral body

Investigations

Plain spinal X-rays. Increased interpedicular distance with or without erosion of the pedicles suggests a spinal tumour. Enlargement of an intervertebral foramen is sometimes seen with a neurofibroma or a neuroblastoma. Developmental vertebral anomalies (hemivertebrae, spina bifida occulta, vertebral fusion or duplication) usually accompany spinal dysraphism with cord tethering and may sometimes be seen with developmental tumours. A bony diastematomyelic peg may be clearly demonstrated.

Spinal imaging. This is best done as a spinal MRI scan but if not available, CT assisted myelography is necessary. It will be normal in hereditary spastic paraparesis. In hydromyelia the whole cord is enlarged and this is seen to be a dilated central canal on MRI scan. An abnormally low-lying conus medullaris is the hallmark of spinal dysraphism with cord tethering. A spinal tumour will be demonstrated and seen to be intramedullary, extramedullary or extradural.

Management

There is no curative treatment for hereditary spastic paraplegia, the recessive type of which progresses slowly so that walking is usually no longer possible by the third decade. Laminectomy is usually required if spinal imaging demonstrates a spinal tumour. Total or partial removal, biopsy or just decompression may be carried out depending on the operative finding. The prognosis depends on the kind of tumour, its operability and the amount of cord damage present before operation. Generally the extramedullary benign tumours (lipomas and dermoids) have an excellent prognosis following removal. The prognosis for intramedullary 'benign' tumours (astrocytoma and ependymoma) is not so good as excision can be difficult. The metastatic extramedullary tumours and lymphomas generally have a bad prognosis. Postoperative radiotherapy and/or chemotherapy is indicated in some cases.

In spinal dysraphism with cord tethering, laminectomy with division of the filum terminale, release of congenital bands and excision of any diastematomyelic peg or band usually prevents any further deterioration and there may be some improvement postoperatively.

ABNORMAL MOVEMENTS

Abnormal movements or postures suggest dysfunction of the extrapyramidal system.

Problem

- Shaking limbs.

Diagnosis — Tremor ? Cause
Tremor is an involuntary oscillating movement with a fixed frequency. It may be present with a limb relaxed (rest tremor), with a limb outstretched (postural tremor) or seen increasingly as a limb moves towards a goal (intentional tremor).

Physiological tremor is seen in most people under conditions of anxiety, fatigue or excitement. It is largely a postural tremor but is accentuated on movement and therefore has an intentional element.

Drug-induced tremor is very similar to physiological tremor and may be produced by adrenergic drugs given for asthma or attention deficit disorder, and it is also an uncommon but recognised side effect of the anti-epileptic drug sodium valproate. The tremor of hyperthyroidism is identical and can also be produced by overdosage with thyroxine.

Head injury. A largely postural tremor with intentional accentuation is seen quite commonly in children recovering from a concussional head injury.

Essential tremor. This is a common cause of tremor in childhood but is rare before the school years. There is often a family history of a similar disorder suggesting inheritance as an autosomal dominant with varying expression. It is a postural tremor with intentional accentuation and may cause problems with writing legibility. It is worse at times of anxiety. Some adults with essential tremor find it is improved with alcohol and there is a danger of alcoholism in such families. Schoolteachers may need to make allowances for written work, and in some affected children this is so bad as to require a word processor. The tremor can be improved considerably with a beta-adrenergic blocker such as propranolol, although it is not usually justified to have such a child on medication long term.

Cerebellar tremor. This is not present at rest or with a limb outstretched but is only seen during activity (intentional tremor). It may be seen with any cause of cerebellar ataxia.

Parkinsonian tremor. Parkinson disease is extremely rare in childhood but is one of the few causes of a coarse tremor present at rest which is reduced with posture and activity.

Problem

- Abnormal posturing of the limbs, trunk and face.

Diagnosis — Dystonia ?Cause

This is a disturbance caused by varying simultaneous contraction of agonist and anatagonist muscles. It may be focal or generalised. Dystonia may occur alone or together with choreoathetosis.

Dystonic cerebral palsy. This is sometimes known as cerebral palsy with variable muscle tone and may be associated with athetoid writhing movements. The commonest cause used to be damage to the basal ganglia from kernicterus due to hyperbilirubinaemia in the newborn period but with better treatment for rhesus incompatibility and neonatal jaundice, this cause is now very rare. Most cases seen nowadays have been due to an acute hypoxic ischaemic episode in the last trimester of pregnancy or during delivery, causing damage to the basal ganglia (status marmaratus).

Drug-induced dystonia. Some children are very sensitive to the extrapyramical side effects of phenothiazines (particularly the fluorine-containing compounds), haloperidol and metoclopramide. Possible reactions include trismus, opisthotonos, torticollis, difficulty with swallowing and oculogyric crisis. These acute reactions can be alarming but are usually self-limited or respond readily to treatment with an anti-cholinergic drug such as benztropine.

Idiopathic torsion dystonia is usually inherited as an autosomal dominant condition and is more common in Jewish children. The majority of gene carriers have developed symptoms before 30 years of age and in many of these the symptoms have started in childhood. Some cases are sporadic. It is a progressive disorder with increasing disability and most cases commencing in childhood are non-ambulant by middle age. CT and MRI scans show no abnormality and the diagnosis is clinical. Therapy with anticholergics may reduce the severity of the dystonia.

Dopa-sensitive dystonia (Segawa disease). This is a kind of idiopathic dystonia in which symptoms become progressively worse throughout the day and are much improved after a night's sleep.

Symptoms often start before school entry. It is important that this condition is recognised, as small doses of L-Dopa produce a dramatic improvement which is maintained.

Wilson disease is associated with the accumulation of copper in liver, brain and cornea. Hepatic involvement is the predominant presentation in the first decade but thereafter it may present as largely a neurological disorder with or without liver involvement. Dystonia, dysarthria and tremor are the commonest neurological features. The finding of Kayser–Fleischer rings is pathognomomic of Wilson disease. Low serum caeruloplasmin and copper with high urinary copper provides support for the diagnosis. Treatment is with copper chelating agents, such as penicillamine, which have to be given long term. Early treatment is associated with resolution of neurological manifestations in a proportion of children.

Problem	• Repeated jerking and writhing.

Diagnosis — Choreoathetosis ?Cause

Chorea is rapid, irregular, repetitive jerking either generalised or affecting any part of the body. Athetosis refers to slow writhing movements of the limbs and is often associated with dystonia. Chorea and athetosis commonly occur together and are also referred to collectively as dyskinesia.

Sydenham chorea. This is a manifestation of rheumatic fever and is quite rare in western countries now. The onset is insidious with restlessness, emotionality, chorea and hypotonia. The chorea is often asymmetrical and may even be unilateral in a few cases. Tendon jerks are characteristically 'hung-up'. When holding the examiner's fingers the child's grasp fluctuates (milk maid grasp). Up to 30% of children with chorea have rheumatic carditis but an associated arthropathy is unusual. Evidence of recent streptococcal infection is uncommon perhaps because the period from onset to diagnosis is often long. If necessary the restlessness and chorea can be treated with drugs like haloperidol or diazepam. Children should be given a full 10-day course of antistreptococcal chemotherapy and certainly those with evidence of carditis require prophylactic penicillin therapy indefinitely.

Huntington chorea is a dominantly inherited disorder due to an expanded trinucleotide repeat on chromosome 4p. Symptoms begin in childhood in only about 5% of cases but early onset is associated with inheritance of the disease from the father (genomic imprinting). When Huntington chorea commences in childhood, it tends to do so with rigidity as much if not more than chorea. Prognosis is poor with increasing dyskinesia and slowly progressive dementia.

Benign familial chorea is inherited as an autosomal dominant and the abnormal movements often start in early childhood. The family history is helpful for diagnosis and there is a tendency to show improvement in adolescence. There is no associated rigidity or dementia and all investigations are normal. Treatment is not usually required.

Drug-induced chorea. Phenytoin and carbamazepine may rarely produce chorea which improves with reduction of dosage. Neuroleptic drugs can produce what is called tardive dyskinesia which comes on months or years after commencing therapy and may be permanent despite prompt discontinuation of the drugs. The involuntary movements tend to affect the mouth and face (oro-buccal dyskinesia).

Lesch–Nyhan disease is an X-linked disorder caused by deficiency of the enzyme hypoxanthine-guanine phosphoribosyltransferase (HGPRT). Massive uric acid overproduction occurs and is responsible for renal calculi and gouty arthritis in later childhood. However the neurological manifestations become apparent in infancy with delayed development and hypotonia followed shortly by the appearance of athetosis and later spasticity and self-mutilation. Diagnosis is suggested by finding a high level of serum uric acid. Treatment with allopurinol helps renal function and arthritis but has no effect on the neurological manifestations.

Problem	• Repeated twitching.

Diagnosis — Tics (habit spasms)
These are sudden, brief, purposeless, stereotyped movements which can be suppressed to some extent by voluntary effort.

Simple motor tics may occur at any time in childhood but are usually seen during the school years. One, or at the most two, different motor tics are present and one may succeed another. Up to 10% of children may have tics at some time or another. Duration is usually less than a year.

Tourette syndrome. This condition is said to exist when there are multiple motor tics which have been present for more than a year and are associated with one or more vocal tics. The syndrome is often familial

Characteristics of the various abnormal movements

	Tremor	Dystonia	Choreoathetosis	Tics
Rhythmic	+	−	−	−
Stereotyped	+	±	−	+
Oscillatory	+	−	−	−
Voluntary suppression	−	−	−	+
Jerky	−	−	+	−

and is much more common in boys. Obsessive compulsive behaviour is a common association. The condition is probably lifelong but there may be periods of relative remission. When symptoms are very troublesome treatment with a dopamine receptor blocking drug such as haloperidol may be helpful in suppressing the involuntary movements.

ATAXIA

Ataxia denotes a disturbance of co-ordination and is clinically associated with a wide-based staggering gait, difficulty in balancing as shown when attempting a heel toe walk, difficulty with rapid repetitive movements (dysdiadochokinesis), a tremor that is only present on movement (intentional tremor) and past-pointing (dysmetria). Fine motor tasks such as doing up buttons, using cutlery and writing, are clumsy. Nystagmus may be associated. Unilateral ataxia affecting mainly fine motor activities suggests a lesion of the ipsilateral cerebellar lobe. Predominant truncal ataxia with minimal fine motor ataxia suggests a midline or vermis cerebellar lesion. Cerebellar ataxia cannot be compensated for significantly by visual input. However the ataxia associated with lesions of the posterior columns and their connections (sensory ataxia) can be so helped. This is the basis of the Romberg test. The child is asked to stand with the feet just sufficiently apart to become steady with his/her eyes open and then the effect of eye closure is ascertained. In cerebellar ataxia this has little effect, but with a sensory ataxia eye closure produces marked deterioration in balance.

Romberg test

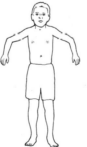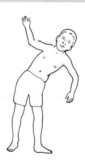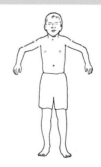

Steady with eyes open   Unsteady with eyes closed = Sensory ataxia   Steady with eyes closed = Cerebellar ataxia

Problem

• Sudden onset of clumsiness and loss of balance.

Diagnosis — Acute ataxia ?Cause
There are a number of conditions to consider when ataxia commences abruptly in a previously healthy child. *Drug toxicity* would be

suspected if the child or anyone in the house was being treated with carbamazepine or phenytoin for epilepsy or piperazine for thread-worms. Loss of hair might suggest thallium poisoning. Lead poisoning is another possibility. One of the commonest causes is the condition known as *acute post-infectious ataxia* which usually occurs in preschool children following sudden non-specific respiratory or gastrointestinal virus infection a week or two previously. Chickenpox is also well-known preceding viral infection. Some children with *Guillain–Barre syndrome* have quite a marked sensory ataxia as part of their symptoms but would be expected to show absent tendon reflexes. A variant of Guillain–Barre syndrome known as *Miller–Fisher syndrome* comprises ataxia, ophthalmoplegia and absent reflexes. *Epilepsy*: after a seizure some children may be ataxic as a temporary post-ictal phenomenon. The condition known as *minor epileptic status* is associated with ataxia but there would also be associated myoclonic jerks and fluctuating responsiveness. Migraine involving the posterior cerebral circulation (*basilar migraine*) often produces ataxia and/or vertigo and would usu-ally be associated with vomiting, prostration and headache. Some *metabolic conditions* can present as acute ataxia, e.g. mitochondrial encephalopathies, maple syrup urine disease. An unusual syndrome with bizarre jerky eye movements (opsoclonus), polymyoclonus of the limbs and ataxia is known as *the dancing eyes syndrome* and may sometimes be associated with an occult neuroblastoma. *Multiple sclerosis* is uncommon in childhood but might present as an episode of acute ataxia. The sudden onset of an ataxic gait in an older child, particularly if bizarre and not associated with any objective neurological findings, raises the possibility of a *hysterical gait disorder*.

Investigations. Drugs causing ataxia may be detected on a toxicology screen of blood and urine or assayed for specifically if an individual drug is suspected. CT or MRI scan would help to exclude brain tumour (an unlikely cause of acute ataxia) and multiple sclerosis. Lumbar puncture and nerve conduction studies might be necessary to clinch a diagnosis of Guillain–Barre syndrome or Miller–Fisher syndrome. Elevated urinary VMA excretion would suggest an occult neuroblastoma. Blood lactate and urine amino acids screen may detect a metabolic disorder. EEG would verify a clinical diagnosis of minor epileptic status.

Problem

• Long standing clumsiness and unsteadiness.

Diagnosis — Chronic non-progressive ataxia ?Cause

This may be congenital or represent incomplete recovery following an acquired ataxia. It is sometimes difficult to distinguish between a very slowly progressive ataxic disorder starting early in life (e.g. ataxia telangiectasia) and congenital non-progressive ataxia. Also distin-guishing between the severer grades of developmental dyspraxia (clumsy child syndrome) and ataxic cerebral palsy may sometimes be difficult. Congenital non-progressive ataxia presents as delayed motor

Dandy Walker syndrome

increased ear to occiput distance

- dilated lateral ventricle
- dilated III ventricle
- hypoplasia or compression atrophy of cerebellum
- grossly dilated IV ventricle

milestones and hypotonia. Intentional tremor may or may not be present on reach to grasp. When the child eventually walks he/she is seen to fall frequently and have a wide-based gait. The term *ataxic cerebral palsy* would be applied to chronic non-progressive ataxia which was congenital or present before school entry. *Ataxic diplegia* is a recognised form of cerebral palsy in which there is spasticity as well as ataxia. The presence of an enlarged head circumference would raise the possibility of *Dandy Walker syndrome*. The presence of a panting respiratory pattern, jerky eye movements and severe developmental delay suggests *Joubert syndrome*.

Investigation. A CT or MRI scan is usually required. A majority of cases will show a degree of hypoplasia of the cerebellar hemispheres or vermis. Vermis agenesis is seen in Joubert syndrome. A posterior fossa cyst extending from the fourth ventricle associated with vermis hypoplasia is characteristic of the Dandy Walker syndrome and often occurs with hydrocephalus.

Management. Physiotherapy encourages improved balance reactions and progress with motor development. Ventriculo-peritoneal shunting might be required in the Dandy Walker syndrome for associated hydrocephalus. Ataxic cerebral palsy is inherited as an autosomal recessive condition in about 50% of cases whether or not there is associated learning difficulties or evidence of cerebellar hypoplasia on scanning. Genetic counselling is usually indicated.

Chronic progressive

The presence of progression is always more difficult to detect if it starts in infancy than if it commences in later childhood. Some children who turn out to have a non-progressive ataxia may therefore have been investigated to exclude a progressive ataxia.

Problem

- Progressing clumsiness and unsteadiness.

Diagnosis — Chronic progressive ataxia ?Cause

Brain tumour. The presence of headache, vomiting and papilloedema would suggest the presence of a **posterior fossa tumour**. Medulloblastomas originate in the midline and cause gait and trunk ataxia and

Tumour in posterior fossa: CT scan

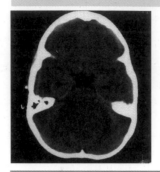 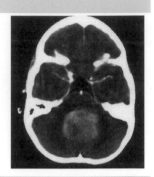

usually early hydrocephalus from obstruction to the aqueduct. Cerebellar astrocytomas usually arise in one lobe of the cerebellum and produce a lateralised cerebellar syndrome without hydrocephalus or clinical evidence of raised intracranial pressure at presentation. Ependymomas of the fourth ventricle produce early hydrocephalus and often only slight ataxia. Haemangioblastoma of the cerebellum may be associated with a positive family history and angiomatous lesions of the retina (**von Hippel–Lindau disease**).

Investigations. Lumbar puncture is strictly contra-indicated if brain tumour is suspected. CT or MRI scan will demonstrate the posterior fossa tumour and any associated ventricular dilatation.

Management. Dexamethasone given in a dose of 0.2–0.5 mg/kg/day reduces oedema surrounding the tumour and often dramatically improves symptoms of headache and vomiting until more definitive treatment can be given. With medulloblastoma, total tumour removal is usually impossible but surgery can often restore cerebrospinal fluid flow and may avoid the need for shunting. The cerebellar astrocytoma is often cystic and may be removed in total. Ependymomas can only be partially removed. Craniospinal radiation is required for all cases of medulloblastoma and most ependymomas, as these are usually malignant tumours. Trials of chemotherapy are also being carried out. Radiotherapy or chemotherapy is not usually required for cerebellar astrocytomas provided total removal has been achieved by the neurosurgeon.

Prognosis. The 5-year survival rate for medulloblastoma treated with surgery and radiation is about 50%. However the prognosis for cerebellar astrocytoma should be excellent provided total removal has been accomplished.

Ataxia telangiectasia. The presence of small telangiectatic lesions in the bulbar conjunctivae or around the ears would suggest ataxia telangiectasia. However these lesions often do not start to appear until about 5 or 6-years of age, long after the ataxia has been noted. Progressive ataxia occurring in a child with leukaemia, lymphoma or recurrent sinopulmonary infections would also suggest this diagnosis. Sometimes a degree of choreoathetosis may occur in addition to the ataxia.

Investigations. Serum alphafetoprotein is elevated in most cases. The response of chromosomes to ionising radiation is reduced and forms the definitive diagnostic test. Immunoglobulins may be reduced, particularly IgA, and there are usually disorders of T cell function if these are looked for.

Management. Physiotherapy will help the child to use his/her motor skills to the best, but this is a progressive condition and ambulation is often lost before the end of the second decade. Infections need to be treated promptly with antibiotics. Annual influenza immunisation should be considered. Routine X-rays should be avoided because of the risks of ionising radiation. Children with this condition need to be watched for the development of leukaemia or lymphoma.

Friedreich ataxia. A slowly progressive sensory ataxia coming on in a school aged child with a positive Romberg sign, absent tendon reflexes, pes cavus, extensor plantar responses and possibly nystagmus on lateral gaze and dysarthria, strongly suggests Friedreich ataxia. This is a slowly progressive spinocerebellar degenerative disorder inherited as an autosomal recessive and shown recently to be due to a homozygous expanded trinucleotide repeat on chromosome 9q. The symptoms arise from degeneration of the posterior columns, spinocerebellar tracts and pyramidal tracts in the spinal cord. In addition there is a mild associated peripheral motor and sensory neuropathy and a cardiomyopathy.

Investigations. CT scan is usually normal. Mild dennervation changes may be seen on EMG and needle sampling of peripheral muscles. Motor nerve conduction velocities are normal or only borderline slow. Sensory nerve action potentials are very reduced and may be absent. CSF is normal. ECG may show conduction defects with bundle branch block and T wave changes. Echocardiography shows thickening of the interventricular septum.

Management. Formal physiotherapy is not usually helpful but children should be encouraged to remain active for as long as possible with participation in PE and games at school. Surgery may be required for scoliosis. Genetic counselling will be required and prenatal testing may be possible looking for the triple repeat expansion. Routine regular tests for glycosuria are recommended as diabetes occurs more commonly in patients with Friedreich ataxia.

Prognosis. Most children may manage to remain ambulant until middle teenage years. Cardiorespiratory symptoms may become troublesome in early adulthood because of myocardial fibrosis and increasing scoliosis and life expectancy is not usually beyond 35 years.

Other rare causes of progressive ataxia include *Refsum disease* (phytanic acid storage with peripheral neuropathy, deafness and retinitis pigmentosa), *late infantile Batten disease* (presents at about 3 years of age with intractable epilepsy), *vitamin E deficiency* (isolated or as part of abetalipoproteinaemia) and *Marinesco–Sjögren disease* (associated congenital cataracts, severe learning difficulties and myopathy).

Site of pathology	Hereditary causes	Acquired causes
1. Anterior horn cell	Spinal muscular atrophies	Poliomyelitis
		Arthrogryposis multiplex
2. Nerve trunk	General muscular atrophy	Guillain–Barré syndrome
		Toxic polyneuropathies
3. Neuromuscular junctions	Congenital myasthenias	Myasthenia gravis
		Infantile botulism
4. Muscle	Muscular dystrophies	
	Congenital myopathies	

MRC scale of muscle strength

0	No contraction
1	Flicker or trace of contraction
2	Active movement with gravity eliminated
3	Active movement against gravity
4	Active movement against gravity and resistance
5	Normal power

FLACCID WEAKNESS

Weakness is associated with hypotonia and diminished or absent tendon reflexes. Causes may be hereditary or acquired and due to pathology involving the anterior horn cells, peripheral motor nerves, neuromuscular junctions or muscle cells.

Problem

- Symmetrical flaccid paralysis affecting the legs first but then ascending to involve the trunk and arms.

Diagnosis — Guillain–Barré syndrome

Associated facial weakness and sometimes bulbar palsy may occur. It may occur at any age after 6 months but is most common between the ages of 5 and 9 years. A history of an acute febrile illness in the preceding 3 weeks is common. Distal sensory losses may be detectable and sensory ataxia can occasionally dominate the picture. Tendon reflexes are absent but occasionally extensor plantar responses are found. Headache, neckache, backache and limb pains are common in the acute phase. It is an acute autoimmune demyelinating polyneuropathy. Whenever the condition is suspected the child must be admitted to hospital, as further progression with the risk of respiratory involvement may occur.

Investigations. CSF shows an elevated protein with little or no pleocytosis. These changes support the clinical diagnosis and help rule out poliomyelitis. Sometimes the CSF is normal during the first few days of the illness but then shows typical changes if repeated in the second week. Nerve conduction studies show markedly delayed motor nerve conduction velocities in most cases. Viral studies may give a clue to the preceding illness. Spinal MRI scanning would be indicated if the clinical features suggest the possibility of a spinal cause for the acute flaccid weakness (e.g. spinal angioma, hydromyelia, spinal trauma, epidural abscess or spinal tumour). Acute dermatomyositis rarely causes diagnostic confusion but if there is doubt, the blood creatine kinase would usually be raised in dermatomyositis. A toxicology screen is indicated if the polyneuropathy might be due to chemical ingestion (lead, arsenic, thallium, mercury, triorthocresyl phosphate).

Management. Respiratory reserve needs to be estimated frequently. In older children this can be done by measuring the forced vital capacity (FVC) 4 hourly in the initial stages when the paralysis is spreading. If the FVC is less than 50% of predicted, blood gases should be measured regularly. Artificial ventilation is only required for a minority (less than 10% of cases). Indications would include an FVC less than 25% predicted, cyanosis at rest, hypoxia and hypercarbia on blood gas estimation, undue tachycardia or exhaustion during nursing procedures. Autonomic involvement may be associated with retention of urine and systemic hypertension. Blood pressure should be measured regularly.

Steroids are known not to have any effect on the course of the disorder. More severe cases used to be treated with plasmapheresis but intravenous gamma globulin 400 mg/kg body weight daily for 5 days has been shown to be as effective. Gentle passive exercises during the acute phase reduce the risk of contracture formation. Prolonged rehabilitative physiotherapy is necessary after the acute phase has passed.

Prognosis. Acute phase mortality is now less than 5% and is mainly due to complications of artificial ventilation and respiratory paralysis. Approximately 80% of survivors make a complete recovery but this may take any time between 3 and 30 months to achieve. Approximately 20% of survivors are left with a varying degree of permanent muscle weakness. Evidence of improving muscle strength occurring before 18 days after the onset of the illness is associated with an excellent prognosis for full recovery. The severity of the initial weakness does not correlate with the long term prognosis. Even children who have required ventilation support usually go on to make a full recovery.

Problem

- Acute onset of asymmetrical flaccid weakness affecting one limb preceded by fever and evidence of neck stiffness.

Diagnosis — Poliomyelitis
In the UK this may be vaccine related or due to an enteric virus other than polio virus. CSF shows lymphocytic pleocytosis with a normal or only slightly raised protein.

Management. The paralysis may worsen and careful observations of respiratory function are required and, if necessary, artificial ventilation. Some permanent paralysis is the rule after acute paralysis.

Problem

- Progressive bulbar and skeletal muscle weakness with loss of tendon reflexes occurring after a few days prodromal symptoms of constipation and anorexia in an infant below 6 months of age.

Diagnosis — ? Infantile botulism

Typical features include ptosis, dysphagia, weak cry and dilated pupils. The condition is due to colonisation of the intestinal tract with *C.botulinum*, the toxin produced being absorbed and producing neuromuscular blockade.

Management. Diagnosis is confirmed by the isolation of the organism from the stool. Supportive therapy is required as the condition is self-limiting with full recovery within 6 weeks. A few infants require ventilation.

Problem

- Recurrent attacks of generalised flaccid weakness affecting limbs and trunk but not extraocular or facial muscles and lasting several hours.

Diagnosis — Familial periodic paralysis

Attacks may be brought on by a period of exercise or a meal with high carbohydrate content. Hypokalaemic periodic paralysis is due to a defect in the calcium channel, hypernatraemic periodic paralysis is due to a defect in the sodium channel. Both are inherited as autosomal dominant conditions.

Treatment of hypokalaemic periodic paralysis during an acute attack is with repeated oral doses of potassium. Surprisingly both hypokalaemic and hyperkalaemic periodic paralysis are improved with prophylactic acetazolamide.

Problem

- A child presenting with variable ptosis, squint and facial weakness often with general fatigueability of muscles in the arms, legs and trunk and the weakness fluctuates being best in the morning and becoming progressively worse as the day goes by.

Diagnosis — Myasthenia gravis

This is an autoimmune disorder in which blocking antibodies are produced to acetyl choline receptors on the postsynaptic membrane. Girls are affected five times more frequently than boys. Age at onset may be as early as 2 years but it is usually in later childhood.

Investigations. The edrophonium (tensilon) test is diagnostic and unequivocally positive in the vast majority of cases. 0.2 mg/kg body weight of edrophonium produces marked improvement in the ptosis,

Motor end plate

ACh = acetyl choline
ChE = choline esterase
CA = choline acetylase

Axon terminal

Synaptic cleft

Ch ← ACh
ChE

Skeletal muscle

receptor site

Curare: competes with ACh at receptor site
non-depolarizing relaxant

Succinyl choline: acts like ACh but is only broken
down slowly by ChE
depolarizing relaxant

Myasthenia gravis: receptor site block with IgG antibody

Neostigmine: a reversible ChE inhibitor

squint and other muscle weakness within a minute of injection and lasts about 6 minutes. Circulating acetylcholine receptor antibodies can be measured and are usually but not invariably elevated. Electromyography shows a decrimental response to repetitive motor nerve stimuli. This is an unpleasant test for young children and is rarely required for diagnosis. Thyroid studies should be done as approximately 10% of children with myasthenia gravis have an associated hyperthyroidism.

Management. Pyridostigmine (mestinon) is a long acting anticholinesterase drug given in a dose of 1 mg/kg body weight three to four times daily and controls symptoms in many cases. Steroids may be helpful if symptoms are severe and not fully controlled with pyridostigmine. Thymectomy is sometimes required in childhood if medical treatment is not producing satisfactory improvement.

Prognosis. In 40% the weakness remains confined to the ocular muscles. Generalised weakness may be present from the outset in 40% or develop within 12 months of an isolated ocular presentation (20%). Myasthenic crises with profound weakness and danger of respiratory paralysis can occur in some children. A minority of children with myasthenia gravis undergo spontaneous remission.

Problem

• Longstanding flaccid weakness which is not progressing.

Diagnosis — Chronic non-progressing flaccid weakness ?Cause
This may be congenital or represent incomplete recovery following an acute illness. The majority of babies born with *arthrogryposis multiplex congenita* have a non-progressive anterior horn cell hypoplasia of pre-natal origin as the underlying problem. *Congenital muscular dystrophy* is usually a non-progressive disorder. It varies in severity and more severe cases tend to be identified in the newborn period as 'floppy babies'. Others present later in infancy because of delayed motor development. Blood CK may be raised in the first year of life but thereafter is usually normal. Muscle biopsy shows increased fibrosis and an abnormal variation in fibre size. In the UK congenital muscular dystrophy is usually associated with normal mentality but the

Japanese type is often associated with cerebral malformations of the neuronal migration type. As this is usually a non-progressive disorder, intensive rehabilitation is justified even in severely affected infants, as they may have a reasonable life span.

Hypotonia and generalised weakness, which is often more proximal than distal and sometimes associated with facial weakness, are symptoms that are seen in the majority of *congenital myopathies*. These are usually non-progressive disorders. Creatine kinase levels are often normal. Diagnosis is dependent on the findings on muscle biopsy and is important for genetic counselling (central core disease and congenital fibre type dysproportion are autosomal dominant and nemaline myopathy is autosomal recessive). Central core disease is one of the few myopathies known to predispose to *malignant hyperpyrexia*.

Problem

- Progressive proximal muscle weakness affecting pelvic and shoulder girdles with early loss of tendon reflexes.

Diagnosis — Spinal muscular atrophy (SMA)

Three main phenotypes are recognised. In *Werdnig–Hoffman disease* progressive weakness commences before 6 months of age and in a few it is present at birth. Infants never achieve independent sitting and fasciculation of the tongue may be seen. Because the chest wall muscles are affected more than the diaphragm, paradoxical ('see-saw') respiration is a feature. Death invariably occurs before 18 months of age. *Intermediate SMA* is characterised by insidious onset of proximal muscle weakness between 6 months and 18 months of age. Independent sitting is achieved but not standing or walking. Fasciculation may be seen in trunk and limb muscles. Rate of progression often slows after 2 years of age and there may be long periods without deterioration. Life expectancy can be into middle age. *Juvenile SMA* commences between 18 months and 15 years of age. Independent walking is acquired and the first symptoms are those of waddling gait and difficulty climbing stairs. A positive Gower sign may cause confusion with muscular dystrophy in boys.

Investigations. Blood creatine kinase levels in spinal muscular atrophy are normal or borderline elevated. Motor nerve conduction velocities are normal or only very slightly prolonged. EMG shows large polyphasic motor unit potentials on volition and spontaneous fibrillation potentials at rest. Muscle biopsy shows the picture known as group atrophy. There are large groups of uniformly atrophic muscle cells with large groups of normal sized muscle cells in between. Histochemical staining shows individual groups of atrophic fibres to be of all the same fibre type.

Genetics. All three types are inherited as autosomal recessives but recently have been shown to be allelic and mapped to 5Q13. About 95% of children in all of the three types show deletion of the Survival of Motor Neurones (SMN) gene at this locus. These recent findings have made it possible to test for all three kinds of SMA prenatally.

Management. No curative treatment is available. In all types respiratory infection should be treated energetically as they represent a particular danger for patients with reduced respiratory reserve. In Werdnig–Hoffman disease, tube feeding is often required terminally as bulbar muscles are affected. In the two more chronic forms regular physiotherapy is required and children need to be encouraged to remain active. Careful regulation of weight is essential as obesity adds to their burden. Orthopaedic treatment may be required for scoliosis. In the later stages, advice on wheelchairs and other equipment will be required.

Problem

- Slowly progressive weakness of the dorsiflexor and evertor (anterior tibial and peroneal) muscles of the ankle and intrinsic muscles of the feet, presents as gait disorder (steppage gait) and foot deformity (pes cavus) with absent ankle and knee jerks.

Diagnosis — Peroneal muscular atrophy (Charcot–Marie–Tooth disease)

This is a dominantly inherited progressive peripheral neuropathy. Significant sensory loss is difficult to demonstrate in childhood but impairment of position and vibration sense may be found if looked for carefully. Scoliosis and moderate ataxia are sometimes associated.

Investigations. In the demylinating kind, motor nerve conduction velocities in both arms and legs are very slow even when the clinical findings are minimal and limited to the feet. In the so-called axonal kind, motor nerve conduction velocities are normal or borderline but sensory nerve action potentials are of low amplitude or absent and EMG sampling shows evidence of denervation. Muscle biopsy is not usually required for diagnosis.

EMG patterns

	Normal	Spinal muscular atrophy	Muscular dystrophy
At rest	silence	fibrillation potentials at rest	silence
Maximal contraction	good amplitude, full interference pattern	baseline visible between large motor unit potentials	low amplitude, full interference pattern
Minimal contraction	biphasic or triphasic motor unit potentials	high amplitude, long polyphasic motor unit potentials	low amplitude, short polyphasic motor unit potentials

Management. There is no curative treatment. Special shoes and an ankle-foot orthosis improve gait and prevent foot drop and contracture formation. Operative treatment for foot deformity and to stabilise the ankle may be required in late childhood in some cases.

Genetics. Usually one parent will be found to be affected clinically or show abnormalities on nerve conduction studies and dominant inheritance can then be assumed. Molecular genetics studies have shown that in the common demyelinating type a duplication at 17P11–12, which contains the peripheral myelin protein gene, is found in 70% of cases. If both parents are found to be clinically and electrically unaffected, the disorder may sometimes be recessively inherited or sporadic.

Prognosis. Is very variable even within the same family. Some may have the disorder but show little or no disability even in later adult life. Some patients have become quite severely disabled by late teenage. The majority fall somewhere in between these two extremes. Progression of the distal muscle weakness eventually affects the lower thighs (inverted champagne bottle sign) and hand and forearm muscles. Disability may be more related to the associated sensory ataxia or scoliosis in some.

Problem

- Pelvic girdle weakness presenting in a boy usually between 3 and 5 years of age who has difficulty climbing stairs and getting up from lying.

Diagnosis — Duchenne muscular dystrophy
Gait is waddling and stance lordotic and there is often a history of delayed motor milestones particularly walking and frequent falls. There is a tendency to walk up on the toes and calf muscles are prominent (pseudohypertrophy). Ankle jerks are brisk but knee jerks are very sluggish. Because of the seriousness of the diagnosis, confirmatory investigations are mandatory before the diagnosis is made. Duchenne muscular dystrophy may be mimicked clinically by chronic spinal muscular atrophy, dermatomyositis, limb girdle and Becker muscular dystrophies and some rarer disorders.

Investigations

Blood creatine kinase is massively elevated with levels usually above 10 times the upper limit of the normal range. Electromyography shows typical myopathic changes; a normal interference pattern, no spontaneous activity at rest and low amplitude short duration polyphasic motor units on volition. Muscle biopsy shows a wider than normal variation in fibre diameter, internal nuclei, opaque fibres and increased fat and connective tissue. Special stains show the complete absence of dystrophin, a cytoskeletal protein normally present in all muscle cells. Electrocardiography demonstrates minor abnormalities in 70% of cases. Molecular genetic techniques can demonstrate a deletion in the dystrophin gene at Xp21 in approximately 60% of boys with Duchenne dystrophy. The remainder are assumed to have a point mutation.

Management	There is no curative treatment. The diagnosis of muscular dystrophy can have a devastating effect on a family and parents should be given ample opportunity for discussion. Some parents find membership of the local muscular dystrophy group invaluable. In the early stages formal physiotherapy is unnecessary but advice on activities is helpful. Affected boys should be encouraged to take part in most activities including PE, swimming, sports, etc. provided they do not become fatigued. Regular passive stretching of the tendo Achilles and the wearing of dorsiflexion splints at night help to delay the development of equinus deformity. When more severe weakness has developed, regular physiotherapy including use of a standing frame, can reduce the progression of scoliosis and other orthopaedic deformities. Intermittent prednisolone therapy given for 10 days of each month starting when severe weakness threatens continued walking, will prolong ambulation on average for about a year. Progressive scoliosis develops in over 90% of boys with Duchenne dystrophy, usually after ambulation has been lost. Bracing is not an effective treatment and surgical correction is usually offered. This has to be done before respiratory function declines to an unacceptable level for anaesthetic.
Appliances	A hand-propelled wheelchair is provided by the disability services centre but sooner or later an electric wheelchair will be required. Wheelchair inserts to maintain spinal lordosis help to prevent progressive scoliosis. Ball and socket arm rests can be fitted to a wheelchair and allow a boy to use his hands when the shoulder girdle muscles have become very weak. Home adaptations are usually required, e.g. a ramp for wheelchair access, a downstairs extension for bedroom and bathroom or a lift to allow the use of upstairs bedroom and bathroom, hoists to enable transfer from wheelchair to bed or bath. These are normally provided by the local social services department.
Education	Most boys continue at ordinary primary school. More mainstream comprehensive schools are now adapted for wheelchair users with the result that fewer boys with muscular dystrophy are attending special schools for physically handicapped children. Employment is uncommon as by school leaving age most boys are very severely physically handicapped. Many boys go on to a college of further education and it is important that appropriate activities or hobbies are encouraged if boredom and depression are to be minimised.
Genetic counselling	When a woman has more than one affected son or an affected brother as well as an affected son, she can be assumed to be a carrier and appropriate counselling given. The risk of carrier status can also be calculated for her daughters and sisters taking into account their creatine kinase levels as well as the pedigree. More commonly the index case is the only one in the family and in this situation it is known that only 66% of such mothers are carriers and would therefore be at risk of having a further affected boy. In the other 33% a new mutation has

occurred and the mother is not a carrier. Unfortunately creatine kinase estimation only identifies 60% of carriers with certainty and so a woman with a normal creatine kinase can still be a carrier. Formuli are available to calculate the risk of carrier status for a woman who has a normal creatine kinase and is related to an index case. A prenatal test is available if the index case has a deletion of Xp21 but not otherwise at present.

Stages of deterioration in muscular dystrophy

		Performance	Stage
Walking	Can climb stairs	Without railings	I
		With railings with mild exertion	II
	Cannot climb stairs without assistance	Slowly and cumbrously with railings	III
		Can stand up independently from chair	IV
		Cannot stand up independently from chair	V
	Predominantly in wheelchair but can walk a little		VII
Wheelchair	Independent in transfer activities (from wheelchair to bed, toilet, etc.)		VIII
	Dependent in transfer activities	Can sit up independently	
		(a) cannot sit up independently	IX
		(b) cannot raise arms up off arm rests	
Bed	Cannot use wheelchair		X

Prognosis

Duchenne muscular dystrophy runs an inexorable course with loss of walking occurring at 6–12 years of age. It is fatal between 13 and 21 years of age from pneumonia in the presence of severely reduced respiratory reserve or congestive heart failure due to progressive cardiomyopathy.

Problem

- Gradual onset of proximal muscle weakness affecting predominantly the pelvic girdle muscles associated with malaise, lethargy and skin rashes.

Diagnosis — Dermatomyositis

This is an autoimmune angiopathy affecting muscles and skin predominantly. The skin rash takes the form of a violaceous discoloration of the upper eyelids, an erythematous eruption on the upper cheeks and telangiectasia over the knuckles and nail folds. Because of the wide variation in presentation, dematomyositis may be confused with Duchenne and limb girdle muscular dystrophies, psychiatric disorders and collagen diseases. Investigations are not always helpful and the diagnosis is essentially a clinical one. It is not associated with underlying malignancies in childhood.

Investigations. Erythrocyte sedimentation rate is usually normal even in the active phase of the disease. Blood creatine kinase may be normal, moderately increased or massively elevated. Antinuclear factor is occasionally positive and blood immunoglobulins are elevated in some cases. Electromyography typically shows a mixture of myopathic (small, short, polyphasic units on volition) and denervation changes (fibrillation and positive sharp waves at rest). However electromyography may be normal, particularly if only limited sampling is carried out. Muscle biopsy typically shows muscle fibre degeneration and regeneration, inflammatory round cell infiltration and perifascicular atrophy. These changes are often focal and patchy which may explain why muscle biopsy can occasionally be negative. Muscle ultrasound shows patchy high signal changes and may be used as a guide for the best site for muscle biopsy.

Management. Prednisolone 1 mg/kg body weight/day is given until improvement begins. The dose is then gradually tailed off over a 3- to 6- month period. Most children will go into complete remission with this regimen. Response to treatment is best judged by improvement in muscle strength and disappearance of general malaise. Changes in blood creatine kinase levels should not be used to monitor treatment as they are unreliable. If it proves impossible to wean the child off prednisolone without repeated relapses, long term alternate day steroid therapy may be required to maintain remission. Failure to respond to steroid therapy adequately or unacceptable steroid side effects would require the use of immunosuppressive drugs such as cyclosporin. Children with dermatomyositis are at risk of developing contractures. Encouragement of active movements and the wearing of night splints help to reduce contracture formation.

Prognosis. Before the advent of steroid therapy, childhood dermatomyositis carried a high mortality (usually from respiratory failure or perforation of the gastrointestinal tract). With steroid therapy the majority of children make a full recovery. A small group remain handicapped by varying degrees of muscle weakness and contracture.

FLOPPY BABY SYNDROME

It is helpful to look at the problem of the newborn baby or young infant who is hypotonic separately as it is a common diagnostic problem. Clinically it is very useful to try to decide whether the hypotonia is associated with obvious muscle weakness or whether the hypotonia is present alone.

Problem	**Hypotonia with obvious muscle weakness**

This strongly suggests some disorder of the lower motor neurone system. *Werdnig–Hoffman disease, congenital myopathies* and *congenital muscular dystrophy* have already been discussed. *Pompe disease* is a progressive lysosomal glycogen storage disorder due to acid maltase deficiency. There is increasing muscle weakness and cardiomyopathy but the liver is not enlarged. Diagnosis is by showing glycogen storage on muscle biopsy and finding low levels of acid maltase in peripheral white cells. *Congenital myotonic dystrophy* is a cause of severe hypotonia in the newborn period sometimes associated with respiratory distress and usually with the need for tube feeding. The mother is always affected but often very minimally so and the demonstration of myotonia in hand and facial muscles may be quite subtle. The hypotonia and weakness shows a lot of improvement over the first few weeks of life and tube feeding can be discontinued. However most affected infants show significant generalised developmental delay.

No myotonia is found however until later childhood or early adulthood. The disorder is due to an expanded trinucleotide repeat on chromosome 19 and this may be used as a diagnostic test in doubtful clinical cases. There should always be a low threshold for suspecting the condition known as *transient neonatal myasthenia*. This arises from passive transfer of acetylcholine receptor antibodies from a myasthenic mother to the baby's circulation. The newborn baby shows weakness of cry and facial movements, feeding difficulties and generalised hypotonia and weakness. The mother does not always have symptoms of myasthenia or may not have been diagnosed. Diagnosis is by showing reversal of weakness with subcutaneous edrophonium and high concentration of circulating acetyl choline receptor anti-bodies. Full recovery occurs within 2 or 3 weeks but injections of neostigmine may be required prior to feeds for this period.

Problem	Hypotonia without obvious weakness

A number of central nervous system disorders can present as profound hypotonia in the newborn period. These include Down syndrome and some other chromosomal abnormalities. Infants who have suffered significant hypoxic ischaemic cerebral insults just before or during delivery are likely to show profound hypotonia for the first day or two. Many of these babies will be found to have cerebral palsy in later infancy. Some infants who are later diagnosed as having cerebral palsy show marked hypotonia at this time in the absence of a hypoxic ischaemic encephalopathy. This is particularly true of dystonic and ataxic cerebral palsy. Prader–Willi syndrome is responsible for marked hypotonia in the newborn period, usually with the requirement for tube feeding and associated cryptorchidism. The hypotonia and feeding difficulties improve but overeating, obesity, short stature, learning difficulties and behaviour problems become apparent later. The condition is due to a deletion on chromosome 15q or uniparental maternal disomy of that chromosome. A newborn baby with marked hypotonia, large fontanelle, high forehead, poor sucking, hepatomegaly and generalised seizures is suggestive of Zellweger syndrome due to absence of cytoplasmic peroxisomes. Some connective tissue disorders such as Ehlers–Danlos syndrome can be associated with infantile hypotonia and an excessive range of joint movements. A number of metabolic disorders may produce a centrally mediated hypotonia in infancy, e.g. maple syrup urine disease, proprionicacidaemia, hypercalcaemia.

FURTHER READING

Aicardi J 1992 Diseases of the nervous system in childhood. MacKeith Press with
      Blackwell Scientific Publications, Oxford
Brett EM 1991 Paediatric neurology, 2nd edn. Churchill Livingston, Edinburgh
Dubowitz V 1995 Muscle disorders in childhood, 2nd edn. Saunders, London
Fenichel GM 1988 Clinical paediatric neurology. Signs and symptoms approach.
   WB Saunders, Philadelphia.
Newton RW 1995 Colour atlas of paediatric neurology. Mosby Wolfe, London
Stephenson JBP King MD 1989 Handbook of neurological investigations in children.
      Wright, London

19 Brain and special senses

Disorders of the nervous system present with wide ranging symptoms and signs including seizures, altered awareness, raised intracranial pressure, retarded development and developmental regression. Neurological diseases may be congenital or acquired, they may be inflammatory, toxic, degenerative, demyelinating or neoplastic, and they may be static or progressive. Evolution of a progressive illness can take many years, particularly in the context of neurodegenerative diseases, and one needs to be constantly aware of this possibility in children with chronic neurological problems. The pace of human brain growth is maximum in prenatal life, with neuronal proliferation and migration taking place in the first and second trimesters of pregnancy with further complex organisation in dendritic proliferation, synaptic connectivity and myelination taking place in the third trimester and the first 2 years of postnatal life. Deleterious influences be they genetic or environmental during early brain growth and organisation, may result in brain abnormalities causing neurological disorders.

SEIZURES

The term seizure (synonyms: convulsions, fits) is non-specific meaning an unusual episode of altered conciousness, abnormal movement or sensory perception. Seizures can be epileptic and non-epileptic and obtaining a competent history, particularly the immediate events before the attack, is helpful in their differentiation. Non-epileptic events in childhood are common and their recognition is important preventing harm to the child by initiation of inappropriate antiepilepsy drug therapy.

The original definition of epilepsy credited to Hughlings Jackson (1873) is as follows: 'Epilepsy is a name for occasional, sudden, excessive, rapid and local discharges of grey matter'. Clinical manifestations depend on the part of the brain from where this abnormal discharge originated from, for example, discharges from the frontal lobe give motor manifestations and those from the temporal lobe psycho-motor phenomena. Sometimes the site of origin can be identified on the EEG. The discharge frequently spreads and generalises to other parts of the brain.

The diagnosis of epilepsy has major educational and social implications for the child and it is important to get it right. To diagnose epilepsy there has to be more than one unprovoked attack. A child who has had a single seizure cannot be said to have epilepsy. The population incidence of a single non-febrile seizure is 5% as against the incidence of epilepsy which is 0.5%. There is an age dependent vulnerability for seizures in children.

Problem

- A 12-month-child is brought to casualty and is reported to have had a fit.
- On examination the child is a little sleepy but behaves normally.
- The child has a fever.

Diagnosis — Probably febrile convulsion

Young children between 1 and 5 years of age are particularly prone to febrile convulsions, they occur in 3% of the normal childhood population. The high temperature acts as a trigger on a background of genetic vulnerability. A family history of febrile convulsions is not uncommon in parents or other siblings. The cause of the fever is from an extracranial source, usually a viral infection of the upper respiratory tract. A typical febrile convulsion is usually a brief generalised tonic clonic seizure associated with loss of consciousness lasting under 5 minutes and has usually stopped by the time the child is seen by a medical practitioner. The child has no residual neurological deficit. Often the convulsion is the first indication that the child is ill and parents find them frightening.

A lumbar puncture will be necessary if there is a clinical suspicion of meningitis and may have to be routinely performed in children under 18 months after a first febrile convulsion. The child's birth and developmental history, family history of febrile convulsions, previous seizures and any focal features, evidence of infection of the upper respiratory tract, urinary tract, skin rash, meningism, etc. should be sought.

Individual susceptibility to febrile seizures in a significant proportion of families is transmitted as an autosomal dominant trait, with boys outnumbering girls in most series. This is explainable on the basis of differential cerebral maturation between the sexes with slower maturation in boys. Atypical features in febrile convulsions include unilateral seizure, multiple convulsions in the same febrile illness, Todd's paralysis and presentation with status epileticus. In fact febrile convulsions are the commonest cause of status epilepticus in children.

Management

Most febrile convulsions have stopped by the time the child has arrived at casualty. If still convulsing, the child is put in the recovery position, an oral airway inserted, oxygen administered by face mask and rectal diazepam 0.5 mg/kg given as the drug of choice. If it is to be given intravenously the dose is 0.25 mg/kg. Intravenous diazepam should be injected very slowly at the rate of 1 mg per min. There is a risk of causing apnoea if injected rapidly. An effective alternative would be to use rectal paraldehyde 0.3 ml/kg mixed with an equal volume of an arachis oil. After a variable postictal period, most children recover completely.

Febrile convulsions may recur and the risk of this happening can be minimised by advising parents in measures of temperature control when the child is ill, including prompt administration of antipyretics and the use of minimum clothing. About 25% of children with one febrile convulsion may subsequently develop further attacks, with the highest risk in those with a family history of febrile convulsion and in the very young child. Parents should be given an explanation of the condition and taught how to manage their child in a future febrile convulsion. This includes lying the child in the recovery position, loosening tight clothing, not thrusting any objects between their teeth. In children with recurrent febrile convulsions parents can be instructed on the administration of rectal diazepam for convulsions lasting longer than 5 minutes.

Prognosis

This is excellent for benign febrile convulsions. One-third of children with the first febrile convulsion have one or more further febrile convulsion and risk factors for recurrence include young age, male sex and a positive family history. Overall the frequency of non-febrile seizures later is twice as high in those who have recurrences as among those who do not. About 2% of children who have had one or more febrile convulsion are at risk of long term epilepsy. Often the febrile convulsion has been atypical and possibly is the first true epileptic attack precipitated by fever.

Problem

- Child is brought to A&E because it is thought that he/she has had a fit.
- Sleepiness but no fever.

Diagnosis — ? Epilepsy

Epilepsy is predominantly a childhood disease, in 75% of sufferers the fits begin before 20 years of age. The prevalance of epilepsy is four per 1000 children. The incidence is greatest in the first year of life, remaining high until 4 years of age and then declines towards adolescence and adult life. Age, growth and development are important factors in the development of epilepsy, its evolution and ultimate prognosis. The challenge is to determine if the child has had a fit and if so what is its nature. It is essential to know the various forms of epilepsy and to take a detailed history.

The aetiology of epilepsy is heterogeneous and sometimes unknown. Causes of symptomatic and cryptogenic epilepsy include prenatal, perinatal and postnatal brain insults. Gross and subtle brain malformations like cortical dysplasias, neuronal migration abnormalities, neurocutaneous disorders like tuberous sclerosis and neurofibramatosis, brain damage from prenatal viral infections, birth anoxia, meningitis, accidental and non-accidental brain trauma are all well recognised causes of childhood epilepsy.

There has been a move towards categorisation of childhood epilepsy into 'epileptic syndromes'. This encompasses clinical features along with their electroencephalographic (EEG) correlates which are consistently associated. Some of these syndromes have been shown to have specific, pathological, chromosomal or biochemical markers.

Aicardi's four main epochs in childhood and adolescent epilepsy with particular aetiological factors obtaining in each

Birth to 3 months	When seizures are related to structural pathology and prognosis is poor
3 months to 4 years	When seizure threshold of the brain is low and reactive seizures, especially febrile convulsions, are common. Serious epileptic syndromes including infantile spasms and the Lennox–Gastaut syndrome occur in this period
4 to 10 years	When there is a predominance of primary or idiopathic generalised and partial epilepsy. For example, childhood absence epilepsy and benign partial epilepsy with centro-temporal spikes. Complex partial seizures secondary to structural brain abnormality become better defined in this period
10 years and beyond	When primary generalised epilepsies occur and complex partial seizures are more frequently encountered

Several descriptive terms are used in epilepsy. A distinction is drawn between generalised epilepsies from those characterized by partial seizures, which imply a focal cortical origin. The second subdivision is between epilepsies which are idiopathic (synonyms primary, genetic, non-lesional) from those which are symptomatic of an underlying brain lesion. The term cryptogenic is used to refer to an epilepsy which has a hidden cause, and in general cryptogenic epilepsy is presumed to be symptomatic, even though no precise aetiology is identified.

Classification of epileptic seizures — International League against Epilepsy (1989)

Partial seizures (seizures beginning locally)
A) Simple partial seizures (consciousness not impaired):
    With motor symptoms
    With somatosensory or special sensory symptoms
    Autonomic symptoms
    Psychic symptoms.
B) Complex partial seizures (with impairment of consciousness):
    Beginning as simple partial seizures and progressing to impairment of consciousness
    With impairment of consciousness at onset.
C) Partial seizures becoming secondarily generalised.

Generalised seizures (bilaterally symmetrical and without local onset)
A) 1. Absence seizures.   2. Atypical absence seizures.
B) Myoclonic seizures
C) Clonic seizures
D) Tonic seizures
E) Tonic clonic seizures
F) Atonic seizures.

Unclassified epileptic seizures

Primary epileptic syndromes occur in otherwise normal children, sometimes with a positive family history and no demonstrable underlying pathology and in whom the EEG shows a normal background interictal activity. Such patients respond well to anti-epilepsy medication with a good prognosis for remission.

In contrast, secondary or symptomatic epilepsy syndromes are usually associated with underlying cerebral disease which may also concomitantly cause learning difficulties or motor disorders. The family history is often negative. The syndromes are associated with abnormal neurological findings in the child. Response to medication is variable and spontaneous remission is unlikely. In some of these conditions affected children suffer multiple seizure types. The following clinical types of epileptic seizures are commonly recognised.

Problem

- Attacks start with sudden loss of conciousness and an initial tonic phase with stiffening of the limbs and body, progressing to a clonic phase associated with generalised jerking of the limbs. Cyanosis, excessive salivation, tongue biting and incontinence may be seen. Most attacks are brief and cease after a few minutes and are followed by a postictal phase, when the child is either irritable or sleepy for a variable period from a few minutes to several hours.

Diagnosis — Generalised tonic clonic seizures

A generalised tonic clonic seizure is associated with generalised high voltage spike and waves, seen symmetrically on the electroencephalogram.

Problem

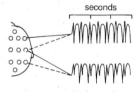

seconds

3-second spike-and-wave discharges

- Attacks consisting of impaired consciousness, when the child becomes still and vacant for periods lasting from 3 to 20 seconds. There is a sudden onset and offset to the attacks. The child often carries on as though nothing has happened after the cessation of the attacks.

Diagnosis — Typical absence seizures

This condition is seen in children between the ages of 5 and 10 years with a female proponderance. Attacks can be brought on by getting the child to hyperventilate for a minute or two. The EEG is associated with bursts of generalised 2.5–3 Hz spike and slow wave discharges. This form of epilepsy has a strong genetic contribution. It responds well to medication and has an excellent prognosis for eventual remission.

Problem

- Sudden shock like contractions affecting either one part or the whole of the body. They may take the form of flexor or extensor spasms or head nodding or a drop attack. The child may be thrown forwards or backwards to the ground, causing injury.

Diagnosis — Myoclonic seizures

They often have their onset in early childhood and are usually seen in symptomatic or cryptogenic epilepsy, usually associated with other abnormal neurological finding, like learning difficulties or cerebral palsy.

Problem

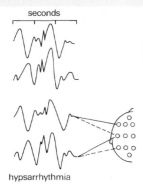

seconds

hypsarrhythmia

• Infant with flexor spasms ('salaam' seizures) and rarely extensor, occurring in clusters several times a day, usually as the infant is awaking or falling asleep. They are often associated with a high pitched shrieking cry. In between spasms most infants show irritability and do not behave normally (epileptic encephalopathy).

Diagnosis — Infantile spasms

This is a rare and distinctive myoclonic epilepsy syndrome seen in early infancy, usually having its onset between 4 and 8 months of age. It is associated with developmental arrest/regression, with a bad prognosis for future intellectual development. In approximately 50% of children who have infantile spasms it is symptomatic of an underlying serious brain disorder. The attacks are difficult to control with anticonvulsant medication and the prognosis is uniformly poor. Such infants may display pre-existing developmental problems before the onset of their spasms. The other 50% may show preceding normal development until the onset of the spasm and have a better prognosis compared to the previous group for both seizure remission and eventual outcome.

Treatment is with vigabatrin (particularly for symptomatic forms) or steroids in the form of ACTH. A minority of children resume normal developmental progress once the spasms cease with initiation of treatment. The EEG shows a typical, electrical pattern called hypsarrhythmia, with chaotic almost continous spike and wave epileptiform discharge present bilaterally. The abnormalities are usually present during sleeping and waking. Infantile spasms are a non-specific reaction of the immature brain to a wide variety of insults and are age specific, tending to be replaced beyond infancy by other seizure types. The insult may be prenatal, include brain malformations, neuronal migrational defects, intrauterine infection, severe perinatal anoxic brain injury, neonatal meningitis and rare neurometabolic disorders. Infantile spasms are a common early manifestation of tuberous scelerosis and this diagnosis should be diligently sought in all infants presenting with the condition.

Problem

• A sudden and temporary loss of postural muscle tone and slowly crumple to the floor (drop attacks).

Diagnosis — Atonic seizures

The EEG shows generalised epileptiform discharges and is more often seen in symptomatic epilepsy.

Problem

- Twitching and jerking involving one side of the body which can progress to involve the whole body ('Jacksonian march').

Diagnosis — Partial epilepsy: frontal lobe
The EEG show focal origin of epileptiform discharges. Magnetic resonance imaging of the brain is indicated in all forms of partial epilepsy except the following specific syndrome:

Problem

- Attacks mainly nocturnal with hemifacial and oropharyngeal contractions causing gurgling noises, can progress to involve one side or the whole body.

Diagnosis — Benign partial epilepsy of childhood with central temporal (rolandic) discharges
This is the commonest partial epilepsy in childhood seen between 5 and 10 years of age with a peak onset around 9 years. It occurs in both sexes with a male preponderance. Sufferers show no neurological or intellectual deficit and they spontaneously remit during adolescence. The typical EEG pattern shows spike discharges unilaterally or bilaterally over the central-mid temporal leads of the conventional EEG. Brain imaging is invariably normal. Genetic factors are thought to play an important role in the causation of this type of epilepsy which has an excellent prognosis.

Problem

seconds

- Attacks of altered awareness with altered perceptions of smell, taste, visual and/or auditory hallucinations.
- A strong psychic element with altered perception of the environment, for example, excessive familiarity in an unfamiliar environment (*dejà vu*), a sense of de-personalisation, etc.
- Commonly lip smacking, sucking or swallowing movements are seen. The speech content is abnormal.

Right mid-temporal spike focus

Diagnosis — Complex partial seizures: temporal lobe epilepsy
Localisation related epilepsies which cause complex partial seizures may be subdivided into those which arise in the temporal lobe area and those which arise extratemporally. Such seizures occur in up to 25% of children with epilepsy and can begin in early infancy. The child may repetitively fidget or show complicated stereotyped movement repertoires. Some show fear or other abnormal emotions. In up to 60% of children with complex partial seizures of temporal origin an underlying structural lesion may be identified on an MRI brain scan. The seizures often run an intractable course to medication and may be amenable to temporal lobe surgery. Generalized tonic clonic seizures are often associated and are a representation of the spread of the seizure discharge throughout the brain. Associated problems include specific learning difficulties and behaviour problems. First line drugs used in

control are carbamazepine and sodium valproate, though newer anti-convulsants like vigabatrin and lamotrigine are also helpful.

Problem

- Seizures lasting longer than 20–30 minutes or serial seizures lasting this duration without recovery of conciousness in between.

Diagnosis — Status epilepticus

Generalised tonic clonic status is an emergency and will have to be speedily terminated with appropriate drug treatment.

Investigation of epilepsy

A competent history is vital but investigations help.

Blood. Fasting blood sugar and calcium estimation should be done, particularly in children having generalised tonic clonic seizures.

Electroencephalogram. This is the most useful investigation. The standard EEG is recorded by 16 electrodes placed on the unshaven scalp, with eight electrodes covering each hemisphere. A single routine normal EEG is not evidence against epilepsy nor indeed is the finding of epileptic discharges in the EEG evidence that the patient's symptoms are necessarily epileptic in nature. A normal EEG may be seen in children with true epilepsy and an abnormal EEG in children who have never had an attack of any kind. The EEG is helpful in categorisation of the epilepsy syndrome. High voltage spikes and slow waves are seen in a generalised distribution and accompany tonic clonic epilepsy, childhood absence epilepsy and myoclonic epilepsy. Focal EEG changes are helpful in localisation in partial epilepsy. Hypsarrhythmia is a typical EEG pattern seen in children with infantile spasms. In children in whom the suspicion of epilepsy is strong, but who have a normal standard EEG, a recording obtained after sleep deprivation or a prolonged ambulatory 24–48 hour EEG may help.

Brain imaging has an important place in children with symptomatic generalised epilepsy and those with partial epilepsy. MRI is the method of choice as it can identify even subtle brain abnormalities.

Drug treatment

The choice of the antiepilepsy drug (AED) depends on the epileptic syndrome being dealt with. The first line drugs in childhood epilepsy are sodium valproate (VPA) and carbamazepine (CBZ) which are effective in most situations. Sodium valproate is very effective and is useful in both generalised and partial epilepsies. The second line AEDs include ethosuximide, phenytoin, lamotrigine, vigabatrin and benzodiazepines. The following table illustrates the usual AEDs chosen in the different childhood epilepsy syndromes and their dosages. Vigabatrin is presently the drug of first choice in symptomatic infantile spasms.

Adverse effects from AEDs may be acute, chronic and occasionally idiosyncratic. They can be divided into central nervous system (CNS) and non-central nervous system side effects. The common CNS side effects which are common to most AEDs include drowsiness, behaviour disturbances in the form of mild irritability and aggression, diplopia, etc. Non-CNS effects include gastrointestinal effects like

Drugs for epilepsy

Type of epilepsy	Drug of choice	Alternatives
GTCS	VPA	CBZ, LTG
Typical Absences	VPA, ethosuximide	LTG
Myoclonic	VPA	LTG, clonazepam
Infantile spasms	Vigabatrin	ACTH, VPA, clonazepam
Simple partial	CBZ	VPA, phenytoin
Complex partial	CBZ	VPA, phenytoin
Secondary general	CBZ	VPA, vigabatrin, LTG
Benign rolandic	CBZ	VPA
Photosensitive	VPA	CBZ
Status epilepticus i.v.	Diazepam p.r./i.v.	Paraldehyde, phenytoin

nausea, vomiting, reversible liver dysfunction and occasional blood dyscrasias.

In patients in whom it has been effective AED treatment is usually continued for 18–24 months from the last documented seizure. There is no need to perform an EEG study before withdrawing AEDs.

The dosage and side effects of the commonly used AEDs

Drug and dose (mg/kg/day)	Adverse effects	
	Common	Rare
VPA (20–40)	Nausea, wt gain	Hair loss, reversible liver dysfunction, thrombocytopenia
CBZ (10–20)	Diplopia, dizziness	Blood dyscrasia, skin rash
Phenytoin (4–8)	Gum hyperplasia	Ataxia (toxicity), hirsuitism, facial coarsening, rickets
Vigabatrin (40–100)	Aggression	Psychotic reaction
Lamotrigine (5–15)	Drowsiness	Skin rash, liver dysfunction
Lamotrigine (combined with VPA) (1–5)	Higher incidence of skin rash	

Over the last decade surgical treatment for epilepsy has become a viable proposition for a minority of children with intractable drug resistant epilepsy. It is particularly helpful in temporal lobe epilepsy and in partial epilepsy with an underlying lesion. Paediatricians should consider surgery sooner rather than later, so that children can make the most of their educational opportunities to enhance future career prospects. Surgery can cure up to 60% of children with temporal lobe epilepsy, with a significant reduction in the frequency of seizures in the other 40%. Palliative surgical procedures are available for children with other forms of chronic intractable epilepsy.

Prognosis

The prognosis of childhood epilepsy tends to be better in the primary generalised epilepsies as there is no cerebral damage or structural abnormality. It is excellent for childhood absence epilepsy and benign partial epilepsy with central temporal spikes. Prolonged febrile convulsions contribute to one-third of intractable temporal lobe epilepsy seen in adults. Children who promptly stop having seizures on medication have a good prognosis. Poor prognosis is associated with chronicity, occurrence of multiple seizure types, association of mental defect or cerebral palsy and young age of onset.

We should do our best to limit the secondary social and educational handicap which may result from the diagnosis of epilepsy and its drug treatment. Children with epilepsy should be allowed to take a full part in all activities at home and school and should not be overprotected. Activities where contact with water is involved are fraught with risk and these children should be encouraged to have showers rather than baths. They should be supervised while swimming and pursuing leisure pursuits near water. Cycling should not be permitted in busy traffic. Athletic and gymnastic activities need supervision. Children who have photosensitive epilepsy should watch television from a distance of not less than 3 metres with background illumination in the room. If they have to approach the television set they should use the remote control or close one eye. Sodium valproate is the drug of choice in photosensitive epilepsy.

The diagnosis of epilepsy and its treatment has a significant impact on the educational and social life of the child and his family. In making a diagnosis of epilepsy, it is better to err on the side of 'not epilepsy' and subsequently to correct one's mistake than to make a wrong diagnosis of epilepsy, which will be doing a great disservice to the child.

There are a number of non-epileptic mimics of epileptic seizures in childhood and these include the following:

Breath holding attacks. Common in toddlerhood, particularly when frustrated or hurt unexpectedly. The child cries, holds his/her breath and becomes cyanosed. It may progress to transient loss of consciousness. These attacks resolve spontaneously as the child grows older.

Reflex anoxic seizures. These are mediated by a sensitive vago cardiac reflex which is particularly prominent during toddling years and is brought on by sudden unexpected trauma. It results in reflex bradycardia, sometimes progressing to transient cardiac asystole manifest as deathly pallor, collapse and floppiness. Attacks are self limiting.

Fainting attacks. These are fairly common in adolescence, particularly in girls, usually brought on by anxiety, fear and prolonged immobility. They recover quickly without a postictal phase.

Benign paroxysmal vertigo is seen in children between 3 and 5 years of age and presents with sudden attacks of abnormal behaviour with collapse, unsteadiness. Consciousness is preserved. Attacks are self limiting.

Day dreaming, night terrors and self stimulatory masturbatory behaviour are other conditions which may be mistaken for epilepsy.

Tics or habit spasms.

Hysterical pseudoseizures are seen in unhappy and emotionally disturbed children, particularly adolescents.

ALTERED AWARENESS

Normal conciousness is a state characterised by awareness of self and environment and associated with the ability to respond appropriately.

Problem

- Disturbed arousal, manifest by changes in normal sleep–wake cycle, eye opening and motor activity.
- Disturbed content of conciousness, self-awareness and reaction to the surroundings.

Diagnosis — Encephalopathy? Cause

Encephalopathy is a state of disturbance of normal conciousness and is characterised by reduced awareness of self and environment and an inability to express thought clearly. Memory is faulty and drowsiness is common with reversal of the sleep–wake cycle. Acute encephalopathy may be due to systemic as well as brain diseases. By far the two

Causes of encephalopathy in children

Traumatic brain injury
   Accidental
   Non-accidental
Intracranial infections
   Meningitis
   Encephalitis
Hypoxic ischaemic brain injury
Acute intracranial hypertension
   Mass lesions
   Acute obstruction to CSF pathways
Epileptic seizure with postictal state
Poisoning
Hypertensive encephalopathy
Respiratory failure
Hepatic failure
Renal failure
Disorders of temperature regulation
   Hypothermia
   Hyperthermia
Inherited metabolic disorders

commonest causes of acute encephalopathy are intracranial infection and hypoxic ischaemic brain injury.

The mechanisms of acute encephalopathy include diffuse and widespread cortical dysfunction, raised intracranial pressure from mass lesions, cerebral oedema — diffuse and or focal compressive lesions of the brainstem.

Assessment of coma

Make a rapid general assessment of the patient's condition with a view to providing immediate cardiorespiratory and circulatory support. A nasogastric tube should be passed and stomach contents aspirated and kept for analysis. A quick and competent history needs to be obtained and needs to include ingestion of likely poisons, trauma, recent foreign travel, exposure to infectious disease, pre-existing neurological disease (epilepsy), metabolic disease (e.g. — diabetes mellitus or inborn errors of metabolism), signs of injury, skin rash, meningism, fundoscopy for haemorrhages, papilloedema, etc. Consider the social context to see if it could be non-accidental injury. The patient should be examined for level of consciousness using the Glasgow Coma Scale (GCS) and evidence of pyrexia, skin rash, hydration, meningeal irritation, obvious signs of trauma, CSF leaks, optic fundi for haemorrhages (NAI in infancy), papilloedema, etc. and evidence of systemic disease.

Glasgow Coma Scale (GCS): based on the behavioural components of normal consciousness

Best motor response	Best verbal response	Eye opening
Oboyo 6	Orientated 5	Spontaneous 4
Localises 5	Confused speech 4	To speech 3
Withdraws 4	Inappropriate words 3	To pain 2
abnormal flexion 3	Incomprehensible sounds 2	Nil 1
Extension 2	Nil 1	
Nil 1		

Note: For a fuller version, see Chapter 3.

Monitoring

Children with GCS 15 are normally oriented and those with 3 are deeply comatose. Children with GCS of less than 8 should be admitted to a paediatric intensive care unit (PICU). The child's vital signs including pulse, temperature, respiration, blood pressure, transcutaneous oxygen saturation and neurological observations including epileptic seizures and abnormal posture should be monitored. Decerebrate posturing with generalised extension and opisthotonus is suggestive of brainstem dysfunction.

Investigations

Urine should be obtained and look for glucose, acetone, protein, toxicology analysis, amino acids and organic acids. A urine sample should be deep frozen for some of the characteristic metabolites seen in some inborn errors. Bloods should be done for FBC, blood cultures, acid–base status, U&Es, LFTs, sugar, toxicology analysis, ammonia, lactate and clotting studies. In those under 18 months of age a lumbar puncture should be done. In older children if there is evidence of raised intracranial pressure (deep coma, pupillary asymmetry, papilloedema, lateralised neurological deficit) the performance of lumbar puncture needs to be a considered decision and a prior CT scan should be obtained. If there are difficulties in obtaining a scan, blood cultures are sufficient.

Treatment

Prevent hypoxia and hypercapnia. Respiratory support may be necessary. Maintain normal acid–base status. Obtain venous access and restrict fluid to two-thirds of maintenance requirements. In suspected intracranial infection start broad spectrum antibiotics, for meningitis, and acyclovir (to cover the possibility of herpes meningoencephalitis). Treat epileptic seizures with anticonvulsants. Intracranial hypertension may become obvious by alterations in vital signs in the form of bradycardia, systemic hypertension, periodic breathing and decerebrate posturing.

A tentorial pressure cone causes herniation of the upper brainstem through the tentorial incisura leading to dilated and fixed pupils, respiratory abnormalities and paralysis of upgaze. A foramen magnum pressure cone causes the cerebellar tonsils to herniate through the foramen magnum compressing the medulla leading to head tilt, neck stiffness, lower cranial nerve palsies, respiratory irregularities including stridor as well as sudden cardiorespiratory arrest.

Intracranial pressure should be monitored with a pressure transducer placed by a neurosurgeon and the cerebral perfusion pressure maintained at greater than 50 mmHg. The need for intracranial pressure monitoring in traumatic encephalopathy is well established but not so in non-traumatic coma except in Reye encephalopathy.

Intracranial hypertension is treated by a variety of approaches, including passive hyperventilation keeping the arterial P_{CO_2} between 3.3 and 3.4 kPa, osmotic agents like mannitol and steroids like dexamethasone. Induced barbiturate coma with thiopentone and hypothermia with artificial cooling and decompressive craniotomy are some of the other approaches available to control intracranial hypertension.

The child's general clinical condition and coma scale rating determine the degree of support necessary. The majority do not require ventilation. Careful attention to fluid balance, blood sugar and blood pressure is necessary. Regular neurological observation by trained nursing staff is very important.

Parents need sensitive counselling and emotional support.

Prognosis

This depends on the cause of the encephalopathy and the duration of coma. Seshia and colleagues have provided valuable information in their series of 177 children with non-traumatic coma. Forty-eight per cent made a complete recovery, 22% recovered with handicap and 30% died. Conditions associated with hypoxic ischaemic brain injury and intracranial infection had a poorer prognosis than children with metabolic coma. All children surviving an acute encephalopathy should undergo careful neurological follow up.

Persistent vegetative state

This is a term suggested by Jennett and Plum to describe patients who recovered the arousal component of consciousness, but not awareness. Many seriously brain injured patients develop a chronically unresponsive state in which they look awake but give little or no evidence of possessing any cognitive mental content to their thought process or recognition of their environment. Some workers regard them as a form of coma. Others consider them as examples of profound dementia and restrict the term coma to sleep like states in which the eyes remain closed.

Brainstem death

When the brainstem is irreversibly damaged the heart stops beating, respiration ceases and the patient can be declared dead. Somatic death follows on brainstem death after a short period even in patients who are on artificial life support. The diagnosis of brain death should be considered in all deeply comatose children who are mechanically ventilated and where there is evidence of brainstem damage. With brainstem death most clinicians agree that mechanical support must be withdrawn. The currently accepted UK criteria by the Royal Medical Colleges emphasise that the permanent functional death of the brainstem constitutes brain death. The diagnosis is made when there has been an absence of brainstem function for 24 hours, in the presence of irremediable structural brain damage after hypothermia, drug and metabolic intoxication have beeen excluded. It is a clinical diagnosis and does not require EEG or other evidence of absent cortical function. In the UK diagnosis of brain death is provided by two doctors who work independently. At the time of assessment the patient's rectal temperature should be greater than 35°C and should be normovolaemic with normal biochemical and acid–base status. Metabolic, toxic and endocrine causes of coma should be excluded. The absence of brainstem function can be reliably determined by careful neurological examination and by the additional specific manoevures to determine cessation of spontaneous respiration, the absence of pupillary reflexes to light with the pupils either in the mid or dilated position, the absence of doll's eye oculocephalic reflexes, corneal reflexes and absent response to a suction catheter passed down the trachea.

The presence or absence of spontaneous respirations is determined by preventilating the patient with 100% oxygen for 10 minutes before the test begins and the $Pa\text{CO}_2$ should be in the normal range of 3.5–5 kPa. The child should be disconnected from the ventilator and oxygen administered at 6 litres per min via a tracheal catheter and the patient observed for 10 minutes. With this procedure the $Pa\text{CO}_2$ should rise sufficiently to trigger normal spontaneous respirations if the respiratory centre is functional. If no spontaneous respiration appears brain death is established. Whether the test should be repeated is a matter of clinical judgement. When parents have difficulties in accepting termination of intensive care a repeat test will be done 24 hours later. However if the situation is hopeless, a repeat test may be performed 4–6 hours later. If brain death is confirmed, mechanical ventilation should be terminated. If organ donation is agreed then artificial ventilation should be continued until donor organs have been removed.

HEADACHE

Like adults, children get headaches for many reasons, including infections especially in the eyes, ears, sinuses and teeth; inflammatory diseases like rheumatoid arthritis; and arterial hypertension. The commonest reasons are migraines and tension headaches. Here we are only concerned only with the most worrying, those due to raised intracranial pressure.

Normal intracranial pressure in children varies with age, mean values are between 2 and 4 mmHg in the neonatal period and 6 and 12 mmHg in the older child. With closure of the sutures and fontanelle the intracranial volume of the brain, the extracellular fluid space and the cerebrospinal fluid compartment are restricted. An expansion of any of the three components rapidly exhausts the compensatory mechanisms and a rise in intracranial pressure follows. Intracranial pressure in excess of 15 mmHg is significant and can reduce cerebral blood flow (CBF) with resulting brain dysfunction and may cause various brain herniation syndromes through the tentorium or the foramen magnum. CBF is maintained by cerebral perfusion pressure (CPP) which is the difference between the mean arterial pressure (MAP) and the mean intracranial pressure (ICP). CPP will decrease when there is systemic hypotension or a rise in intracranial pressure. In acute encephalopathy there is evidence that if the CPP is maintained over 50 mmHg the prognosis for neurological outcome is good and this worsens if CPP is under 40 mmHg. The symptoms and signs of raised intracranial pressure in young infant differ from those in later childhood, because of the compliant skull of infancy with open sutures and fontanelles. The symptoms and signs of intracranial hypertension depend on the rapidity with which it develops.

Problem

- Young infant with a gradual increase in head circumference and sutural separation and enlargement of the anterior fontanelle.
- Engorging scalp veins.
- Irritability and poor feeding (an infant with a headache).
- Older child with nausea, early morning vomiting and headaches.

Diagnosis — Raised intracranial pressure ?Cause
Acute severe rise in intracranial pressure in older children gives rise to herniation syndromes causing pressure on the brainstem leading to bradycardia, systemic hypertension and periodic breathing.

Hydrocephalus

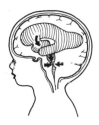

No communication with 'LP'

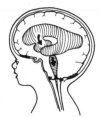

Communication with 'LP'

Causes of raised intracranial pressure

Hydrocephalus
Space-occupying lesions, including brain abscess, posterior fossa, tumours, intracranial haemorrhage
Dural venous sinus thrombosis
Intracranial infection, with brain swelling — meningitis, encephalitis
Acute metabolic encephalopathy, including Reye syndrome, meningeal leukaemia

Hydrocephalus: CT scan

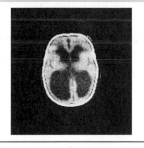

Pinealoma: CT scan

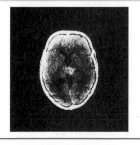

Hydrocephalus implies an excess of cerebrospinal fluid within the skull under increased pressure with an enlargement of the ventricular system. Hydrocephalus may be obstructive/non-communicating when there is an obstruction to its normal flow from the ventricular system to the subarachnoid space and non-obstructive/communicating when there is either an overproduction of the CSF or failure of its reabsorption. The causes of hydrocephalus include congenital and acquired disorders. *Congenital aqueductal stenosis*, accounts for 10–15% of hydrocephalus. *Arnold–Chiari malformation* is a varying degree of downward displacement of the caudal brainstem and cerebellar vermis through the foramen magnum and the severest form is associated with an open myelomeningocele. The malformation obstructs the free flow of CSF either directly or indirectly through arachnoiditis and adhesion causing hydrocephalus. *Dandy Walker syndrome* is a malformation resulting from occlusion of the exit foramina of the fourth ventricle with a greatly distended fourth ventricle and an enlarged posterior cranial fossa with a hypoplastic cerebellum. Obstructive hydrocephalus and cerebellar ataxia are seen in all cases, with severe learning difficulties in up to two-thirds of children. Cerebellar and pyramidal signs are common. The CT scan shows a large cystic fourth ventricle, occupying most of the posterior fossa. Obstructive hydrocephalus may also be produced by a vascular malformation of the posterior fossa such as the *aneurysm of the great vein of Galen*, which acts as a space occupying lesion, obstructing CSF pathways. The space occupying lesions including neoplasms of the posterior fossa cause obstruction to the flow of CSF and cause hydrocephalus and ataxia. Obstructive hydrocephalus can also result acutely from pyogenic and tuberculous meningitis as a result of inflammatory adhesions causing obstruction to the flow of CSF in the basal cisterns. Periventricular haemorrhage is fairly common in preterm infants having multiple neonatal complications including hydrocephalus. Communicating hydrocephalus from overproduction of CSF by a choroid flexus papilloma is known but rare. Defective absorption of CSF can be seen in children who show evidence of dural venous sinus thrombosis from severe dehydration.

Infants with hydrocephalus show failure to thrive, irritability, vomiting and delayed motor and social development. On examination the

Epidural haematoma: CT scan

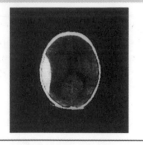

Brain abscess: CT scan

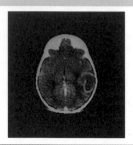

head circumference is greater than the 97th centile. Other signs include sunsetting and a sixth nerve palsy causing a convergent squint.

Investigations include ultrasonic and CT brain imaging. Dexamethazone 0.5 mg/kg/day is particularly helpful in children with brain swelling in association with tumours. Children with hydrocephalus usually require insertion of a ventriculoperitonial shunt. Further additional management depends on the cause of the hydrocephalus.

Brain tumours are considered in Chapter 15.

Intracranial haemorrhage may be intracerebral, subarachnoid, subdural or extradural. It can follow accidental and non-accidental trauma. Extradural haemorrhage is a neurosurgical emergency as it tends to cause shift of midline structures with brainstem herniation, usually across the tentorium. It is often due to a torn middle meningial branch of the superficial temporal artery from trauma. Intracranial haemorrhage is rarely seen in bleeding disorders, for example in the haemorrhagic disease of the newborn. CT scan demonstrates the presence of intracranial bleeding very well. Central nervous system non-accidental injury in infancy gives rise to *chronic subdural haemorrhagic effusion* which presents with progressive increase in head circumference, tense fontanelle, retinal heamorrhage and an infant who is failing to thrive, anaemic and vomits repetitively.

Brain abscess presents insidiously with irritability, failure to thrive, vomiting, fever and lateralised neurological deficit. There may be an association with ear infection mastoiditis, sinusitis, cyanotic congenital heart disease, etc. CT scan shows the abscess well, particularly after a contrast injection when ring enhancement is well seen. Often the pathogenic organisms are anaerobic. It is treated with broad spectrum antibiotics and metronidazole and neurosurgical treatment in the form of aspiration/excision of the abscess. Brain abscess is a potential cause of epilepsy. Anticonvulsant drugs are used prophylactically.

Dural sinus thrombosis is often seen in association with severe dehydration, middle ear infection and mastoiditis. Infective dural sinus thrombosis is associated with otitis media and mastoiditis and mainly affects the lateral sinus. Primary sagittal sinus thrombosis is seen following severe dehydration. The infant presents with irritability, seizure and occasional hemiplegia. Isotope brain imaging shows the site of thrombosis.

Benign intracranial hypertension. In this condition there is raised intracranial pressure in the absence of an obstructive lesion to the CSF pathways. It causes a communicating hydrocephalus and is commonly seen in obese pubertal girls. It has an association with various drugs, including tetracycline, hyper vitaminosis A, use of the contraceptive pill and steroid treatment. It may also be seen in association with hyper- and hypocalcaemia. CT scan is normal and a lumbar puncture confirms the elevated CSF pressure on manometry. The composition of the CSF is normal.

Management. The performance of a lumbar puncture often relieves the recurrent headache associated with this condition. Despite the terminology, there is nothing benign about the condition and there is a serious threat to vision from pressure damage to the optic nerve. Visual acuity and fields need to be monitored serially. Treatment is with steroids or acetazolamide is helpful in most situations. Rarely optic nerve fenestration may be needed if medical treatment fails to arrest sight deterioration.

Raised intracranial pressure is commonly seen in association with meningitis, encephalitis, Reye syndrome and meningeal leukaemia.

RETARDED DEVELOPMENT

Normal child development follows a well ordered sequence in a craniocaudal direction. An infant first develops head control before learning to sit, stand and walk. The normal developmental progress is conveniently separated into four main areas, namely gross motor development, vision and fine motor development, hearing and speech development and social and emotional development. Normal developmental progress may be adversely affected by a wide variety of brain disorders. The delay in development may be global affecting all areas, or specific affecting only a particular area, for example, speech and language development. The assessment of childhood development includes the quantification of delay in relation to the child's chronological age, the pattern of retarded development, i.e. whether global or specific, and seeking the underlying cause.

Common causes of developmental delay	
Prenatal factors	Disordered brain development, e.g., neuronal migration faults, brain malformation, fetopathy, severe intrauterine growth retardation, exposure to teratogens like alcohol, chromosomal aberations, etc.
Perinatal factors	Severe birth asphyxia and birth injury
Postnatal factors	Intracranial infection, e.g. meningitis, encephalitis, accidental and non-accidental trauma, hypernatraemic dehydration, etc.

Seek a family history of developmental delay — suggests a genetic cause, like the fragile X syndrome, neurocutaneous disorders (tuberous sclerosis, neurofibromatosis). A perinatal and postnatal history may indicate a brain damaging event. On examination look for dysmorphic appearance, head circumference, neurocutaneous features, and evidence of evolving spasticity or hypotonia. A 'cause' is more often found in a child showing profound developmental delay and severe learning difficulties. It is less likely in children with mild to moderate developmental delay. In about one-third of children with developmental problems no precise aetiology is found.

Investigations: thyroid function test, serum calcium, TORCH serology, chromosomal studies and molecular genetic screen for fragile X genotype, blood creatine kinase, urine amino acids, organic acids and screen for mucopolysaccharides and blood lactate.

Management

A multidisciplinary team will be needed for assessment and ongoing management of the child and the family. A sympathetic and sensitive explanation should be given to the parents. Aspects of management include the following:

Physical therapy. Regular contact with a physiotherapy department is helpful in promoting a full range movements, optimal movements of different joints, prevention of deformities in contracture.

Developmental stimulation or portage. Parents are given guidance in stimulation and ways of encouraging the development in a severely handicapped child. A developmental team based at the child development centre and including doctors, child psychologists and therapists, should be involved. Early placement in a nursery is often helpful.

Families appreciate expert genetic counselling and to be told about the chance of recurrence of the condition in their future offsprings. This is often empiric as only a minority of children are identified to have a heritable condition.

Educational provision. Children with mental handicap should undergo a formal statementing of their special educational needs to provide appropriate resources in the class room. The current practice is to integrate children with learning difficulties with their normal peer group with provision of additional support of areas of need as far as possible. Only profoundly handicapped children with an IQ under 50 attend schools for children with severe learning difficulties.

Respite care provision to lighten the burden of parents should be provided for families with children who have learning difficulties. They must also be given guidance on the provision of appropriate financial and other benefits, which may help to make the task of caring for the child easy.

Prognosis

This depends on the child's profile of abilities. Children with severe learning difficulties remain dependent throughout life and need to be cared for in a sheltered environment. The emphasis of education in such children is to teach them self care ability and to let them attain limited independence. Those children with mild to moderate learning difficulties, with appropriate help, are capable of independent existence.

HEARING IMPAIRMENT, SPEECH DELAY AND VISUAL IMPAIRMENT

Parents are very good at suspecting deafness in their children and their concerns must be taken seriously and investigated. Neonatal screening using auditory cradles employing evoked response audiometry is currently used for high risk groups and leads to the early detection of deafness. Routine health visitor screening is carried out in infants between 8 and 10 months of age using distraction testing. The pick up rate is low. In later infancy and toddlerhood a child thought be to deaf can be investigated with free field and pure tone audiometry.

Problem	Suspected deafness

Children learn to speak by imitation and unless they can hear normally, speech acquistion will be profoundly delayed. Such infants babble, like normal children, around 5–6 months of age, but without the reinforcement from hearing their own voice and that of others, this ceases by 9–10 months of age. There may be a history that the child does not respond to loud noises. Deafness may be conductive and/or sensorineural.

Conductive deafness. Serous otitis media/glue ear is one of the commonest causes of mild to moderate hearing loss. In children of school age there may be a history of recurrent ear infection or catarrh. The ear drums appears dull and retracted and impedance audiometry shows diminished compliance. Such children usually have eustachian tube dysfunction from adenoidal enlargement. It is treated with myringotomy, insertion of grommets and adenoidectomy (see Ch. 8)

Sensorineural deafness. This usually produces severe or profound impairment of hearing and results from genetic as well as acquired disorders. Such children need the help of a team including an ENT surgeon and an audiologist. Deafness of genetic origin may be isolated or part of a range of other developmental disabilities in a child. The deafness may be static or progressive and all patterns of inheritance, including autosomal dominant recessive and X-linked, are known. Acquired sensorineural deafness results from prenatal, perinatal or postnatal disease. Prenatal viral infection from CMV, rubella and toxoplasma, as well as birth trauma, birth asphyxia, hyperbilirubinaemia, meningitis and encephalitis, may produce significant hearing loss, either alone or in combination with other handicap.

Investigation

All children with delayed speech and language acquisitions or suspected deafness should be referred to a children's hearing assessment service for comprehensive assessment. Further tests may be necessary, including impedance audiometry and electrocochleography.

Degrees of hearing loss:

Mild	20–40 dB loss
Moderate	40–60 dB loss
Severe	60–90 dB loss
Profound	> 90 dB loss

Deafness may be a part of a dysmorphic syndrome. There may be other diagnostic clues like the white forelock seen in Waardenburg syndrome, facial coarsening and corneal clouding as in Hurler syndrome. A child with severe congenital sensorineural neural hearing loss, but without family history, significant past history without abnormalities on examination and negative investigation is usually assumed to have autosomal recessive inherited deafness.

Investigations of deaf children:

Thyroid function tests, karyotype, TORCH serology looking for evidence of prenatally acquired fetopathy
Urine examination for protein considering Alport syndrome
Cervical spinal X-ray considering Klippel–Feil syndrome
ECG looking for the prolonged QT syndrome

Management

Amplification using a hearing aid should be provided as early as possible. The peripatetic teacher for the deaf provides valuable guidance to families on how to communicate with their child and encourage development of speech. Communication by using sign language is to be encouraged so that total communication is possible using both sign language and speech. The British Sign Language and Paget Gorman are the most usually used signing systems. For children with learning difficulties with cognitive impairment, a simplified system of signing like Makaton is helpful. Children with profound hearing loss usually attend a special school for the deaf. Children with lesser degrees of deafness attend partial hearing units attached to an ordinary school. Parents of the deaf child need counselling. When the deaf youngster grows up, he/she also needs to be separately counselled.

Language is the generation and transmission of symbolic communication. Speech is spoken language which includes both the production and transmission of comprehensible coded sounds. Children with deafness and visual impairment are late to acquire language. Human speech has a receptive and an expressive component. Disorders of speech and language may affect only the expressive component or, rarely, both the receptive and expressive forms of speech.

Problem

Suspected delay in speech and language acquisition

Speech problems in general are commoner in boys than in girls. The common causes of delayed speech are deafness, mental handicap, psychosocial deprivation from lack of stimulation and the so called developmental speech and language disorder. The more common expressive speech delays improve gradually with time and speech therapy. Children with the more profound receptive and expressive speech disorders are more severely affected and may need to be taught non-verbal forms of communication and long term input from speech therapists and specialist teachers. Such children have significant reading retardation. Local factors like cleft palate, bulbar palsy, etc. will also cause disorders of speech. There needs to be ongoing speech therapy involvement. In the rare condition called Landau Kleffner syndrome (acquired epileptic dysphasia), the child has a history of epilepsy and language regression after a period of normal development. The epileptic seizures may be infrequent, but the EEG shows frequent epileptiform discharges. The prognosis is poor for speech development.

Vision forms an important link between the child and his/her environment and consequently severe visual impairment will interfere with all aspects of development, particularly manipulative abilities and social skills. Visual impairment may occur alone or be associated with other co-existing problems. Unilateral visual impairment does not affect general development in a healthy child. Bilateral visual impairment always retards general development.

Most visual development is completed in the pre-school years. Amblyopia is the term used to denote visual loss without organic signs. It is produced by cortical suppression of image from one of the two eyes and is reversible if the duration of sight deprivation is short. Irreversible damage can occur if treatment is not started before school entry.

When visual acuity can be measured accurately and it is 6/60 or worse in the better eye, the child is eligible to be registered blind and will need education as a blind child. When it is 6/24 or worse in the better eye the child is referred to as being partially sighted.

Problem	Visual impairment ?cause

Disorders of the eye. These include anophthalmos, cataracts, high myopia, retinal disorders like retrolental fibroplasia, optic nerve hypoplasia, optic atrophy, etc. Some of them may run a progressive course.

Ophthalmic abnormalities with other disability. Examples include eye abnormality seen in association with other conditions like metabolic disorders, retrolental fibroplasia in a baby with perinatally acquired handicap.

Blindness of cortical origin. In this group of children there is no significant ophthalmic abnormality. They have additional disabilities including severe learning difficulties. Nearly two-thirds of children who are visually handicapped have additional disability.

Delayed visual maturation. Some normal children and some with learning difficulties are visually unresponsive in the early months of life only to develop normal vision later. This group of children are said to have delayed visual maturation.

Leber amaurosis is a congenital degenerative condition in which there is profound visual handicap. On clinical examination there is no retinal abnormality but electroretinogram (ERG) and visual evoked response (VER) are both totally absent.

Assessment

The child will need to be assessed by a multidisciplinary team including ophthalmological, paediatric neurological, genetic and educational professionals. Electrophysiological tests in the form of ERG and VER will be helpful in separating retinal causes of blindness from those of visual structures beyond the retina, e.g. in Leber amaurosis, both ERG and VER are totally absent, whereas with cortical blindness the ERG is normal and the VER usually flat. Investigations to determine the cause of visual handicap include exclusion of galactosaemia by appropriate blood tests, serology for congenital infection, pituitary function tests and brain imaging — CT or MRI scan.

Management

Ophthalmic assessment and treatment for treatable disorders.

Parental guidance. Parents need regular advice on their child's development to ameliorate the effect of visual handicap. The blind child will need specialised developmental assessment and specially tailored remedial programme with parents as the main teachers, guided by a peripatetic teacher for the blind from the Royal National Institute who visits the home and school and advises parents and teachers. Learning by modalities other than vision is encouraged. Motor development is abnormal with delayed walking. Children often do not crawl at all. Speech and language acquisition follows an unusual pattern in view of the difficulty in acquiring symbolic concepts.

Education of blind children with normal cognitive abilities. These children need to learn Braille. Partially sighted children can use low vision aids and perhaps manage in a mainstream school. Completely blind children may need to attend a school for the blind.

Genetic counselling. Genetic causes are implicated in a high proportion of children with visual handicap, e.g. in children with congenital choroido-retinal degeneration, high myopia and congenital cataracts. Altogether about 50% of all blind and partially sighted children have a genetic cause for their visual handicap.

DEVELOPMENTAL REGRESSION

Regression is present in children who have shown previously normal development but then lose their acquired skills from a dementing process. It usually suggests a progessive neurodegenerative disorder. These include a wide variety of neurological, neurometabolic disorders and slow viral diseases affecting the brain. Neurometabolic disorders affecting the brain present with a variety of symptoms, including developmental delay, or a period of normal development followed by regression. These include disorders of amino acid, organic acid metabolism, mucopolysaccharidoses, inborn errors of the urea cycle, mitochondrial, peroxisomal and lysosomal disorders. These disorders have major genetic implications and a poor prognosis. The provision of a diagnostic label is often helpful to families. Most of these conditions run a progressive course with death following after variable period. A minority may be amenable to treatment.

Certain features from the history and examination may help narrow down the diagnostic possibilities. A useful way to approach neurodegenerative diseases in childhood is to see whether or not they are associated with epilepsy and other clinical discriminators like age, sex, racial origin, positive family history and some of the important clinical symptomatology. Often a battery of screening tests is necessary. The following clinical situations are possible:

Deterioration in infancy with no obvious clues

Hypothyroidism.
Phenylketonuria.
Homocystinuria.
Organic acid disorders.
Biotinidase deficiency.

Regression in infancy with epileptic seizures

West syndrome.
Tuberous sclerosis.
Glycine encephalopathy. CSF glycine may be elevated despite normal plasma levels.
Menke kinky hair disease. The clinical clue of pili torti is not always obvious.
Molybdenum cofactor deficiency. Plasma uric acid is elevated. Ocular lens dislocation may be seen.

Irritable and extending infants

Krabbe disease. Infant shows severe irritability and neck retraction, absent deep tendon reflexes. Other confirmatory investigations include slow nerve conduction studies and high CSF protein. White cell enzyme analysis shows deficiency of galactocerebrosidase.
Glutaric aciduria type I. The typical story is of acute onset of dystonia during the course of a febrile illness followed by regression. Diagnosis may be missed by organic acid analysis and the enzyme glutaryl coA dehydrogenase must be measured in fibroblast culture.
Infantile Gaucher disease. Splenomegaly may be a clinical clue as well as the loss of rapid pursuit movements of the eyes (saccades).
Tay–Sachs disease. An excessive startle response to noise, and a cherry red spot on the macula are helpful.
Molybdenum cofactor deficiency. This presents with intractable epilepsy and lens dislocation.
Lesch–Nyhan disease. This is seen in boys and regression commonly begins in the first year of life. Extrapyramidal signs supervene beyond the first 2 years of life.

Niemann-Pick disease. This presents with hypotonia, cherry red macular spots, and hepatosplenomegaly and areflexia. Nerve conduction is dramatically slow, suggesting demyelination. Bone marrow examination shows foamy lymphocytes. White cell enzyme analysis is diagnostic.

Pelizeus-Merzbacher disease. The presence of early nystagmus is a clue to this diagnosis. MRI of the brain shows typical white matter changes.

Presentation in 2–3-year-old children with no obvious clues

Rett syndrome. This is usually seen in girls with progressive loss of purposeful hand use with hand wringing/weaving frequently seen.

Autism spectrum disorders.

Regression in 2–3-year-old children with seizures

Progressive neuronal degeneration of childhood (PNDC). Synonyms — *Alper/Huttenlocher disease.* Presents with intractable epilepsy, with gradual liver failure, high blood and CSF lactate.

Batten disease. Late infantile neuronal ceroid lipofuscinosis. Ataxia, intractable epilepsy, dementia and progressive blindness are the cardinal features of this condition. ERG is flat with giant visual evoked potentials on EEG with slow flicker. Electron microscopy of white cells in buffy coat or biopsy of skin, conjunctiva, or rectal mucosa show curvilinear bodies.

Lennox–Gastaut syndrome. Presents with the triad of tonic seizures, drop attacks and atypical absences associated with developmental arrest and regression.

Disorders in the young child with neurological signs

Metachromatic leucodystrophy. Shows evidence of peripheral neuropathy, loss of reflexes, spasticity, ataxia and dementia. Helpful tests include raised CSF protein, metachromatic deposits on renal tubual cells in urinary sediment and deficient aryl sulphatase A in white cells.

Leigh disease. This is a mitochondiral disorder presenting with encephalopathy, seizures, impaired eye movements, respiratory irregularities and ataxia. Blood and CSF lactate are raised and on brain imaging low density lesions are seen in the basal ganglia.

Ataxia telangiectasia. Children present with striking ataxia, choreoathetosis and eye movement disorder (oculomotor dyspraxia). There is raised alpha fetoprotein in plasma and DNA repair defects in fibroblasts.

Regression in the school child

Subacute sclerosing panencephalitis. This is a slow viral infection of the human brain with the measles virus. EEG shows classical polyphasic periodic complexes. MRI brain scan shows white matter hypodensities. Excessive intrathecal synthesis of measles antibodies can be demonstrated.

Adrenoleucodystrophy. This presents with school failure. CT scan shows leucodystrophy. Raised plasma very long chain fatty acids.

Wilson's disease. This is eminently treatable if diagnosed early and must be considered in any child with unexplained regression from 5 years and upwards. Early on, it presents with hepatocellular dysfunction. Kaiser–Fleischer rings in the cornea on slit lamp examination are characteristic.

San Filippo disease. Dysmorphic features may be mild.

Moya Moya disease. Progressive occlusion of the blood vessels of the circle of Willis

Management

A thorough and detailed search for the underlying condition is necessary. The prognosis for most neurodegenerative diseases of the brain is poor, and they run a progressive course with increasing physical and mental disability. The children often die of hypostatic pneumonia. The families need a lot of support and genetic counselling must not be forgotten.

FURTHER READING

Aicardi J 1992 Diseases of the nervous system in childhood. Clinics in developmental medicine No. 115/118. Mac Keith Press

Brett EM 1991 Paediatric neurology, 2nd edn. Churchill Livingstone, Edinburgh

Chadwick D, Bates D, Cartlidge N 1990 Medical neurology. Churchill Livingstone, Edinburgh

Holten JB 1994 The inherited metabolic diseases, 2nd edn. Churchill Livingstone, Edinburgh

Hosking G, Powell R 1985 Chronic childhood disorders. Wright, Bristol

Newton R W 1996 Colour atlas of paediatric neurology

Newton RW 1995 Colour atlas of paediatric neurology. Marby-Wolfe, London

O'Donohoe NV 1995 Epilepsies of childhood, 3rd edn. London: Butterworth Heinemann

Plum F, Posner J B 1982 The diagnosis of stupor and coma, 3rd edn. FA Davis

Roger J, Bureau M, Dravet C, Dreifuss F, Perret A, Wolf P 1992 Epileptic syndromes in infancy, childhood and adolescence, 2nd edn. John Libby, London

Seshia SS, Johnston B, Kasian G 1983 Non-traumatic coma in childhood: clinical variables in outcome. Development Medicine and Child Neurology 25: 492–501

Stephenson JBP, King MD 1992 Handbook of neurological investigations in children. Wright, Bristol

Wallace S J 1996 Epilepsy in children. Chapman & Hall, London

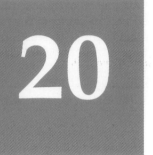

20 Skin

Skin conditions are important for two reasons. First, some skin diseases such as atopic eczema, warts and mollusca are very common in childhood and most cases are usually quite easy to manage. Second, skin lesions sometimes provide us with a vital clue to the diagnosis of an underlying systemic disorder such as systemic mastocytosis or Langerhan cell histiocytosis. In these circumstances, consultation at an early stage with a dermatologist is important.

As with all disorders, first take a history and determine how long the lesion/eruption has been present, where it is and if it has changed in appearance and distribution. Is it itchy and how is it interfering with the child's development and family life? Then describe the lesion/eruption. For an eruption, it is useful to start *macro* and end up *micro*. Begin by describing the overall *distribution* for example, mainly extensor for psoriasis, and whether it is *symmetrical* which implies an endogenous cause. Then describe how individual lesions *associate* with each other — do they form a herpetiform cluster or do they seed along a line of trauma like the Koebner phenomenon seen in psoriasis and lichen planus, or do they form a line (e.g. bites) or a circle (e.g. tinea)? Then finally describe the individual lesions — are they papules (pimples), flat macules (marks), vesicles or plaques. Even if the presenting complaint in a child is not a skin problem always make a note of any skin lesions; do not make the mistake of looking through the skin as if it were an inert covering!

Lesions

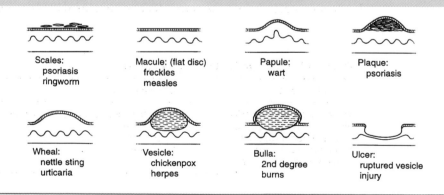

Scales:
  psoriasis
  ringworm

Macule: (flat disc)
  freckles
  measles

Papule:
  wart

Plaque:
  psoriasis

Wheal:
  nettle sting
  urticaria

Vesicle:
  chickenpox
  herpes

Bulla:
  2nd degree
  burns

Ulcer:
  ruptured vesicle
  injury

RED SPOTTY RASHES WHICH ARE NOT VERY ITCHY

Causes of a relatively non-itchy macular-papular rash (morbilliform eruption)

Viruses	Drug eruptions	Others
Measles	Penicillins	Guttate psoriasis
Rubella	Salicylic acid	Graft vs. host disease
Fifth disease	Barbiturates	Erythema multiforme
(Parvovirus B19)	Isoniazid	Pityriasis rosea
Infectious mononucleosis	Phenothiazine	
Exanthema subitum	Thiazide diuretics	

Children commonly have red spotty rashes and most are harmless and self limiting. They are usually easily distinguished from each other by establishing whether the child is systemically well and whether any drugs have been given recently. Drug reactions are usually morbilliform and symmetrical, starting on the inner aspects of the proximal limbs and progressing to the trunk. Peeling of the skin 2–3 weeks after an viral exanthem/drug rash is quite common.

Pityriasis rosea. This may be a reaction to a recent viral infection. It often begins with one large oval patch on the trunk (the herald patch) and then spreads to form many other scaly, oval patches and small red spots on the trunk and proximal limbs. It takes around 6 weeks to clear and although it looks quite alarming, the child is usually quite well. If itching is a major component, then a mild topical corticosteroid preparation such as 1% hydrocortisone ointment plus a soothing emollient such as aqueous cream may be used for symptomatic relief.

A SPOTTY RASH DUE TO BLEEDING INTO THE SKIN

Another type of red spotty rash which does not itch very much is that due to small bleeds into the skin. Most erythemas will blanch if a glass

Causes of purpura and/or bruising into the skin

Normal platelet	Low platelets
Meningococcal meningitis	Idiopathic thrombocytopenic purpura
Henoch-Schönlein purpura	Leukaemia
Certain haemorrhagic viral	Aplastic anaemia
rashes [occasionally]	Septicaemia
Trauma from scratching	

slide is pressed against the skin but if a rash is due to extravasated red blood cells, then it will still be visible when the slide is pressed against the skin surface.

Meningococcal purpura is a sign never to be missed — these lesions may be present in small numbers on the distal limbs in a sick child. They imply significant septicaemia. Henoch–Schönlein purpura can also appear quite dramatic with palpable purpura on the limbs, buttocks and lower abdomen along with a variable degree of arthralgia, gut symptoms and associated renal problems. Treatment is usually symptomatic. Leukaemia can present as spontaneous bruising in the skin. Traumatic bruising due to child abuse should be suspected in any unusual distribution of bruising, especially if the shapes of individual bruises appear 'un-natural', e.g. linear or finger shaped.

RASHES OF VESICLES AND SMALL BLISTERS

Some rashes start as red spots (papules) and then quickly develop into spots containing clear fluid (vesicles). These may then rupture to form ulcers like cold sores or the clear fluid may turn cloudy as in a pustule. Larger blisters (1 cm and above) are usually called bullae.

Common vesicular/pustular rashes in childhood

Cause	Features
Varicella/zoster virus	Simple chicken pox is characterised by polymorphic lesions, i.e. papules, vesicles and pustules, will usually be present at the same stage. Shingles usually has a dermatomal pattern, or it may be widespread in the immunocompromised
Herpes simplex	Neonatal herpes simplex may present as blisters and pustules in the newborn and requires urgent treatment with acyclovir. Primary herpes simplex usually presents as mouth ulceration and systemic upset. Secondary herpes simplex presents as clusters of vesicles
Hand/foot/mouth disease	Vesicles or grey pustules on palms, soles and back of mouth (Coxsackie A 16)
Scabies	Vesicles/pustules usually on feet and axillary region in young babies. Finger webs in the older child. Excoriations +++ and secondary infection common. Others usually affected
Eczema	Eczema has many causes but acute eczema is characterised by vesicles, especially on the sides of the fingers and palms of the hand
Impetigo	Clusters of 1–2 cm flaccid blisters quickly rupture and dry with honey coloured crusts

Impetigo. This is characterised by flaccid blisters which quickly rupture to form erosions. These erosions are covered by dried serum, producing the characteristic honey coloured crusts. Impetigo usually presents as a few lesions around the nose or mouth but occasionally it can spread to involve the whole trunk and involve deeper layers of the skin (ecthyma). The commonest cause of impetigo in developed countries is *Staphylococcus aureus* but in developing countries, nephritogenic strains of streptococci may also be found. Impetigo can also complicate scabies and lice infestations and impetigenisation of atopic eczema with *Staph. aureus* is also common. In such secondary impetigo, it is important to treat the underlying cause as well as the secondary infection. Systemic antibiotics (flucloxacillin or erythromycin in a penicillin allergic subject) are preferred in widespread impetigo but some localised lesions can be treated with simple antiseptics or topical antibiotic ointments such as mupirocin.

Acne is occasionally seen in infancy. In the first 3 months, it is usually a transient phenomenon due to maternal androgens. Infantile acne may also be present after this time, especially in boys. The acne lesions look the same as teenage acne with inflammatory papules, occasional pustules and even scarring. Treatment with topical erythromycin lotion or long term oral antibiotics (not tetracyclines) may sometimes be needed. Children developing acne between the ages of 2 and 10 should be investigated to exclude an endocrine disorder. Acne treatment in the older child/young teenager should be directed at removing the keratin plugs, e.g. with 5% topical benzoyl peroxide or a topical retinoid and suppression of lipolytic bacteria with long term topical or low dose oral antibiotics. Acne causes considerable morbidity in young people and now that effective treatment is available, acne scarring should be a thing of the past.

Acne

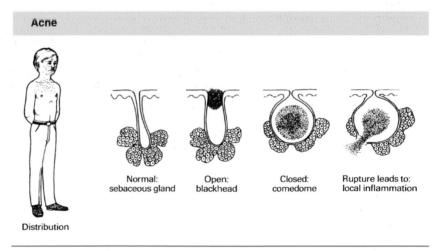

Normal: sebaceous gland   Open: blackhead   Closed: comedome   Rupture leads to: local inflammation

Distribution

Fungal infections are quite common in childhood and take on many forms according to the infecting agent and site of infection. The commonest are due to candida infections of the mouth and napkin area. Here, small circinate erosions on a red background are commoner than the classical milky white superficial satellite lesions. Swabs should be sent to confirm the diagnosis and topical nystatin along with measures to dry the affected areas should be instituted. Tinea pedis (athletes' foot) often presents as scaling and itching in the third and fourth toe clefts. It is commoner in the older child and can be treated with topical imadizoles. Forefoot dermatitis (a glazed persistent erythema with cracking) is not due to fungus infection and may be associated with occlusive foot wear. Occasionally, toe and finger nail fungal infection is seen in the older child and this should be treated with oral griseoful-vin. Tinea corporis (ringworm on the body) can be treated with topical therapy but hair involvement (tinea capitis) should always be treated with oral griseofulvin at a dose of 10 mg per kg for 6–10 weeks because the hair roots are infected below the surface of the scalp. Occasionally, tinea capitis due to animal fungus can produce an intense inflamma-tory reaction covered by a boggy mass (kerion). This usually responds to soaking with antiseptics.

RASHES WHICH ITCH

Causes of itching	
Eczema	Scabies
Contact dermatitis	Papular urticaria
Some drug reactions	Animal mites
Conjugated hyperbilirubinaemia	Flea bites
Kidney failure	Lice infestations (pediculosis)

The division of skin rashes into itchy and non itchy is arbitrary, one as some so-called 'non-itchy' rashes such as pityriasis rosea can occasion-ally itch a lot and, conversely, some young infants with widespread scabies do not appear to itch very much. Itchy rashes often indicate a primary skin disorder, whereas itching without any visible rash often indicates a systemic problem such as liver or renal disease.

Problem
• Red itchy rash.

Diagnosis—Atopic eczema
This is the commonest itchy skin eruption in childhood affecting 10–15% of 7–11-year-old children in Europe. It is associated with asthma and hay fever and a family history of such atopic disease is found in around 70% of families. There may be a slight female prepon-derance in early childhood and over 70% of cases begin before the age of 2 years. Around 65% of children with atopic eczema go into long term remission by the age of 16 but such children are always prone to irritant dermatitis because of their generally dry skin. Early onset and severe disease in childhood are bad prognostic factors.

The distribution of atopic eczema varies with the age of the child. Typically, it presents on the cheeks and outer forearms and legs in the infant and may quickly spread to involve the trunk. Eczematous lesions are characterised by poorly defined erythema with surface change — the surface change may be in the form of oozing, crusting, vesicles or thickening in response to scratching (lichenification). After about the age of 2, atopic eczema normally has a predilection for the skin flexures, especially behind the knees, fronts of the elbows and around the neck.

Eczema through the ages

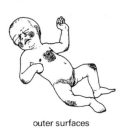 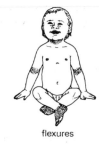 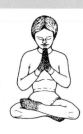

outer surfaces   flexures   Hands and feet

A generally dry skin (atopic xerosis) is also common. Atopic eczema is a chronic intermittent condition and the chronic pruritus frequently leads to sleep loss, emotional upset and an exhausted family. Other complications can include secondary impetigenisation with *Staph. aureus*. Occasionally, primary herpes simplex infection can spread rapidly on an area of eczematous skin (eczema herpeticum). This requires urgent treatment with oral or intravenous acyclovir.

The cause of atopic eczema is probably due to a combination of genetic and environmental factors, ranging from perinatal nutrition through to specific allergy against house dust mite. Allergic factors are often overemphasised in atopic eczema and non-specific irritants such as wool, soaps and climatic factors may be just as important. Dietary factors may be important in the early infant for both disease incidence and chronicity but these are rarely implicated in the older child.

Treatment

Given that atopic eczema is a chronic relapsing condition, for which there is no 'cure' at present, time taken to explain the background and natural history to the parents is essential. All children probably benefit from emollients such as white soft paraffin/liquid paraffin 50/50 mixture and oily bath additives are sometimes helpful. The correct emollient is that which the child will use. Use of soap substitutes, keeping the nails short and avoidance of wool or rough clothing is also recommended. Secondary infections due to *Staph. aureus* should be treated with oral flucloxacillin (or erythromycin if penicillin allergy is present). Pustules may not always be present and secondary infection should always be considered if a child's atopic eczema suddenly deteriorates and becomes very red and sore. Topical corticosteroid preparations are quite safe to use in children with atopic eczema, providing that the weakest possible strength which is effective is used. Most children with atopic eczema have mild disease and can be controlled with 1% hydrocortisone ointment twice daily for a period of 7–10 days followed by an emollient 'holiday'. Children with more stubborn lesions or discoid lesions may require 5–7-day bursts of more potent corticosteroids but these should not be applied to the face or moist areas such as the napkin area without a dermatologist's supervision. Side effects such as skin thinning are now extremely rare but 'corticosteroid phobia' is now firmly instilled in the public's mind. Although it is true that topical corticosteroids probably do not alter the natural history of atopic eczema, they produce very effective relief from symptoms, allowing the child to lead a normal and happy life and treatment should not be withheld from children who are suffering. The use of bandaging techniques such as 'wet wraps' can also be helpful for children with very excoriated limbs. Reduction of house dust mite levels at home is helpful in some children. Children in whom there is a clear parental account of their child reacting to certain foods may benefit from exclusion from that particular food. Skin and blood tests are not especially helpful because of their poor positive predicative value. Antihistamines are quite popular but should only be given as a short term adjunct during a severe relapse. Tar treatments are quite messy and most children do not appreciate their smell or consistency. Evening primrose oil has been used widely to treat atopic eczema in childhood but the benefits, if any, are probably quite small. Third line measures such as photochemotherapy, cyclosporin A and Chinese medicinal herbs are sometimes used and these are best initiated in liaison with a dermatologist. The management of atopic eczema is reviewed by Henry et al. (1996). Parents may also gain valuable support from self help groups such as the National Eczema Society (whose address is shown at the end of this chapter).

Discoid eczema. This is characterised by coin-shaped eczematous patches on the trunks and limbs. Usually, there is associated atopic eczema in the flexures at some time when this pattern of eczema occurs in childhood. It responds to potent topical corticosteroid preparations.

Allergic contact dermatitis. This is rare in childhood but should always be considered in any dermatitis not responding to normal measures, especially when it occurs on sites such as the feet, where, for example, shoe dermatitis can occur.

Cheilitis. This can occur as part of atopic eczema or as an isolated phenomenon. Constant licking of the lips perpetuates the condition and soft paraffin will help protect against further damage.

Juvenile plantar dermatosis. JPD is characterised by a glazed erythema of the soles, especially the forefoot, seen typically in pre-pubertal school children. There is a possible link with atopy. Although JPD has been blamed on synthetic footwear, allergic contact dermatitis has not been consistently demonstrated. Regular emollients to prevent cracking and the occasional use of potent steroids under polythene occlusion for short periods have been helpful. It usually clears spontaneously at around puberty.

Blepharitis. This may be an isolated phenomenon or it may be part of seborrhoeic dermatitis which also affects the scalp margin and external ear canal. It usually responds to 1% hydrocortisone ointment.

| Problem | • Itchy rash in creases. |

Diagnosis — Scabies

This typically presents as erythematous papules on the axillary folds, hands and soles of feet together with non-specific excoriations elsewhere on the limbs and trunk. Small linear, grey burrows, 1–3 mm may occasionally be seen, especially around the wrists, ankles and finger webs, and genital lesions are common on boys. Intense itching is characteristic, especially at night, and usually more than one family member is affected. Where possible, the acarus should be removed with a clean pin and examined under the microscope to confirm the diagnosis (and sometimes to convince the parents!). However, one should have a high index of suspicion for scabies in a child who is itching, especially if vesicular or pustular lesions are present on the feet. Benzyl benzoate is not suitable for children as it is quite irritating but aqueous malathion or permethrin cream are suitable alternatives. Two applications, 1 week apart, is all that is required. The most important thing is to treat all family members and close physical contacts *at the same time* to avoid reinfection. In babies, the face and scalp should also be treated but in older children and adults, only areas below the neck need to be treated.

SCALY SKIN AND OTHER DISORDERS OF KERATINISATION

Causes of a scaly skin

Condition	Clinical feature	Inheritance
Collodian baby	Rare, severe, present at birth	
Ichthyosis vulgaris	Commonly widespread, spares flexures	Autosomal dominant
Sex-linked ichthyosis	Coarser with brown scales and not sparing flexures	sex-linked
Keratosis pilaris	Around hair follicles, upper thighs, arms and buttocks, onset puberty	
Darier's disease	Rare, follicular, greasy scales, neck and upper trunk	Autosomal dominant
Psoriasis	Guttate or extensor	family history+
Pityriasis rosea	Herald spot, body rash, ?infection	

Problem

- Scaly rash.

Diagnosis — Psoriasis

Most commonly, psoriasis in childhood presents as an eruption of small (1 cm) and slightly scaly, red lesions in a 'shower' over the trunk. This appears quite abruptly and is known as guttate psoriasis. It is usually preceded by a streptococcal sore throat in childhood which should be treated accordingly with penicillin or an alternative. Guttate psoriasis usually clears spontaneously in around 6–10 weeks but some children benefit from an emollient, or a combination of a mild topical corticosteroid/tar preparation.

Treatment. Some children with florid guttate psoriasis may also require a course of ultraviolet therapy under a dermatologist's supervision. Chronic plaque psoriasis is not very common in childhood but when it does occur, it can be difficult to treat as many of the more potent adult measures cannot be used safely. Mild topical corticosteroid/tar preparations are commonly used and for thick plaques limited to extensor areas, topical short contact dithranol cream can be used with caution. Thickened psoriasis in the scalp can be treated by Ung Cocois Co massaged into the scalp at night and washed out with a tar shampoo in the morning. Once the scaling in the scalp is clear, this may need to be repeated on a weekly basis. Occasionally, phototherapy is used and in such cases, referral to a dermatologist is recommended.

Psoriasis and pityriasis

Common Psoriasis (66%)   Guttate Psoriasis (33%)

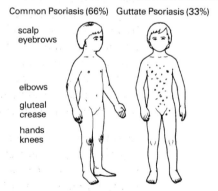

scalp
eyebrows

elbows

gluteal
crease

hands
knees

Pityriasis rosea can resemble guttate psoriasis but the oval patches of pityriasis rosea are larger and the herald patch may be characteristic. Another type of pityriasis, called *pityriasis lichenoides*, can also look like psoriasis but the course is far more chronic and individual lesions are smaller with a characteristic collarette of scale. Pityriasis lichenoides may have a variety of acute and more chronic lesions present at any one time and it can lead to quite marked hypopigmentation, especially in the darker skin child.

LARGE BLISTERS

Epidermolysis bullosa. The skin is fastened together, one layer upon the other. Occasionally by genetic default, the layers are not fastened sufficiently and the skin become detached in sheets, just as it does after a second degree burn. This occurs in epidermolysis bullosa, the various forms of which are shown in the illustration below.

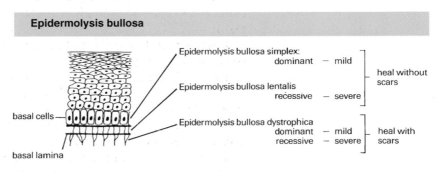

Epidermolysis bullosa

Epidermolysis bullosa simplex:
dominant – mild

Epidermolysis bullosa lentalis
recessive – severe

heal without scars

basal cells

Epidermolysis bullosa dystrophica
dominant – mild
recessive – severe

heal with scars

basal lamina

The severe forms present at or soon after birth and may involve the nails and upper gastrointestinal tract. Complications such as scarring, fusion of the digits (syndactyly) and oesophageal strictures may require surgical intervention. There is no effective treatment apart from general supportive care, preferably by an experienced team.

Staphylococcal scalded skin syndrome. Some strains of staphylococci produce a potent toxin called exfoliatin which produces a widespread toxic erythema and eventually superficial necrosis of the epidermis. This can occasionally be life threatening and the child should be treated with flucloxacillin as well as supportive care for the erythroderma, i.e. attention to temperature control, fluid loss and electrolyte disturbance. Another condition, called *toxic epidermal necrolysis*, can sometimes look similar but this is usually caused by drugs and the level of split is at the dermo-epidermal junction. A skin biopsy is sometimes required to distinguish between the two.

Incontinentia pigmenti. This is an X-linked condition and occurs only in girls. The gene is assumed to be fatal in the male. Blisters may appear in streaks on the trunk during the first few months and these are eventually replaced by warty lesions which slowly resolve to leave whorls of brown pigmentation following Blaschko's lines on the trunk. There may be some associated minor dental, ocular and CNS abnormality.

Chronic bullous disease of childhood. This is a rare immuno bullous disorder characterised by circles of large blisters, most typically occurring on the upper thighs. Immunoflorescence reveals a linear deposition of IgA at the basement membrane zone. Systemic immunotherapy in the form of oral prednisolone or sulphonamides is usually necessary. Referral to a dermatologist with an interest in immunobullous disorders is recommended.

NAPKIN RASHES

There are four basic causes of an eruption in the napkin area: chemical irritation, napkin candidiasis, infantile seborrhoeic eczema and atopic eczema.

Problem

- Widespread eczematous change confined to the napkin area with pronounced surface damage (i.e. scaling and oozing).
- Convexities of the skin in maximal contact with the nappy are most affected whereas the deeper inguinal creases are usually spared.

Diagnosis — Chemical napkin dermatitis

This is simply due to the irritant effect of ammonia and moisture being held in prolonged contact with the skin. It has probably become less common with the highly absorbent disposable nappies available today but occasional cases are still seen. Frequent changing of the nappies along with liberal quantities of an emollient such as white soft paraffin/liquid paraffin 50/50 mixture are usually all that is required but occasionally a 5-day course of 1% hydrocortisone ointment is needed.

Problem

- Onset in the first 2 months of life.
- Well demarcated, non-itchy areas of erythema and scaling.
- Happy looking child.
- Similar satellite lesions 1–3 cm in diameter spreading to the lower parts of the abdomen.
- Prominent cradle cap in scalp.

Diagnosis — Infantile seborrhoeic dermatitis

We are still unsure as to the exact cause of this eruption but the child always appears remarkably unperturbed despite the distressing appearance of the rash to the parents. This eruption clears spontaneously within 6–10 weeks but a 1-week course of 1% hydrocortisone ointment applied twice daily will usually speed its resolution.

Problem

- Erythema in the napkin area characterised by a sore exudative area around the genitalia and anus.
- Circinate erosions or superficial white pustules around the edge of the erythema.

Diagnosis — Napkin candidiasis

This commonly follows an acute GI upset or recent antibiotic therapy. It is usually treated by topical nystatin. Occasionally a course of oral nystatin may be needed to remove the gut reservoir if heavy candidal overgrowth has occurred.

| Problem | • Very itchy, eczematous rash in the napkin area.
• Generally dry skin.
• Patches of eczema elsewhere on the body, especially in the flexures. |

Diagnosis — Probable atopic eczema

This may present for the first time in the napkin area and is probably a form of irritant dermatitis superimposed on an atopic background. Caution should be made in making this diagnosis on one visit alone and in the absence of typical atopic eczema lesions elsewhere. Treatment with regular nappy changes, emollients and mild topical corticosteroid preparations in short courses are beneficial.

COLOURING AND ABSENCE OF COLOURING

Causes of pigmentation

Type	Description	Onset
Racial	Generalised	Birth
UVL exposure	Light exposed	Any age
Freckles	1–4 mm pale brown macules on light exposed areas	2 years onwards
Lentigines	1–4 mm dark macules. Generalised. Often after light exposure	Later childhood
Café au lait spots	1–4 cm oval macules. Less than 6 total	2 years onwards
Neurofibromatosis	Numerous café au lait spots. Steady increase in number. Axillary accentuation	2 years onwards
Post inflammatory	At site of injury or other skin disease	Later childhood
Acanthosis nigricans	Pale pigmentation and velvety thickening in flexures. Autosomal dominant	2 years onwards
Urticaria pigmentosa	Pale brown 0.5–1 cm macules which urticate on scratching. Increase in number	Birth onwards

| Photosensitivity | The commonest form of photosensitive eruption in a child is due to contact with plants containing psoralens during sunny periods — the so-called *phytophoto dermatitis*. Lesions usually present as linear whip-like streaks of erythema and blisters and these rapidly resolve to form pigmented streaks which eventually clear. Polymorphic light eruption can also occur in childhood as papules and vesicles occurring within 12–24 hours on exposed areas such as the arms and legs, usually in the beginning of spring. Occasionally, phototoxic eruptions due to drugs, such as thiazide diuretics, are seen. Porphyria may also present in childhood and, occasionally, this can be very subtle. The pressure of tiny scars on the nose in a child complaining of a burning sensation as soon as he/she goes outside should alert one to the possibility of erythropoietic protoporhyria. |

Causes of depigmentation

Type	Description	Onset
Albinism	Generalised total absence of pigmentation	Birth
Piebaldism	Patchy total loss	Birth
Vitiligo	Patchy symmetrical total loss	Any
Halo naevus	Aura of vitiligo around a naevus	4 years onwards
Pityriasis alba	Slight depigmentation and scaling on cheeks	4 years onwards
Post inflammatory	Following dermal injury Usually in dark skins	Any
Pityriasis versicolor	Patchy-light depigmentation and scaling on trunk	Later childhood
Tuberose sclerosis	Scattered white macules on trunk	A few months

SOLITARY SKIN LESIONS

Birth marks. Vascular birth marks are quite common in childhood and are a source of considerable distress to many parents. It is important to distinguish between the permanent mature capillary haemangiomas (port wine stains) and the immature capillary haemangiomas (strawberry marks), as the latter regress spontaneously within a few years. Port wine stains are present at birth and underlying intracranial venous malformations may occur for very extensive lesions, especially when this involves the orbital area. Port wine stains can give rise to significant morbidity in later life and can be treated by pulsed tunable dye lasers at specialist units. Strawberry marks develop as bright red swellings a few weeks after birth and grow rapidly for the first 9 months. Occasionally, they may ulcerate or bleed but spontaneous regression is the rule. This can take anything from 2 to 10 years. Currently, intervention by laser therapy for uncomplicated strawberry naevi is not justified.

Pigmented lesions. The differential diagnosis of pigmented lesions is centred around excluding melanoma. Malignant melanoma is fortunately extremely rare in childhood and, when it does occur, it is often seen in conjunction with giant bathing trunk naevi. Children may be born with a few naevi and these are termed congenital melanocytic naevi. Most naevi are acquired in the first 20 years of life until the adult compliment of 40–60 naevi is achieved. Benign naevi are characterised by a uniform colour, symmetrical shape and smooth outline. Any lesion developing an irregular black pigmentation or irregular border should be seen by a dermatologist. Itch per se is not a serious sign as many benign moles itch, especially when rubbing against clothes.

Warts and mollusca. Both of these lesions are caused by viruses, namely human papilloma virus and a pox virus respectively. Warts are typically hard, horny papules 2–6 mm in diameter, usually on the hands and soles of the feet (verrucae). Occasionally filiform lesions

Rare skin lesions

Disorder	features	treatment
Infections		
Kawasaki disease [presumed virus infection]	General spotty rash, may be urticarial, cracked lips, sore mouth, desquamation of fingers and toes	
Erythema multiforme reaction to infection ? herpes	Symmetrical more evident on extensor surfaces of arms and legs, maculopapular, blisters, annular target lesions	Symptomatic
Stevens–Johnson syndrome	Severe form of above with mucosal lesions and toxaemia	? Short course of steroids
Erythema nodosum (reaction to infection? strep., ?TB ?others)	Red tender lumps on shins, may occur on thighs and arms as well	Symptomatic
Inherited disorder		
Erythropoietic protoporphyria	Photosensitivity	Protection. Autosomal dominant
Incontinentia pigmenti	Males lethal, girls have widespread small blisters appearing soon after birth, develop into warty lesions with pigmentation, associated bone, skeletal and CNS abnormalities	X-linked dominant
Anderson–Fabry disease	Small red spots on lower back, buttocks and genitalia. Pain in hands and feet. Alpha-galactosidase deficiency	X-linked recessive
Peutz–Jegher syndrome	Pigmented macules on lips, face, hands and feet, associated with bowel polyposis	Autosomal dominant
Acrodermatitis enteropathica	Eczematous lesions around mouth and in napkin area but also on limbs	Zinc administration Autosomal recessive
Ectodermal dysplasia	Smooth polished skin, inability to sweat, alopecia, pointed teeth	Treat fevers vigorously with antipyretics and cooling X-linked recessive
Ehlers–Danlos syndrome	Many forms, minor cuts leave gaping wounds with residual scars and keloids	Most are autosomal dominant
Neurofibromatosis [von Recklinghausen disease]	Soft skin lumps of neural origin at many sites, pigmented macules areas of depigmentation. Many associations including acoustic neuromas and optic nerve gliomas	Autosomal dominant
Tuberous sclerosis [epiloia]	Red-brown papules on cheeks, ashleaf macules from birth, fibroma under the nail, 'shagreen' orange peel patch on lower spine. Epilepsy, low intelligence	Autosomal dominant Mutations common
Others		
Dermatitis herpetiformis	Burst and scratched vesicles on knees, elbows and buttocks. Itching ++	Dapsone and ?gluten-free diet
Langerhan cell histiocytosis	Slightly haemorrhagic plaques with greasy scales few mms across, affect scalp and trunk	Like histicytosis X

may be present on the face. Mollusca on the other hand are smaller (1–5 mm in diameter) and are shiny. Larger lesions contain a central umbilication. 90% of childhood warts probably resolve spontaneously within 2 years but if treatment is needed, topical proprietary wart gels containing glutaraldehyde or salicylic acid are effective if they are used for a few months. Freezing with liquid nitrogen is probably more effective but this is painful for children and is usually unnecessary for such a self limiting condition. Mollusca resolve more quickly than warts. Spontaneous resolution is usually heralded by a sudden enlargement and redness of the affected lesion which is often confused with secondary bacterial infection. Usually all the mollusca disappear in one go never to appear again but unusual solitary and persistent lesions can be treated by breaking the top of the lesion and expressing the contents or alternatively cryotherapy if the child is in agreement.

DIAGNOSTIC CLUSTERS

There are a number of rare diseases in which the skin lesions may be prominent which do not fit easily into the above categories.

FURTHER READING

Champion RH, Burton JL, Ebling FJG Textbook of dermatology, 5th edn. Blackwell Scientific, Oxford

Cohen BA 1994 Atlas of pediatric dermatology. Wolfe, London

Frieden IJ 1989 Blisters and pustules in the newborn. Current Problems in Pediatrics 19: 549–614

Hay RJ 1995 Management of scalp ringworm. Drugs and Therapeutics Bulletin 35: 5–6

Hogan PA 1996 Viral exanthems in childhood. Australasian Journal of Dermatology 37 (Suppl 1): S14–16

McHenry PM, Williams HC, Bingham EA 1996 Management of atopic eczema. British Medical Journal 310: 843–847

Moss C, Savin J 1992 Dermatology and the new genetics. Blackwell Scientific, Oxford 1995

USEFUL ADDRESS

National Eczema Society, 163 Eversholt St, London NW1 1BU. Tel: 0171 388 5651

Index